"It's time to make some basic improvements in the way we live. Society, in its hunger for high technology, has warped our external and internal environments. This book is presented to inform you about internal yeast overgrowth, a disease running rampant in the 1980s. Experts estimate that about thirty-three percent of everyone living in the industrialized West is afflicted with the yeast syndrome.

"We will help you confront the yeast assault on your immune system. We will furnish you with the newest research about this high-tech disease and its devastating symptoms. We hope you will be motivated to find answers for your family, and to act on what you discover."

—the authors

John Parks Trowbridge, M.D., is an international leader in the holistic-preventive medicine movement. As president-elect of the American College of Advancement in Medicine, he is at the forefront of research into alternative approaches to improve health and treat diseases inadequately handled by conventional care. Schooled at Stanford, Case Western Reserve, the University of Texas/Houston, and the Medical Research Institute of the Florida Institute of Technology, he is also board-certified in chelation therapy for heart and blood vessel diseases. At his Houston, Texas, clinic—The Center for Health Enhancement—he is pioneering new methods of treating arthritis and degenerative diseases, digestive ailments, and other persisting problems using innovative approaches with nutrition, medications, health enhancement and life extension techniques.

Morton Walker, D.P.M., has been a professional medical journalist and author for over twenty-one years, specializing in holistic medicine, orthomolecular nutrition, and alternative methods of healing. The author of forty-nine books and 1,400 magazine articles, he has received twenty-two professional awards for his work.

The Yeast Syndrome

John Parks Trowbridge, M.D.
and
Morton Walker, D.P.M.

BANTAM BOOKS

NEW YORK · TORONTO · LONDON · SYDNEY · AUCKLAND

This book is not intended to replace your own physician with whom you should consult before taking any medication or considering treatment.

THE YEAST SYNDROME

A Bantam Book / November 1986

ISBN 0-553-27751-0

Published simultaneously in the United States and Canada

Bantam Books are published by Bantam Books, a division of Bantam Doubleday Dell Publishing Group, Inc. Its trademark, consisting of the words "Bantam Books" and the portrayal of a rooster, is Registered in U.S. Patent and Trademark Office and in other countries. Marca Registrada. Bantam Books, 1540 Broadway, New York, New York 10036.

PRINTED IN THE UNITED STATES OF AMERICA

*John Parks Trowbridge, M.D., dedicates this book to
Sabrina Lynne Williams*

*Morton Walker, D.P.M., dedicates this book to
Susan Sherr Walker*

This book has been written and published strictly for informational purposes. In no way should it be used as a substitute for your own physician's advice.

While John Parks Trowbridge, M.D., and Morton Walker, D.P.M., are collaborating here as coauthors, Dr. Trowbridge is the physician expert on the Candida (yeast) syndrome and Dr. Walker is the medical journalist reporting on such health care information.

You should not consider educational material in this book to be the practice of medicine, although almost all the facts have come from the files, publications, and personal interviews of informed physicians who diagnose and treat candidiasis and/or their patients who have suffered from the yeast syndrome. Moreover, lecture presentations, audiotapes, case reports, anecdotes, testimonials, patient histories, and other information have been utilized from the three Yeast–Human Interaction Symposiums held in San Francisco, March 29–31, 1985, in Birmingham, Alabama, December 9–11, 1983, and in Dallas, Texas, July 3–5, 1982.

If you, as a potential user of knowledge received from these pages, require opinions, diagnoses, treatments, therapeutic advice, correction of your lifestyle, or any other aid relating to your health, it is recommended that you consult either Dr. Trowbridge, the other physicians contributing to this book, or your own medical expert on the Candida syndrome. A list of such candidiasis experts is appended to this book.

These statements are to be considered disclaimers of responsibility for anything published here. The coauthors provide the information in this book with the understanding that you may act on it at your own risk and also with full knowledge that health professionals should first be consulted and that their specific advice for you should be considered before anything read here.

CONTENTS

ACKNOWLEDGMENTS

Writing a nonfiction book usually is a collective action involving the cooperation of many people, and this one has been no exception. First we want to acknowledge enthusiasm for the subject from our literary agents, Lois de la Haba and Luna Carne-Ross of New York City. They encouraged us to invest in *The Yeast Syndrome* about three thousand hours of research, actual writing time, and extra editing. Rob Fitz helped with the editing, too.

We also want to thank Abram Hoffer, M.D., Ph.D., for his superb foreword. J. J. Wetz deserves a special expression of gratitude for supplying recipes for Section Three. Adhering to our nutritional requirements, he cooked quantities of food for tasting as an adjunct to our four-phase Celebration of Healthy Eating program.

The medical case histories described in the following pages are true and accurate, including quotes taken from recorded or written interviews with patients and physicians. In some cases, when patients have requested anonymity we kept to their stories but changed their names, locations, and other identifying characteristics. Others have provided us with permission to tell their complete health histories, and we affirm the value of their disclosures. Giving service to humanity at large, and in the order of their appearance in these pages, they are: Norma Meyer, Martha E. Mansell, Diane M. Toombs, Jody L. Baccellieri, Juliana Picola, and Carol Wilson.

Numerous physicians have contributed many case studies, only a fraction of which we were able to include. For the patient histories that were used, we followed up with recorded interviews; therefore, we thank the following professionals for taking the time to provide us with candidiasis information: L. Terry Chappel, M.D., John Rechsteiner, M.D., Warren M. Levin, M.D., Leo Galland, M.D., Conrad G. Maulfair, Jr., D.O., Pannathpur Jayalakshmi, M.D., Jonathan Collin, M.D., Pearl A. Coleman, Milan J. Packovich, M.D., Leon Anderson, D.O., Sherry A. Rogers, M.D., David A. Darbro, M.D., Sandra Denton, M.D., T. Daniel Pletsch, M.D., Arthur L. Koch, D.O., Harold C. Walmer, D.O., and William C. Douglass, M.D.

Much current diagnostic and treatment information of high caliber was graciously furnished for general public welfare by the following: Charles Fox, David Roth, Philip Hoekstra, III, Ph.D., J. Alexander Bralley, Ph.D., Roy Kupsinel, M.D., Alfred V. Zamm, M.D., John Thoreson, Ted Loomis, Edward E. Winger, M.D., and Jeffrey Katke. To those who also contributed but aren't mentioned here, we acknowledge that you have advanced health and improved daily living by assisting in bringing forth *The Yeast Syndrome*.

FOREWORD

This is a valuable, timely, and life-enhancing book. The coauthors, John Parks Trowbridge, M.D., and Morton Walker, D.P.M., have done you, me, and the rest of the world a great favor. They have provided us with this single information source for everything known to date about a heretofore unrecognized clinical entity—the Candida (yeast) syndrome.

Polysystemic chronic candidiasis is the new yet old generalized fungus infestation responsible for a vast number of diverse physical, mental, and emotional disorders. Who would have dreamed that a seemingly innocent yeastlike organism, *Candida albicans*, could cause so much misery to the point even of stimulating thinking about shortening one's time on earth? But this state of mind sometimes sets in among those depressed enough by the Candida syndrome. Later, I shall describe one of my patients with psychiatric depression from the Candida syndrome.

Finally we know the truth about chronic yeast infestation. The newest diagnostic techniques and anti-Candida therapy available now, and detailed in these pages, will extend and ameliorate life for millions of people. With approximately one-third of our planet's population victimized by the Candida syndrome, knowledge furnished here has been sorely needed for patients and their physicians, alike.

It happens that I wish *The Yeast Syndrome* to be in public demand, for I had a hand in bringing to light revelations by C. Orian Truss, M.D. In my capacity as editor of the

Journal of Orthomolecular Medicine I was the first to provide a forum for his discoveries. Dr. Truss told me about his studies of *C. albicans* a few years ago at one of our meetings of the Huxley Institute for Biosocial Research. I listened with great interest, especially because he was so enthusiastic. Perhaps unlike most scientists, I find enthusiastic clinicians much more interesting than cold academics.

I am a practicing psychiatrist, and the idea that a mycotoxin (fungal poison) generated in and on the body could cause schizophrenia, depression, and other diseases was, to me, novel and important. It meant that we could pull out another group of patients from the schizophrenias. Those schizophrenics having the Candida syndrome might not respond to other treatment, but they would respond to anti-Candida treatment. This was an exciting concept.

But was Truss right? I know of only one way to determine whether an observation is correct. First, you must think about it and see if it is supported or contradicted by theory and by other observations. The candidiasis work passed this first test. Then, you must repeat the work honestly by duplicating as accurately as possible the original work. I planned on accomplishing this duplication as soon as possible.

One of my psychiatric patients had suffered from depression for many years and had not recovered under my care for two years. I tried every known treatment except electroconvulsive therapy (ECT). As soon as I returned to my office in Victoria, British Columbia, I reviewed her history again. There were a number of leads which suggested that the Candida syndrome could be her problem.

Immediately I started my patient on Truss's program. One month later she was mentally and emotionally normal. Observing her swift progress toward health, it was difficult for me to accept that she could just snap out of her depression. Frankly, I remained unenthusiastic about her recovery. But I could not invoke a placebo response since she had failed to respond to every other treatment I had given her. She then added another piece to solving the puzzle by advising that her depression started a few weeks after she had spread antifungal ointment on a new sheep her farm had purchased.

Indeed, the woman remained well for one year. On my recommendation she then stopped taking the antiyeast medicine, Mycostatin®. One month later she was very depressed again. Again, when anticandidiasis medication was resumed, she recovered and has remained well since.

I then invited Dr. Truss to present his findings at one of our Huxley scientific meetings. He received a tremendously enthusiastic response from the audience, both physicians and laypersons. I had also asked him for his manuscript for publication in the *Journal of Orthomolecular Medicine*. You see, we were ready for the next step in the scientific method—to spread the information widely. This journal has a large number of curious clinicians reading it. I knew it would not take long for others to test Truss's idea because our readers are interested in innovative treatments. "Tissue Injury Induced by *Candida albicans*: Mental and Neurological Manifestations" appeared in 1978 (volume 7, pp. 17–37). It was followed by a second report, "Restoration of Immunological Competence to *Candida albicans*" (1980, volume 9, pp. 287–301). Then his third article, "The Role of *Candida albicans* in Illness" was published by the *Journal of Orthomolecular Medicine* in 1981 (volume 10, pp. 228–238). Finally, Truss's seminal work was self-published in book form, *The Missing Diagnosis* (1982).

As I had hoped, the Truss reports stimulated an explosion of interest, both among orthomolecular physicians and among a few academic physicians. A number of yeast-human interaction symposiums were held which dealt entirely with candidiasis. More recently, William G. Crook, M.D., self-published *The Yeast Connection*, which has had an enormous impact in publicizing the Candida syndrome.

Treatment of the Candida syndrome has taken two paths. One is the more allopathic type followed by physicians who can prescribe antifungal medication such as nystatin. They also utilize Candida-free diets and other anti-Candida measures. Another route is followed by alternative health therapists such as chiropractors and naturopaths, who are legally unable to prescribe drugs. Their treatment techniques are dependent on natural antifungal substances such as taheebo tea, garlic, and yogurt.

The discovery by Dr. Truss that chronic candidiasis can

cause a wide variety of reactions has broad implications for everyone. The mycotoxin from *C. albicans* represents only a small proportion of mycotoxins made by thousands of fungi. We now should be looking for patients who are sensitive to mycotoxins present in mold-contaminated foods. Is this why most people cannot stand the taste of moldy food, why we instinctively reject moldly apples or oranges? Is this why a few patients cannot tolerate bran or whole wheat flour but have no problem with white flour? Few people are aware that modern farming techniques, especially when harvesting is done in wet weather, lead to increased molds and spores on the surface of the grain which are not fully removed by the cleaning and milling process. Bran is then contaminated by these fungal products, whole wheat less so and white flour very little. Fungi hardly invade white flour products because they contain such minuscule amounts of nutrition.

The agricultural/food-processing industry does not like to think about bran or whole wheat dampness. Why? Simply, it would mean changing harvesting methods to make sure grain is thoroughly dried before it is stored and milled. Drying techniques entail more money, time, labor, and inconvenience. If the processors can get away without drying, even at the cost of some mildewing . . . Well?

The discoveries by Dr. Truss described in his book, in Dr. Crook's book, and now in this more extensive and complete book by Drs. Trowbridge and Walker, have ushered in a whole new dimension in maintaining health and treating disease. Our new food rule is not to eat any food infected with mold with the exception of foods such as bread, which is heat-treated, and the cheeses, but even these will have to be avoided by many. Why? More of our populace is ill with candidiasis than anybody ever imagined. The Candida syndrome is rampant all over the world, especially in industrialized countries.

This book contains the needed help and advice that sufferers of candidiasis must possess to be effective partners with their physicians in controlling disease and maintaining health. It will be an educational experience as well for numerous physicians who have remained in the dark about the Candida syndrome. In fact, *The Yeast Syndrome* may be the most important book of this decade.

Abram Hoffer, M.D., Ph.D., Victoria, British Columbia
Editor, *Journal of Orthomolecular Medicine*
President Emeritus, Huxley Institute for Biosocial Research

April 3, 1986

PREFACE

A new medical condition of the 1980s is affecting approximately one-third of the total populations of all Western industrialized countries. The new disease involves a generalized yeast infection produced by the organism once known as *Monilia albicans* but now commonly called *Candida albicans*, which gives rise to a loosely defined syndrome—a series of chronic disorders variably affecting the nine different body systems: digestive, nervous, cardiovascular, lymphatic, respiratory, reproductive, urinary, endocrine, and musculoskeletal. The Candida syndrome manifests itself with symptoms throughout the body, and they can vary over time in one person and in kind and severity among different people.

Candida albicans is a yeast growth present in and on most of us which is normally controlled by our immune defenses and by the usual bacterial flora present in and on the body. But when an ecological change takes place in the internal environment, helpful bacteria tend to be decreased and immune response becomes depressed. Then the yeast begins to increase in the body, especially in the colon (large intestine). These yeast colonies release powerful chemicals (toxins) that may be absorbed into the bloodstream, causing such widely varying symptoms as severe menstrual cramps in women and lethargy, chronic diarrhea, bladder irritations and infections, asthma, migraine headaches, depression, skin eruptions, and many other difficulties in both men and women. Localized areas of Candida overgrowth cause other obvious, recurrent, and persistent infections such as yeast vaginitis, oral thrush, and diaper rash. These problems often herald the insidious beginning of the deeper-seated and more dangerous inner infections. Thus, a myriad of symptoms and signs are the Candida-caused human disorders collectively referred to as "candidiasis."

Fifty years ago doctors identified *Candida albicans* as a frequent cause of vagina, mouth, throat, and gastrointestinal tract infections. Now it's well known to affect almost all body parts, organs, tissues, and cells. Research physicians suspect Candida as a complication in acquired immune deficiency syndrome (AIDS), a contributor to early death in various forms of cancer, a source of infertility in some women, and a mischief-maker in other medical tragedies such as multiple sclerosis, myasthenia gravis, schizophrenia, and arthritis. On rare occasions yeast overgrowth results in pneumonia, meningitis, and similar devastating body invasions.

Candida is a germ that ordinarily lives by eating dead tissue—a saprophyte—rather than living matter. When you consume quantities of animal protein like steaks and chops loaded with antibiotics, or when you are prescribed certain antibiotics for the treatment of bacterial infections, these newly introduced drugs tend to turn the saprophytic organism into a pathogen. A pathogen can thrive on living tissue in your body and is capable of causing infection or disease. Taking cortisone, birth control pills, or other steroid derivatives creates hormonal imbalance in your body. Again, alterations in the yeastlike organism can occur so that the Candida syndrome may begin.

Reading this book you will become aware that the Candida syndrome is a result of frailty of the human body. Virtually everyone in Western industrial societies is susceptible to becoming ill with it. Simply said, the unveiling of symptoms in an affected individual means that his or her immune system finally has succumbed to the unnatural effects of "high tech" lifestyles. Since *Candida albicans* is universally present, any time a person's immunity becomes more than slightly compromised, the yeast can overcolonize.

Candida is an "opportunistic organism." The yeast grows more abundant when your resistance has been lowered because of either nutritional deficiency, infection, or some debilitating agent in the environment. More often than not, such debilitators are manmade, the result of our technological overload.

Furthermore, *Candida albicans* slowly increases its total area of tissue invasion after being converted to pathogen status. Aspects of our lifestyle that foster continuing yeast growth include not only the taking of oral contraceptives, but also administration of anti-inflammatory cortisone medications, multiple pregnancies, eating foods high in mold or yeast content such as bread, brewer's yeast, beer, and mushrooms, and having a diet with excess refined or simple sugar carbohydrates, such as candies, sweets, cookies, chips, pastas, and ever present "junk food." As we shall see in Chapter Two, the increasing number of antigens and toxins overwhelm immune system cells, and your immunity drops. An antigen is any substance that the body regards as foreign or potentially dangerous and against which it produces an antibody or other defense reaction. Absorbed toxins or an excessive antigen load may reduce the effectiveness of your defenses, bring on serious disease symptoms, and—in severely ill patients—occasionally result in generalized Candida septicemia (blood poisoning), and possibly death.

A class of white blood cells (lymphocytes) called "suppressor cells" prevents immunologic responses to your own tissues (discussed in Chapter Three). In other words, you are capable of mounting an immune attack against your own organs but are stopped from doing so by lymphocytes that suppress such a damaging effect. In autoimmune diseases such as systemic lupus erythematosus, rheumatoid arthritis, myasthenia gravis, multiple sclerosis, Hashimoto's thyroiditis, certain hemolytic anemias, and other more rare conditions, both clinical and laboratory studies suggest that *Candida albicans* interferes with immune system cells, actually blocking their suppression phenomenon. Yeast infection can decrease the percentage of natural suppressor cells in tissue fluids and blood—dropping from about 15 percent to as little as 1 percent. When the Candida infection is successfully treated, the percentage of these suppressors rises toward normal and the symptoms tend to clear. This observation was made by the discoverer of polysystemic chronic candidiasis, C. Orian Truss, M.D., Medical Director of the Critical Illness Foundation of Birmingham, Alabama. Dr. Truss, a genius of modern diagnosis and treatment and literally the father of a whole new field of medical practice, may at last have made many of the autoimmune diseases eligible for specific treatment.

Among the infectious organisms studied in bacteriology, mycology, and other microbiological sciences, *Candida albicans* is a most complex agent. It releases a minimum of seventy-nine known chemical substances against which the human body creates an identifiable antibody. Each Candida strain—*Candida albicans* being just one among eighty-one—has about thirty-five antigens, implying that millions of antigens are possible. Different strains can colonize the same person at different stages in life. Treatment might get rid of one or more strains present today, only to have others strike at a later time when defenses are down.

You might live your entire life with yeast growing as a minimal part of your intestinal flora. Such an accommodation simply means that your immune system has been able to manage the organism's presence and cope with its toxins. You are a fortunate combatant in the perpetual struggle between humankind and *Candida albicans*.

There are two other significant characteristics of *Candida albicans* toxin. First, this fungal antigen could stimulate a nonspecific reaction in your body which your doctor is unable to diagnose. It is possible that nothing in your immunological response—signs or symptoms—matches any label the best traditionally thinking diagnostic minds can identify. The result may be a psychiatric referral by your physician. Why is this problem so common in modern medical practice? The reason is both clear and unacceptable.

When a physician schooled in orthodox medicine cannot fit *your* particular pieces of the Candida syndrome into the modern allopathic-osteopathic medical jigsaw puzzle that passes for diagnosis, the doctor may conclude, "It's all in your head." Thousands of people have been branded as mentally or emotionally ill when the true health problem has been infestation and overgrowth of internal fungus.

Second, when one's systemic response involves a particular tissue, organ, or group of cells, the condition can easily—and incorrectly—be labeled with a familiar diagnosis.

For instance, when *Candida albicans* affects the gut with

regional enteritis (inflammation of the intestine), it may be diagnosed as Crohn's disease. When abnormal uterine bleeding during or between menstrual periods occurs, a gynecologist steeped in conventionally oriented medical belief is likely to label the problem metrorrhagia and treat the woman with hormones (or, occasionally, antibiotics). Such treatment could worsen her problem if Candida overgrowth is the true cause. Consequently, a number of different diagnosed local "diseases" may actually be reflections of one common, generalized cause—polysystemic chronic candidiasis (PSCC).

Most patients respond to anti-Candida treatment in as few as ten days. Recovery of immune defense system function, reversal of the effects of Candida toxin, and correction of nutritional deficiencies usually take eight to sixteen or more months. Some victims have taken as long as three years or longer to "get better," if they are quite ill or have failed to be faithful to their therapeutic programs. Major symptoms that usually improve quickly are headaches, diarrhea, constipation, vaginitis, emotional and behavioral difficulties, skin troubles, generalized itching, and several more discomforts. Since the Candida syndrome is frequently well established in its victim before being identified, treatment efforts must be continued as long as necessary to correct underlying problems and to prevent the yeast-related illness from recurring.

As will be discussed in Chapters One, Six, and Seven, medical controversy certainly does surround chronic, generalized candidiasis. Establishment-type doctors who stick to the old traditions in medical practice are at odds with pioneer-type physicians (who proudly refer to themselves as "medical mavericks"). These pioneers utilize the newer complementary medical methods of diagnosis and treatment. The issue centers on whether symptoms are actually caused by the Candida syndrome—and whether treatment directed at yeast and nutritional support can be effective and appropriate. Concepts in medicine evolve as scientists and physicians look at research and clinical data in new ways. In this book, we present you with the most current thinking from pioneers in this exciting, emerging field.

Our book will help you confront the Candida assault on your immune defenses by furnishing you with the newest research and most current information about this technology-caused disease and its devastating symptoms. From what is written here, we hope you will be motivated to look for answers to some complex questions and to act on what you discover.

John Parks Trowbridge, M.D., Humble, Texas
Morton Walker, D.P.M., Stamford, Connecticut

March 5, 1986

SECTION I

Potential Yeast Syndrome Carried Within Us

1

Yeast Disease Arising from Modern Technology

Do you want finally to have a diagnosis made that connects your various disparate symptoms—distressing patterns of illness which you've been experiencing for too long—problems that are not really psychosomatic after all but have actual organic causes?

Are you a victim of vaginal discharge, itching, constipation, excess "gas," abdominal discomfort, headaches, fatigue, diminished sex drive, irritable personality, memory deterioration, lost self-esteem, acne, asthma, and other such troubles?

Would you like to stop suffering with cystitis, bladder inflammation with overly frequent urgency to pass urine—accompanied each time by severe burning that's so awful it has you dreading the next episode of urgency?

Do you have a persistent cramping pain in the lower abdomen after the bladder has been emptied, a condition exceedingly common among women?

Is it your wish to get rid of jock itch, athlete's foot, brittle and brown toenails or fingernails, rectal tickling or irritation, skin rashes, white-coated tongue, blurred vision, sinusitis, types of allergic reactions, chemical intolerances to foods and inhalants and water impurities, any one of which could be the bane of your existence?

Are you the concerned parent of a child who is hyperactive, autistic, who gets and keeps colds one after the other or has repeated earaches, experiences continuous nose congestion, stays restless and grumpy, displays tantrums, or seems addicted to sweets and other carbohydrates?

Are you interested in knowing of a safe, effective, tested, legal, nonsurgical treatment which can eliminate diarrhea, chronic belly pains, inflammation, ulceration, and malabsorption in your gut, even possibly conditions known as colitis, enteritis, ileitis, or Crohn's disease?

Would you want your family physician to know all about a comfortable but complicated series of corrections for your numerous and variable health difficulties and assist you to follow a lifestyle that could improve the quality of your existence, perhaps adding twenty to thirty years more to the time you have to live?

Might you be dubious if an informed person told you that some allergists, immunologists, gastroenterologists, psychiatrists, endocrinologists, internists, and other medical specialists refuse to recognize and have no knowledge of a proven underlying diagnosis for your health problems—and an effective treatment program—despite an informed estimate that at least 80 million Americans (three-fifths of them women, one-fifth each men and children) also join you as victims?

If you have the need for appropriate treatment with a particular remedial program, would you feel frustrated and angered at not being informed of the existence of such therapy, so that you might live more comfortably?

Do you believe that you're alone in your wandering from doctor to doctor, seeking either a cure for or the control of your illness problem?

You are not alone! Many thousands of other victims of nonspecific, undiagnosed illness syndromes have responded to questions such as these, and have then found permanent relief.

THE CASE OF ABBY RAE BENNETT

Born December 20, 1948, Abby Rae Bennett is a teacher in Lake Charles, Louisiana. She won the outstanding teacher award in her school for 1981. Her husband, S.M. "Sam" Bennett, Jr., is a successful insurance agent. On June 1, 1983, Mrs. Bennett visited the offices of John Parks Trowbridge, M.D., of Humble (a suburb of Houston), Texas, requesting assistance with her longstanding ill health.

For a long time the woman had suffered with anorexia and bulimia. She dropped from 170 to 140 pounds before her marriage to Sam. Her menstrual flow stopped completely when food binging alternating with forced vomiting brought her weight down to 115 pounds. For six years she had failed to have any menstrual periods, a condition known as amenorrhea. In 1979 an endocrinologist declared that Mrs. Bennett's amenorrhea was correlated with the anorexia and bulimia. Standing five feet, two and one half inches in stocking feet, the patient now weighed just 102 pounds.

Sniffling nose congestion, "up and down" energy levels, constant fatigue, and addictlike food cravings were additional troubles for Mrs. Bennett, according to the extensive patient history form she filled in. She also described multiple digestive complaints, including stool color changes, watery stools with a foul odor, and lower bowel gas. She invariably suffered with an upset stomach after eating greasy foods as well as abdominal pain, bloating from any food intake, increased pulse rate after meals, and a coated tongue. There were also obvious sugar-handling problems such as hunger between meals, irritability and moodiness just before meals, shaking and dizziness with delayed meals. All of this was combined with frequent melancholia, the repeated onset of the "blues," and nervousness. Remarking that her "get up and go had got up and gone," she also reported traditional low thyroid (hypothyroid) complaints. Further, Mrs. Bennett had joint stiffness, watery eyes, poor circulation in the hands and feet, sensitivity to cold, keyed up feelings, easy exhaustion, brown spots on the skin, and weak nails, and she commonly developed "goosebumps."

The patient's litany of disorders illustrates the *un*characteristic illness patterns that Dr. Trowbridge proceeded to evaluate.

After a series of clinical and laboratory examinations, Mrs. Bennett was found to have a satisfactory chemical profile. Nothing significant in her tests suggested the true source of the numerous abnormalities. Cytotoxic testing—one method of checking for cell poisoning by environmental agents—did reveal allergic reactions or chemical intolerances to twenty-seven different foods. Her hair mineral analysis showed a pattern typically found in people with hypoglycemia (low blood sugar). She had a number of mineral deficiencies as well as receding gums. Attributing her irritable bowel symptoms to recent home stresses, she explained that she and her husband were trying desperately to meet the qualifications to adopt a baby.

The doctor prescribed relief-giving medication and nutritional supplementation and advised other simple remedies for these diverse difficulties. Until he could sufficiently define her underlying problem, the true reason for all of these signs and symptoms, he was treating empirically (based on his observations).

Dr. Trowbridge consulted with Mrs. Bennett bimonthly thereafter, but no spectacular improvement occurred in her condition. She retained all of the same troubles, reported that four nose bleeds had spontaneously come on at different times, and her underarm lymph glands had become swollen and tender.

At her visit on December 12, 1983, Mrs. Bennett described several weeks of intense sugar cravings that had caused her to gobble down many refined carbohydrates—candy, cake, bread—and she was experiencing constipation that she attributed to a mostly dairy diet, including lots of ice cream. In their discussion Dr. Trowbridge drew out the critical fact that the teacher was feeling severe discomfort from the mildew in her classroom, which had accumulated as a result of tornado and hurricane flooding that had affected their area of Louisiana and Texas in the late summer and early fall of 1983. Her nasal congestion was worse than ever.

With a clinical supposition that this mildew from fungal microorganisms was contributing to her problems, Dr. Trowbridge started his patient on an antifungal (anti-Candida) treatment program. When Mrs. Bennett returned for consultation three weeks later, she reported an easing of her constipation, a lessening of the sniffles, and lots more energy. She also asked to eliminate the thyroid medicine, which had been required to lessen her fatigue. Dr. Trowbridge added more antiyeast medication, *Lactobacillus acidophilus* powder (the friendly culture from which yogurt is made), and aged garlic extract and recommended a reduced carbohydrate diet to counteract the worsening mildew situation in which she worked.

She reported gradual improvement at each bimonthly visit. By August 1984, Mrs. Bennett had experienced her first menstrual period in seven years. It lasted five days. It was a harbinger of her return to near normal health and significant because she and her husband had just learned that they did not yet qualify to adopt a baby.

During the months that followed the woman reported the steady reduction of her discomforts. Her sexual desire returned strongly. Her breasts swelled at her regular menstrual cycles, just as they had done when she was in her early twenties.

In October 1985, Mrs. Bennett stated that she remained happy with the treatment she had received to rid her body of various yeast-related illnesses and to restore balance to her biochemical functioning. Poor health was almost entirely gone, and the remaining symptoms were easily controlled by continuation of her diet, supplemental nutrients, a small amount of antiyeast medication, and other activities that had become part of her lifestyle.

THE FINDINGS OF DR. C. ORIAN TRUSS

The treatment prescribed by Dr. Trowbridge for Abbey Rae Bennett was predicated on a discovery made about twenty-five years earlier by C. Orian Truss, M.D., a specialist in internal medicine and allergy, who practices in Birmingham, Alabama. Dr. Truss noted quite by chance that a particular yeast, *Candida albicans*, was capable of causing disorders more severe than were attributed to it by conventional allopathic medicine. At the Eighth Annual Scientific Symposium of the Academy of Orthomolecular Psychiatry held in Toronto, April 30 to May 1, 1977, Dr. Truss first presented his highly significant medical findings. An article reviewing his observations and conclusions was soon published in *The Journal of Orthomolecular Medicine*. The first generalized, chronic candidiasis case ever responding to anti-Candida treatment was described by Dr. Truss in this way:

> An incident that occurred in 1961 was the first indication that this organism perhaps is capable of causing disorders much more severe than conventionally attributed to it. A forty-year-old woman whom I was treating for allergic rhinitis and migraine headaches walked into the office with one of her severe headaches. It was rapidly apparent that she was also quite depressed, which was characteristic of the severe premenstrual symptoms that she experienced for one week each month. *Candida albicans* was one of her allergens, and chronic yeast vaginitis worse premenstrually was a prominent complaint. A small dose of Candida extract relieved the headache, but the most startling result of the injection was the rapid and complete disappearance of the depression. Her initial unsmiling, agitated manner was suddenly replaced by a relaxed smiling countenance. In subsequent months it was possible to duplicate this experience, both in her and in other similar cases of severe premenstrual depression and tension.[1]

During the next sixteen years, following that first case and its publication, Dr. Truss observed many more patients displaying the Candida syndrome. Most of them have gotten well utilizing his prescribed anti-Candida treatment. He has published three additional clinical papers on his significant medical findings.[2,3,4]

Dr. Trowbridge is a medical disciple of Dr. Truss. He has also adapted therapeutic recommendations offered by William G. Crook, M.D., of Jackson, Tennessee. Dr. Crook has withdrawn now from active practice to pursue his media efforts to inform physicians and patients of the emerging and successful therapeutic approach to candidiasis. Until now, his self-published 1983 book, *The Yeast Connection*, has done more than any other information source to popularize knowledge about the Candida syndrome. Dr. Trowbridge has used the Crook book extensively in the past to educate his patients about *C. albicans*.[5]

THE NEW/OLD DISEASE ARISING FROM MODERN TECHNOLOGY

With cancer, heart disease, herpes, AIDS, and so many other problems stalking us, the last thing we need is news of yet another disease spreading at epidemic rates. But that particular predicament is the reality. Almost everyone in the world exhibits some minor complication from the disease, but large numbers of people show signs and symptoms that have them functioning at very low levels of wellness, if not outright sickness. Approximately 30 percent of all persons around the world above the age of twelve—mostly females—are suffering with yeast-related illnesses caused by the fungus within us known as *Candida albicans*.

As illustrated by the patients attended by Drs. Trowbridge, Truss, and others described in later chapters, some of the easily recognizable symptoms and signs of Candida invasion—a common intestinal yeast that has veered out of usual body balance—include vaginitis, vulval itching, cystitis, menstrual disorders, premenstrual syndrome, sexual difficulties, decreased libido, infertility, headaches, stiff joints, arthritis, indigestion, intestinal gas, nausea, bloating, abdominal pain, diarrhea, constipation, dizziness, fatigue, lethargy, white-coated tongue, brittle and brown nails, acne, giant hives and other skin eruptions, blurred vision, rectal itching, inadequate nutrient assimilation, nearly every type of allergic reaction one can think of, chemical intolerances to foods, water impurities, and inhalants such as tobacco smoke, irritable bowel syndrome, chronic grumpiness, autism, minimal brain dysfunction, hyperkinesis, anxiety, depression, and other emotional illnesses, mental illnesses, asthma and other respiratory tract disorders, and many more abnormalities of the human physiology.

If left untreated, *C. albicans* wreaks havoc throughout the human system. It so severely debilitates the body that victims could become easy prey for far more serious diseases such as acquired immune deficiency syndrome, multiple sclerosis, rheumatoid arthritis, myasthenia gravis, colitis, regional ileitis, schizophrenia, and, possibly, death from Candida septicemia. Yet, diagnosis is reasonably straightforward and highly effective therapy does exist. Until now, organized medicine has largely ignored such diagnosis and treatment.

Why isn't treatment being rendered? Simply because orthodox physicians who practice strictly within the medical mainstream are poorly informed about this systemically invading yeast. When establishment-type doctors can't find any recognizable reasons for a patient's persistent ailments, most of them slip into a diagnosis of psychosomatic illness. Candida patients suffer with their clinical problems because little has been published or discussed about the condition, except among the medical mavericks who specialize in diagnosing and treating it.

In the summer of 1985 the American Academy of Allergy and Immunology (AAAI) provided the Candida problem with a label: "candidiasis hypersensitivity syndrome." Nearly a decade before, the medical pioneers routinely attending to this malady named it "polysystemic chronic candidiasis" (PSCC), or generalized, chronic Candida disease. Here we are calling it "the Candida or yeast syndrome."

Unfortunately, although the AAAI has found no way to counteract the devastating disorders of the Candida syndrome, it has disavowed the condition as a clinical entity and calls therapeutic procedures which work against it "speculative and unproven" (see Chapter Seven for full details).

The yeast syndrome is actually an old disease that has become newly predominant in industrialized Western nations largely arising from "high tech" alteration of external environments and the resulting assault on the internal body environments of the resident populations. This yeast disease is increasing and expanding across international borders as a result of modern technology. It is a parasitic disorder at once endemic (occurring in a particular region and/or population) and epidemic (spreading rapidly through the local populace to affect a national population, thus infesting a large proportion of people). It is a major health crisis of the 1980s.

The excessive use of self-administered or professionally prescribed antibiotics, steroids, and birth control pills coupled with a milieu of universal pollution tends to sponsor progression of the local yeast occurrence within all of us to become chronic, invasive, systemic, and differentiated infections. Such infections may cause tissue damage throughout the body. Both men and women can have it, although candidiasis occurs more frequently in women, and with more severe effects. It also strikes many children, especially those receiving an inordinate amount of antibiotic therapy or consuming excessive sugar and "junk foods." Newborns are eligible to acquire *C. albicans* infestation as they come down the mother's birth canal or during diaper changes or feedings. Pregnancy, by its hormonal alteration of a woman's body, tends to stimulate the resurgence of yeast growth in her tissues.

HOW THE YEAST SYNDROME SHOWS ITSELF

Candida symptoms fall into three main areas:

1. problems in the gastrointestinal and urinary tracts
2. allergic reactions
3. emotional and mental difficulties.

Candida overgrowth may also cause women to experience fertility difficulties and can bring about birth defects in newborns.

At this writing, laboratory testing techniques are just being developed, and they are available to physicians who will take the time to understand their complicated rationale. Rather than clinical examination or laboratory tests, however, the patient's history and symptoms are usually the keys to diagnosis. Chronic symptoms in the categories listed above, together with a history of using oral contraceptives, steroids for treating arthritis, relieving allergies, or chemical intolerances, and the misuse or overuse of antibiotics (even for skin conditions such as acne) may all point to a Candida problem being present.

The presence of chronic vaginitis very often indicates that polysystemic candidiasis is an underlying problem, because nine out of ten cases of this one disorder are caused by *C. albicans*. Vaginitis—inflammation of the vagina—often manifests itself with irritation, increased vaginal discharge, and pain on passing urine (cystitis symptoms). Candida-connected vaginitis may be brought on by ill-fitting contraceptive devices, irritation from contraceptive creams/jellies/suppositories, dietary deficiencies, poor hygiene, and other causes, which will be described in Chapter Twelve.

Allergy tests for fungus, yeast, and mold may uncover an unsuspected yeast invasion. Traditional skin prick/scratch/patch testing or blood tests by establishment-type allergists often fail to reveal this serious assailant of the body's defense system. Specialized approaches used by clinical ecologists, those environment-oriented doctors who deal with problems encountered when man fails to adapt to his changing and toxic surroundings, are more likely to give an accurate indication of the presence of the yeast syndrome.

The patient's own response to treatment is considered by medical authorities as "pathognomonic"—unique to Candida, with the pattern of improvement allowing for positive diagnosis—the conclusive step in labeling his or her condition as due to yeast overgrowth.

PARTIAL LIST OF YEAST-CONNECTED ILLNESSES

Agitation

Allergies

Anxiety

Asthma

Body aches

Bronchitis

Chemical sensitivities

Chronic heartburn

Chronic infections

Colitis

Constipation

Cramping in the belly

Depression

Diarrhea

Disturbed senses: taste, smell, vision, hearing

Dizziness

Earaches

Gastritis

Headaches

Hives

Hyperactivity (mostly in children)

Hyperirritability

Impotence

Infections: bacterial, viral, fungal

Insomnia, both chronic and sudden sporadic episodes

Lethargy

Loss of concentration

Loss of libido

Loss of memory

Menstrual irregularities

Premenstrual anxiety/tension

Premenstrual depression/moodiness

Sensitivity to odors, chemicals, fragrances, smoke

Stomach distension/bloating

Swelling/fluid retention or loading

Vaginal yeast infection

Weight changes: gain or loss

TREATMENT TECHNIQUES FOR YEAST OVERGROWTH

Treatment for candidiasis is fundamental yet complicated because of the many organ systems involved in producing symptoms. Nevertheless, treatment is finally effective if the patient will remain persistent with the required regimen. The health professional's goals are first to control the yeast infection in the patient's body and then to build up the defense system's ability to keep it from reexpanding. Doctors are using several techniques to treat yeast overgrowth, based on each patient's history and response to therapy. Following are some of the techniques which will be described in Section Two:

1. the generic antifungal drug nystatin, highly efficacious and well tolerated by the patient

2. special antiyeast diets that exclude foods upon which the yeast feeds, tending to "starve out" the Candida organism

3. avoidance of antibiotics unless their use becomes absolutely mandatory (which, of course, is how all physicians are supposed to practice)

4. discontinuing birth control pills, especially if a vaginal discharge is present or if headaches accompany the menstrual periods

5. a homeopathic remedy which has almost no side effects and is reported to work against Candida in some patients

6. consumption of aged garlic extract (or fresh garlic cloves), an easy, quick, and sometimes efficient way to help control the condition

7. Tricophyton-Candida-Epidermophyton (TCE) vaccine injected into the skin to stimulate immune defense responses (immunotherapy)

8. avoiding drugs that suppress the immune system, such as steroid-based pharmaceuticals

9. eliminating allergies to yeast and mold to help build up the immune system's ability to resist infection

10. drinking tabebuia/la pacho/taheebo tea or decoction (an herbal remedy made from the inner bark of the la pacho tree)

11. regularly taking nutritional supplements to achieve fully integrated nourishment, reduction of free radical pathology, and support for the body's immunity

12. engaging in appropriate testing procedures before, during, and after full treatment is rendered, to make sure the Candida syndrome is defeated.

Patients may show a response to anti-Candida treatment in as few as ten days. Some of the worst victims have taken three years or more to be cured, and a few physicians have reported that even after four years some patients still have symptoms of the disease. Length of the treatment program seems inversely proportional to the cooperation of the patient. In other words, if he or she has failed to be faithful to the therapeutic program, the problem hangs on and longer treatment is needed. Since the yeast syndrome probably was well established before being identified, treatment efforts must be persistent and continued as long as necessary to control the infirmity and to prevent recurrence.

NOTES

1. C. Orian Truss, "Tissue Injury Induced by *Candida albicans*," *Journal of Orthomolecular Medicine*, 1978, 7:17–21.

2. C. Orian Truss, "Restoration of Immunologic Competence to *Candida albicans*," *Journal of Orthomolecular Medicine*, 1980, 9:287–301.

3. C. Orian Truss, "The Role of *Candida albicans* in Human Illness," *Journal of Orthomolecular Medicine*, 1981, 10:228–238.

4. C. Orian Truss, "Metabolic Abnormalities in Patients with Chronic Candidiasis: The Acetaldehyde Hypothesis," *Journal of Orthomolecular Medicine*, 1984, 13:66–93.

5. William G. Crook, *The Yeast Connection*, 2nd ed., Jackson, Tenn.: Professional Books, 1984, pp. 5–7.

2

How *Candida Albicans* Views Jane

I am Jane's yeastlike organism—*Candida albicans*. I live within her gut. Jane is my universe.

My name is Clarissa Candida. I am a one-cell fungus from the phylum of plants with no chlorophyll, and I have the unique characteristic of reproducing without requiring another organism. My way is asexual—I reproduce by budding—and that's why I'm yeastlike. Just one of me can beget billions, which is part of what makes me a danger to poor unknowing Jane.

I have a large, round, thick-walled spore shaped roughly like a tiny chicken egg. I am so absolutely fascinating that large sections of the most authoritative mycology book ever published (*Medical Mycology*, by John W. Rippon, Ph.D.) detail my family tree, my upbringing and lifestyle, and my very special characteristics. Just think, doctors everywhere have had to read all about me and all of my relations.[1]

My aunts, uncles, sisters, and brothers may be found throughout Jane. I dangle with other kinfolk in clusters similar to bunches of grapes. We sometimes hang from threads spread out through and attached to Jane's gut. I love the gut's warm, dark, moist environment. Its five feet of large intestine contain a veritable zoo—upwards of 500 fungal, bacterial, and viral varieties with a total population in the *multitrillions*. There are, for instance, at least eighty-one strains of my fellow yeasts. Often several different strains of us are together in the same gut or living on other parts of the body. Since there are more of my *C. albicans* strain than any other genus of yeast, I am most likely to overpower Jane's immune defensive system.

But she's got something going for her. Many of the bacterial types work in Jane's favor. They control my family of saprophytes and keep them in check, neither helpful nor harmful.

Along with friendly bacteria that compete against me and aid in protecting Jane, antiyeast toxins called hormones and enzymes are also made by my universe. They hold down my family numbers. I try to do mischief by imitating the molecules of Jane's hormones and interrupting the traffic of normal physiological processes. It's easier for me to interact this way when bacteria friendly to her are knocked for a loop by particular foodstuffs and drugs that she puts into her body.

Jane and other male and female universes just like her send materials into and out of my world through nine or ten holes, seven at the top and two (male) or three (female) at the bottom.

Recent human history is full of instances of furthering the existence of me and my Candida family. For example, as soon as a new human universe is born, it has its bottom holes wrapped with a warm, moist, dark, comforting, and yeast-inviting environment referred to as "diapers." Just the time when the new human being is unable to tell whether we yeasts belong inside him or her, parents give us a great chance to set up residence.

Furthermore, the new human's parents mistakenly feed it a food derived from an entirely different animal—a cow. Cow's milk is good for calves but unfavorable to *Lactobacilli acidophilus*, man's friendly bacteria, which ordinarily keep yeasts from invading further up the intestines. So we're able to spread along the human's whole digestive tract. The more cow's milk our young universe is given to drink, the more we Candida thrive. If that's not enough, they dispense to that baby plenty of different kinds of antibiotics for any casual sniffle or earache. This practice also makes more inviting the esophagus, nose, mouth, and the rest of the baby for my Candida relatives to settle in. Oh, do we ever love antibiotics!

There is so much for every budding yeast to know about humans and yeasts that we had to send spies to a medical conference to bring back information. At the second Yeast–Human Interaction Symposium held in Birmingham, Alabama, December 9–11, 1983, Sidney MacDonald Baker, M.D., Medical Director of the Gesell Institute of Human Development in New Haven, Connecticut, gave a perfectly marvelous description of my entire species and the way we view the globe (human being) in which we live.[2] My 4473rd cousin, Corky Candida, who at the time was struggling for survival in the gut of John Parks Trowbridge, M.D., was present in the audience and told me what Dr. Baker said. Alas, Corky is no longer with us. He succumbed to the wholistic lifestyle and proper nutrition advocated by Dr. Trowbridge.

Luckily for me, Jane isn't so knowledgeable. She smokes; drinks coffee, soda pop, cola beverages, beer, and liquor; eats canned fruits, plenty of pastries, and other refined carbohydrates; takes oral contraceptives; and recently had surgery for which immunosuppressive drugs were prescribed. In fact, Jane does lots of things that have me and my family luxuriating throughout her body in Candida overgrowth.

A YEAST'S-EYE VIEW OF HUMANS

Unlike us yeasts, who are all buddies under the skin (hah!), most humans become highly individualistic and do things to themselves such as inhaling tobacco and marijuana smoke, drinking alcohol, snorting cocaine, and popping an endless variety of pills. Actions like these further my family's capabilities and allow us to produce quantities of the highest quality toxins. Our toxins can disarm the most aggressive immune system defenders that Jane or any other human has to throw against us. It's no trouble at all to poison a human being's immune system, especially if she or he lives in an industrialized country.

All *C. albicans* see human beings from a particular point of view. We know that they start out existing in two shapes or forms. One is a single-celled organism shaped roughly like a polywog with a very long tail. It's designated by the fancy name, "spermatazoon." A single deposit of spermatozoa number in the millions, but only one makes it into the more scarce, rounded, and larger biological entity known as an "ovum." It's just an egg which appears on the scene once a month. When the two human organisms come together they form a new fruiting body made up of approximately 80 trillion cells. I witnessed this fruiting when Jane twice became pregnant.

These trillions of cells usually live in harmony in the one human body, communicating through enzymes and hormones that I've described as toxins for me. There are salivary enzymes, pancreatic enzymes, intestinal enzymes, steroid hormones, endocrine hormones, neurotransmitter hormones, plus thousands of others of these nasty toxins. I hate them all and am constantly creating substances called "antigens," which counteract Jane's enzymes and hormones that are dangerous to me.

Hormones are produced by individual human tissue cells to talk with other cells. When this happens, I am provided with a wonderful opportunity to cause trouble. All of us yeasts build molecules disguised to look similar to hormonal molecules. Some of these disguises become our surface antigens; they allow us to enter our universe's cellular communication traffic. I slip into Jane's metabolic process of cell communication and give her sleepless nights, cramp-filled days, and painful sexual intercourse.

CANDIDA OBSERVATIONS OF HUMAN CONSCIOUSNESS

All of a human being's senses—sight, sound, taste, smell, touch, and maybe others—are extremely costly to its metabolism. The expense of consciousness renders a human rather fragile, requiring him or her to eat foods that are almost alive. In contrast to us yeasts, who thrive on dead and decaying substances containing no life and light, human foods must contain a high content of living matter together with its accumulated packaged light energy derived ultimately from the sun through green plant processes.

But my family members have nothing to worry about, for

we have friends in the commercial world of human beings. These benefactors are food-packaging industrialists. The advertising dollars of processed food manufacturers aid us about eighteen hours a day by changing human eating habits. Food refiners persuade their customers to restrict themselves only to dead foods, leaving the human diet much more suitable to yeasts. They sell what consumer advocates call "junk foods." I rather like them myself.

A number of other practices and even some federal and state laws are helping yeasts, too. For example, there are laws that say you have to kill all the food before you can label it with appetizing names or before you may put it on the shelf in grocery stores and supermarkets. Toward this end, preservatives, additives, coloring agents, foaming agents, binders, thickeners, stabilizers, emulsifiers, and other items have been invented that kill or remove nutrition from foods. People who work in the food industry along with those in the pharmaceutical industry assuredly are the best buddies that *C. albicans* and other yeast strains have among humankind.

YEASTS AND THE MAKING OF INTERNAL ALCOHOL

Do you recall that I was talking about human consciousness—the senses—before? Well, my candid observations may be beneficial to you. I have learned that the consciousness of *Homo sapiens* is most active during the daylight hours. It leaves people in the nighttime, when they go to sleep. Yet, it's only in this state of unconsciousness that humans are most alive, at least from my point of view. In periods of unconscious rest they are actually building up molecules. When awake, humans break down molecules in order to achieve a more alert consciousness.

Taking molecules apart during daytime hours has the human producing self-poisoning substances called "catecholamines," which help to keep him conscious. During these daylight catecholamine production periods, my yeastly relatives and I can provide our host with a real dilemma by producing molecules with just two carbon atoms such as acetaldehyde or ethanol. He or she has no place to put those simple two-carbon products.

The critter's metabolism can't turn a two-carbon molecule into pyruvic acid for conversion into sugars. Instead, he or she must metabolize it right away. This obligation is liable to interfere with a human's consciousness in very dramatic ways. It tends to intoxicate the person, giving him symptoms of absent memory, lightheadedness, dizziness, lack of concentration, and even loss of consciousness.

The discovery centuries ago that my yeast family can make these two-carbon fragments has led to the widely advertised and popular purposeful consumption of yeast products for the alteration of consciousness. We can make alcoholic beverages out of ordinary fruit or grain sugars. When humans drink the liquid for purposes of altering the consciousness, you might say that we Candida are happy to go along for the ride.

Why? Well, the Professor and Chairman of the Division of Dermatology at the University of Tennessee Center for the Health Sciences in Memphis, E. William Rosenberg, M.D., explained how we yeasts work on an alcohol imbiber. Dr. Rosenberg was the speaker to appear after Dr. Sidney Baker's talk at that 1983 Yeast–Human Interaction Symposium. Before poor Corky Candida died (may he rest peacefully in yeast heaven), he reported to us on Dr. Rosenberg's lecture. Dr. Rosenberg has written two scientific papers, one of them coauthored with Dr. Baker, reporting on psoriasis and inflammatory bowel disease in the same patients. The two health problems clear up simultaneously when *C. albicans* is treated with that awful stuff, oral nystatin.[2,3,4]

"While you are drinking alcohol, one of the things that it does is make the Küpffer cells in your liver sleepy," said Dr. Rosenberg in his 1983 Birmingham lecture. "The Küpffer cells, lining the hepatic sinusoids of the liver, constitute about 90 percent of all the macrophages in the human body. If the Küpffer cells get sleepy, your portal blood [blood flow from the intestine, loaded with foodstuffs and chemicals in your diet and drinks, headed toward the liver for processing] has access to the general circulation."

The danger to humans is that such intestinal blood has not been detoxified by the liver and can do damage to body cells. We like that! Since the whole object of our existence is to bring about illness and the potential for death in the host, the drinking of alcoholic beverages makes our job a little easier.

The Japanese medical community is aware of internal alcohol production by *C. albicans*. Such knowledge is just beginning to filter into the annals of American medicine. Yes, Candida alone can produce signs and symptoms of human drunkenness without the human ever having to drink a drop of an alcoholic beverage.

Sound fantastic? Fanciful? Unbelievable? Those are the same reactions people had to poor old Charlie Swaart, the "drinkless drunk," when he tried to convince his neighbors and employers that he never touched liquor.

THE MAN WITH A LIQUOR DISTILLERY INSIDE HIM

As recently as eleven years ago, it was not uncommon for Charles M. Swaart, now age seventy-six, a trim, soft-spoken, retired public relations counsel currently residing quietly in Phoenix, to reel, slur his words, fall down, reek of whiskey, and show the blood-alcohol level of a full-blown drunk. This, when he never touched a drop of liquor, beer, wine, or any other form of alcoholic beverage.

For thirty years, from 1945, when Charlie was a public information officer for General Douglas MacArthur in occupied Japan, a strange malady plagued him.

He would pass out on his front doorstep, too intoxicated to find the keyhole.

He would crawl home on payday without a cent in his pocket, all of it handed out to bench-warmers in the local park.

He was picked up for drunken driving following a fashionable dinner hosted by a prominent Arizona politician. He repeatedly swore that he did not imbibe, but nobody believed poor old Charlie. People aren't dumb, and everyone knew there was no such thing as a drinkless drunk.

The truth is that the man, purely and simply, had not been drinking. He was walking around with his own personal distillery lodged in his intestines. It was a still created by *C. albicans* capable of converting refined carbohydrates that he got from food and turning them directly into alcohol. For thirty years Mr. Swaart was condemned as a drunk when he actually was the victim of the mysterious drunkenness disease called *meitei-sho* by the Japanese.

It was only chance that led Charlie Swaart finally to deduce that my fellow yeast organisms were the cause of his drunkenness. A long feature article by Don G. Campbell published in a 1983 issue of the *Los Angeles Times* told how fate intervened against my relatives and won the man his freedom from our grasp.[5]

Charlie's wife, Betty Swaart, had quietly been making tiny marks on the bottles of liquor that they kept in their home for guests. She proved to herself that her husband wasn't secretly imbibing on his own, even though he still frequently gave off alcoholic fumes and reeled when he walked, as though intoxicated. He did this, in particular, after he ate a high carbohydrate meal like fruit salad and spaghetti. The couple brought his nondrinking drunkenness problem to psychiatrists, internists, alcoholism specialists, and other health professionals in search of a solution. They went through the medical literature thoroughly. The man had access to all the clinical journals because, ironically, he became the American Medical Association's first public relations director. Later Charlie was made the public relations counsel for the Colorado Medical Association. No clue turned up. None of the costly physician consultations brought any solution. Nothing in the clinical journals identified his condition. My yeasty cousins really had Charlie and his big deal "we-have-all-the-answers" medical specialists bamboozled.

"The doctors," Charlie recalls, "reported that 'there is nothing in medical literature to support endogenous alcohol.' It was a doctor's way of politely tagging me a sneaky drinker." And for nine years after his first attack in Japan, even the patient wondered about himself.

"It was in the spring of 1954, though," he remembers, "that I realized I could get drunk without so much as a short beer. I was in the hospital for a month recovering from a severe attack of viral hepatitis, and I got drunk there [without imbibing]. Then, my personal physician warned me that, because of the severe liver damage, I must not touch anything alcoholic for at least two years. I followed his advice to the letter. And I still got drunk."

In the mid-1960s Charlie went on a strict high protein, low

carbohydrate diet to reduce his weight from 240 pounds to 170. During the period when his weight was coming down to normal, the intoxication attacks came less frequently and less severely. His Phoenix physician had no medical explanation for the improvement, however, and consuming less carbohydrates did not strike Mr. and Mrs. Swaart as being significant. Therefore, they failed to pick up on the elimination of carbohydrates from his diet as a meaningful factor. The main foods for us yeasts, of course, are sugars and starches . . . carbohydrates!

At a New York City business meeting with a pharmaceutical representative, a few years later, Charlie turned down the offer of a cocktail preceding their meal. "When I told him that I could get drunk on an Italian dinner," he explained,"there was a funny look on his face and he told me that he'd read of a similar case in a medical journal. I became excited, but skeptical, too, and told him he must be mistaken since I recently had dozens of specialists researching medical literature for me for years, and they'd never run across a similar case. The executive promised me he'd dig it out and send it to me in Phoenix.

"I went home with crossed fingers, but the guy was as good as his word and called me long distance the following day," said Charlie. "You can imagine how my hopes were dashed, though, when his first words were: 'You were right, and the doctors were right. There's no record of a case like yours in any scientific medical literature.' "

However, there was a case report published in the July 20, 1959, issue of *Time* magazine. It seems that for twenty-five years, forty-six-year-old Kozo Ohishi of Tokyo had tried to prove he was a teetotaler despite his continuous display of intoxication symptoms. It wasn't until Okkaido University Hospital in Sapporo, Japan, agreed to run him through a series of test diets did Ohishi's digestive juices reveal a flourishing growth of *C. albicans*. Ridding his body of the Candida syndrome was a cure of "alcoholism" for the Japanese national.

On the basis of the *Time* article, Charles Swaart's Phoenix medical doctor, Francis Sierakowski, M.D., ordered laboratory tests on the patient. It looks to me like fate stepped in for Charlie by his consulting a maverick who practices by innovative thinking instead of following the medical mainstream sheeplike.

The lab tests showed massive colonies of my relatives in his intestines.

"Of all the specialists who had examined and treated me over the years no doctor had ever mentioned the existence of Candida," said Swaart. "The detailed medical and hospital records I had amassed showed no specialist had ever ordered a test designed to discover whether or not I had Candida colonies in my intestines."

He got brief relief in 1970 from the prescribing of that obscene material you humans use against my species, Mycostatin®. But since Charlie was being treated without the full anti-Candida program that's utilized today, we yeasts were eventually able to overcome the singular Mycostatin® remedy. We came back strong with intoxication symptoms that were worse than ever.

So then the fellow began to fear that he was staring into the face of death. A paper that he read, written by Rosalinde Hurley, M.D., of Queen Charlotte's Maternity Hospital in London, said, "Untreated systemic candidiasis has a mortality rate approaching 100 percent [from Candida septicemia]. Delay in treatment is dangerous and will almost certainly end in death of the patient." Only rarely do we Candida spread from the gut to involve the deeper tissues, but Charlie sure looked like our man.

Poor Charlie searched everywhere for a solution. He and Betty contacted a London Candida specialist and sent off a letter to a mycology professor in Tokyo who had participated in the treatment of identical cases of *meitei-sho*. The intoxication bouts became more frequent and more severe, inevitably leaving him drained of strength. Old Chuck and his wife finally took off for London. Even after three weeks in a London hospital, no relief, not even confirmation of the diagnosis, was forthcoming.

To the great joy of my yeast relatives fermenting alcohol from carbohydrates inside the man's intestines, the couple returned home to Phoenix terribly disappointed. But then they read their mail. Waiting in their stack they found a packet of medical journal reprints on the Japanese drunkenness disease accompanied by a letter from Kazuo Iwata, Ph.D., Chief Mycologist at Tokyo University School of Medicine. Intrigued by the first reported non-Japanese to be stricken with *meitei-sho*, Dr. Iwata visited the Swaarts' home en route to an American medical meeting. He consulted with Dr. Sierakowski and recommended other more appropriate drugs for the patient.

The recommended medicines were unavailable in the United States. My Candida forces were winning this battle to keep Charlie Swaart sick and finally snuff out his life. The American Food and Drug Administration (FDA) helped us by not allowing the potent anti-Candida drugs into the United States despite evidence from doctors at St. Joseph's Medical Center in Phoenix, where testing showed Swaart had a raging case of the Candida syndrome.

Hearing that the U.S. Veterans Administration (VA) sometimes could obtain drugs not available to civilian medical practitioners, the patient and his wife appealed to VA physicians for help. They turned over to them all of the Japanese medical journals, clinical and laboratory article translations, Dr. Sierakowski's medical records of Charlie, and copies of Dr. Iwata's letters specifying the kinds and use of the drugs. The patient begged for treatment, but the VA would have none of it.

They tested the man for a year, in the hospital and out. Their tests included long periods of bed confinement, and eventually the VA declared that the man was legally drunk. He exhibited intoxication with high blood levels of alcohol even when he was stuck in a hospital bed for a month. To conclude this unrewarding experience, the VA medicrats accused Betty Swaart of smuggling booze in to her husband.

The couple had no choice but to fly to Tokyo, where *meitei-sho* specialists at the city's Junendo University Hospital took him under treatment. Dr. Iwata participated in reaching a definitive and correct diagnosis on the patient's condition within four days. Worse luck for us yeasts, the man received a cure in three weeks. It was delivered by means of a powerful antifungal, chemotherapeutic agent called flucytosine/Roche, under the brand name Ancobon® which had been developed by Hoffman-La Roche of Switzerland.

Ancobon® has potential side effects which must be carefully monitored. It's not your everyday remedy which would be used against the usual discomforts my Candida cousins and I regularly produce in humans. Indeed, flucytosine is the sort of treatment reserved for serious infections caused by strains of Candida, as in septicemia (blood poisoning infection), endocarditis (inflammation of the valves or lining of the heart), and pyelonephritis. infection of the kidneys (urinary system disease), although it is not effective against all Candida strains. Ancobon/Roche® has now been approved for use in the United States.

"From that day to this," Swaart says, "no Candida have been found in me, even though regular medication was discontinued in September, 1975. And I haven't had one symptom of intoxication. The only time I use it now, rarely, is when I feel the symptoms beginning to gang up on me—fatigue, a little wooziness, and when I start developing a cold sore."

To what does Charlie Swaart attribute his being the first non-Japanese to exhibit symptoms of *meitei-sho*? The former U.S. Army officer who became part of Japan's American occupation forces at the end of World War II blames it on high technology. Besides innovations in the areas of medicine, leisure, entertainment, lifestyle, food, personal finance, fashion, personal care products, household appliances, automobiles, education, and childrearing, he was exposed to the residual effects of the highest technology industrialized society has ever developed. He cites the microorganism aftergrowth resulting from the 1945 atomic bombs dropped on Japan.

"The Japanese are convinced that the atomic blast produced mutations in the organism that—in certain people—resulted in a stupendous proliferation of the Candidas to a level never believed possible before," he said. "And the yeast disease is obviously communicable, probably through unsanitary food handling, since it is showing up now in second and third generation carriers." Betty and Charlie Swaart believe that he picked up and brought home some of Japan's mutated *C. albicans*. Other Americans are recently reported to be affected by this strong toxic reaction furnished by my yeast relatives—the Japanese drunkenness disease—including people who have never been to Japan. This shows that my potent yeasty genus, more especially *C. albicans* like me, are spreading their effects from human universe to human universe, encircling the earth.

WHAT CLARISSA CANDIDA IS ACHIEVING INSIDE JANE

Jane has been around for twenty-nine years. I came on board nearly ten years ago, when she began taking birth control pills just prior to her marriage. Before then she had begun to weaken her defenses against my entry when, for several years during her teens, she took tetracycline for acne. But oral contraceptives really opened the door for me. It was then that I began to find life pleasurable and productive. With her eating French fries, pizza, soda pop, cola drinks, and later beer and wine, I was encouraged to give Jane some lovely disorders. She got skin eruptions, joint aches, headaches, and other miscellaneous troubles, according to whichever body systems my toxins and waste products offended.

Jane now has two children. Right after her first vaginal childbirth, I hung on her some vulvovaginal symptoms of discharge and itching. This was before my Grand Aunt Connie Candida went to work on her with painful sexual intercourse. My vaginitis attack bothered her for a while until she consulted an establishment-type gynecologist, who chased my aunt and me deeper into her body—the gut—with his ineffective local vaginal medication approach, particularly antibiotic creams and suppositories.

Next I hit her with bowel discomforts that alternated between constipation and diarrhea. I added excess gas, abdominal distention, bloating, and general cramping discomforts.

But now life is even more fun. She had a second joining of spermatazoon and ovum, then formed and delivered another of those fruiting bodies with seven holes on top and three underneath. Now, a few days a month, I'm able to give Jane abnormalities of her menstrual cycle and flow—sometimes cutting off the flow altogether, other times making her bleed large clots, occasionally producing severe menstrual cramps, and often doing all kinds of other queer things with her menses. I invariably cause Jane to suffer with premenstrual tension and bring on other miserable aspects of the premenstrual syndrome (PMS). She is nearing the edge of her emotional stability—not to mention how frustrated and irritated her husband gets with her constant complaints, lack of energy, loss of enthusiasm for sex, and obvious ill health.

Last year I added heartburn, sour stomach, and regurgitation symptoms when I lined her esophagus with my offspring. And I've just now thrown in an attack of oral thrush with a coating on the tongue, white spots on the gums, and soreness at the corners of her mouth. The long medical name for this thrush is "acute pseudomembranous candidiasis." It hurts Jane even to smile. Watch your smile, Jane, you're on Candida camera. Hah!

By integrating my toxins into her hormonal secretions, I can become part of the lady's nerve and brain neurotransmitters to change her personality. I can help cause various emotional upsets, including depression, extreme irritability, anxiety, and crying jags. Jane's behavior is starting to affect her marriage. Her husband doesn't come home on time anymore. I think that he's found other companionship.

Deterioration in intellectual function for Jane is a predicament I've been working on. My efforts have lost her a modicum of concentration and reasoning power, but my next enterprise is to give her a loss of short-term memory like people suffer with in Alzheimer's disease. It will be a great coup for me to achieve memory deterioration in one so young. With it will come the total destruction of self-confidence, so severe that it will result in her inability to cope with even the simplest problem. Then Jane will want to kill herself, and I will have attained the highest pinnacle of *C. albicans* achievement. Jane dies young, and I conquer my universe.

NOTES

1. John W. Rippon, *Medical Mycology*, 2nd ed., Philadelphia: Saunders, 1982.

2. *The Yeast–Human Interaction 1983: A Symposium*, Birmingham, Alabama, December 9–11, 1983. Cassette tapes, Creative Audio, 8751 Osborne, Highland, IN 46322, (219) 838-2770.

3. F. William Rosenberg, et al., "Crohn's Disease and Psoriasis," *New England Journal of Medicine*, 1983, 308:101.

4. F. William Rosenberg, Sidney M. Baker, et al., "Oral Nystatin in the Treatment of Psoriasis," *Archives of Dermatology*, 1984, 120:435.

5. Don G. Campbell, "The Ordeal of 'Poor Old Charlie,' Drinkless Drunk," *Los Angeles Times*, January 4, 1983.

Yeast Toxin
Attacks Your Immune System

Writing in the *Journal of Holistic Medicine*, John Rinehart, M.D., a psychiatrist practicing in Newton, Connecticut, has classified chronic unwellness as a syndrome—a series of symptoms—that plagues many people living in developed countries. Dr. Rhinehart categorizes these symptoms into the following groups:

Mental Cognitive. The people often complain of mental fogging, a loss of their former alertness, and poor information recall. They perceive a loss of productivity and creativity in job performance, changes that are not necessarily noted early on by their colleagues or supervisors.

Energy. This primarily exhibits itself as tiredness over a period of from nine months to two years (or longer). The person will often say that even after nine to ten hours of sleep, he or she does not feel rested.

Emotional. The patient notices low periods of depression, accompanied by irritability and outbursts of anger. Usually the individual perceives this as an important symptom because it affects others who are close to that patient.

Somatic. Victims report headaches, ranging from mild and fleeting discomfort to severe migrainelike pain. Other somatic symptoms include vague gastrointestinal malfunction, intermittent diarrhea, bloating, indigestion, and discomfort after eating. Menstrual irregularities are common, and many victims claim ill health since the birth of their last child. Sexual function deteriorates in both males and females.

Dr. Rhinehart mentions in his article that these symptoms—the full syndrome—are found quite commonly but don't fit into any traditional disease pattern. Three questions arise then: What are likely causative possibilities that a doctor must discover when presented with a patient having these symptoms? Will he or she be able to diagnose the syndrome? How must it be treated?[1]

Alan Broughton, M.D., Chief Pathologist and Medical Director of the Antibody Assay Laboratories in Orange, California, attempts to answer the questions posed. First Dr. Broughton suggests that the term "chronic metabolic distress," as used by Dr. Rhinehart, be altered to another that is perhaps more subtle and succinct: "chronic unwellness."

Then Dr. Broughton advises that our society's stated preoccupation with health is a misnomer. *The medical mainstream is fascinated with disease, not with health or wellness.* Physicians-in-training are taught to identify disease situations; when a patient's symptom complex does not readily fall into a predefined disease state, the patient is either referred to another physician or told "it's all in your head"—meaning that he or she doesn't have any "real" disease, only what's imagined. Patients with complex and often conflicting symptoms may end up seeing internists, neurologists, gastroenterologists, endocrinologists, allergists, psychiatrists, and many other types of specialists—sometimes all in the same time frame. At this stage the patients really do become convinced they are imagining their symptom complex, all too familiar for people suffering with the yeast syndrome.

Although pervasive throughout developed nations, chronic unwellness is controllable—even reversible—to attain a high level of wellness. Treatment administered uses four main modalities: nutritional, detoxifying, immunological, and antiviral/antifungal. These are the major therapeutic choices, because ecological alteration of the environment is producing four sets of conditions on Earth that human physiology has never before confronted.

First, although people are paying more attention to their nutritional needs today than ever before, "dysnutrition" through bad eating is probably the most common malady in the Western industrialized countries. Certainly dysnutrition is quite apparent in the United States. The perfect example of this is Super Bowl Sunday, when people gather before their television sets to watch football. They gobble hot dogs, potato chips, pretzels, and salted peanuts, all washed down with kegs of beer and jugs of soda pop. Super Bowl Sunday comes but once a year, but some people carry on this same unhealthy practice almost on a weekly basis.

Overindulgence in refined carbohydrates, so popular in the American diet, presents the body with an overdose of "sugar," one of the factors producing gastrointestinal symptoms seen in chronic unwellness. Additionally, "sugar highs" and withdrawal symptoms can occur following excessive intake of refined carbohydrates day after day. C. Orian Truss, M.D., has documented that this type of diet, coupled with excessive use of antibiotics, results in chronic unwellness from the Candida syndrome.

Second, in our modern society we are constantly being exposed to slowly increasing levels of toxic materials to which some of us react much more than others. Examples of such materials include carbon monoxide, ozone, formaldehyde, insecticides, cleaning agents, and myriad pollutants. Individuals with symptoms related to chemical intoxication often find it impossible to avoid these chemicals—they become environmental cripples. These people usually are among the first to display manifestations of the Candida syndrome.

Third, both dysnutrition and chemical intoxication can produce severe immunological changes. The resulting immune dysregulation creates opportunities for further damage by infections with viral and fungal agents. Conditions such as Candida overgrowth, in which the immune system is affected either primarily or secondarily, can easily result in the immunologically ill patient. Hypersensitivity to various foods and fungi (such as that resulting from immunoglobulin-mediated hypersensitivity) frequently is difficult to distinguish clinically from other causes of chronic unwellness.

Fourth, although many patients with chronic unwellness are told that their symptoms are due to obscure "viral" infections, the precise causative agents are seldom known. The true cause quite likely is often fungal. Recent information in the medical literature has shown that many patients with chronic ill health do indeed have serological evidence of persistent Epstein-Barr virus (EBV) disease, a ubiquitous member of the herpes virus group which infects many or most human beings at some stage of their lives. Primary infections with EBV are usually of short duration, self-limiting, and without long-term effect. If they occur in childhood, they are often symptomless or cause only mild "cold" symptoms. In adolescents or young adults, EBV infections present themselves as infectious mononucleosis, which may reactivate later in times of stress. Other viral agents, such as cytomegalovirus (CMV) and Herpes simplex, can be causative factors as well. These viral organisms have been shown to be stimulated by fungal infestation with *C. albicans*.

With this information presented by Drs. Rhinehart and Broughton, we now return to one of our original questions: How should the provider of health care and the patient who suffers with chronic unwellness proceed? Since correction of chronic unwellness is achieved by building up the body's immune response to stressors, we should first know the immune physiology involved.

KNOWING YOUR BODY'S IMMUNE RESPONSE

Immunology is the science of "self" and its invaders. The recognition of "self" by our personal body immunity is what protects us from the likes of *Candida albicans*. When you or I offend our internal environment with ecological changes in our external surroundings, we open the "self" to damage by yeasts and other microorganisms. In addition, we may create "self-damaging" internal situations in the form of both auto-immune diseases and immune deficiency syndromes such as has occurred to sufferers with acquired immune deficiency syndrome (AIDS).

A microorganism is classified as a pathogen if it has the ability to incite disease in susceptible animals, including people. *C. albicans* is such a pathogen. While the body's resistance mechanisms against most pathogens involve physical barriers such as the intact skin and mucous membranes, certain fatty acids and sebaceous secretions, normal body temperature, essential metabolites, protein peptides of tissues, interferon, and other mechanical factors, these don't protect us against the yeast invader. It's within the "self" that we find our champions. Floating in the lymphatics, intercellular fluids, and bloodstream, particular white blood cells referred to as lymphocytes are our deadly immunological weapons against Candida. While phagocytes (primitive white blood cells) devour whatever alien substances cross their path, lymphocytes seek foreign tissue that they recognize as different from "self" and destroy it with the single-minded intensity of an assassin.

There are B-lymphocytes (B-cells) and T-lymphocytes (T-cells). B-cells produce antibodies, the free-floating "humoral immunity" system, which seek out specific invaders for destruction. A different antibody must be made to counteract each type of invader. Antibodies are pure protein products and are not cells. Unlike phagocytic cells or lymphocytes, they can't crawl to the site of foreign product invasion. Indeed, antibodies are not actively involved in protecting us against *C. albicans* pathogenicity. They probably are passively involved with complement fixation. Complement is a heat-sensitive, complex system in blood which, in combination with antibodies, is important in the host defense mechanism against invading microorganisms like yeasts.

The lymphocytic T-cells also respond only to particular matching microorganisms, but not by producing antibodies. Rather, three T-cell varieties exist which perform different immunologic tasks. Type-7 is a microbe killer (T-killer cell) that attacks with potent chemicals consisting of enzymes and hormones. Type-4 is an aid (T-helper cell) to the B-cells and prods them into producing antibodies. Type-8 is a kind of administrator, which works at regulating the immune response. It's an immunity suppressor (T-suppressor cell) that prevents the body from the excesses of its own defense. The work of these three types of T-cells is called "cell-mediated immunity." Obviously, other numbered types exist and play varying roles in the defense system function, but these three are most active in candidiasis.

Any substance that elicits a response from B- or T-cells is an antigen. All kinds of antigens exist. They include fungi, tiny bits of organic matter, inorganic debris, bacteria, viruses, toxins, serum air bubbles, and other assorted junk materials within your tissues and blood. Antigen determinants such as proteins and sugars usually mark the antigen, and the T- and B-cell lymphocytes remember these markings. Individually created lymphocytic defenders are genetically programmed to recognize their targeted foes among the millions that might invade your body.

The *C. albicans* toxin is an antigen and will elicit an antitoxin response by your body. All antitoxins are antibodies. But the yeast itself may or may not bring any antibody response inside your body because even when present as overgrowth the organism can raise disguising antigens and mask its hostility. It has, in fact, as noted in the Preface, at least seventy-nine such antigens. An escaping quantity of yeast organisms with their heavy load of antigens may overburden some cells, a tissue, an organ, or it may be released in the bloodstream and stimulate an immune response that has you sick with a variety of symptoms. This burden is known as the candidiasis "antigen load," which may keep you at a subclinical (just at the point where you're sick but don't recognize it) level of chronic illness or hit you hard with an acute disorder.

Also, "immune response genes" with which you are born have properties that determine the strength of the body's immune reaction to *C. albicans* antigens and/or toxins. If you get candidiasis rather quickly or easily, it could be that your immune response is genetically weak. Weak genes for yeast defense may account for a handing down of mother-daughter susceptibility.

Furthermore, *C. albicans* is commensal, meaning that it lives inside and on the skin surface of nearly everyone without causing harm or bringing benefit. This commensalism continues uneventfully unless you give your yeasts an opportunity to expand their growth. In Chapter Four, you will learn how prescribed antibiotics or those consumed in meat and poultry turn your commensalistic Candida into the sometimes cannabilistic source of the Candida syndrome.

After a time, one's immune system can become nonresponsive or "paralyzed" to the continued presence of pathogens, including *C. albicans*. It's not commensalism but an actual unresponsiveness to antigens that sets in. At first there will be a rise in immunity, and then, with continued increases in antigen load, a critical point is reached beyond which the immune system fails to respond. Dr. Truss describes this "tolerated" antigen load in *The Missing Diagnosis*.[2] The only way immunologic tolerance can be reversed is to discontinue exposure of a person to the yeast antigens and toxins. That's why the Candida syndrome must be treated successfully and completely in anyone who shows its signs and symptoms. The medical problem lies not with the yeast infestation but with the compromised performance of the immune system itself. If normal immune defense function is not restored, dire consequences are later in store for the Candida syndrome victim.

AUTOIMMUNE DISEASE

Acquired immune deficiency syndrome and other very serious health problems comprise the worst possible scenario of a biological nightmare come true. They appear to be among the growing number of otherwise unrelated disorders partially caused by inflammation and destruction of cells, tissues, and organs by the body's own antibodies (autoantibodies). These disorders belong to the autoimmune classification of diseases. Science hasn't explained why the body should lose the ability to distinguish between substances that are "self" and those that are "nonself." An accumulating stack of evidence is pointing the finger of suspicion directly at *C. albicans* as well as at other parasites or infections. How the yeast organism fosters a compromise of normal immune function is the subject of investigation and much speculation by the worldwide scientific and clinical communities.

Medical scientists in the Department of Mycology at the Institut Pasteur, Paris, France, investigated six patients who were suffering with chronic, generalized candidiasis of the skin, nails, and oral and genital mucous membranes. The scientists were looking for the presence of autoantibodies during the course of the patients' yeast infections. As mentioned, the presence of autoantibodies means that the body has launched immune defense reactions against parts of itself. The researchers carried out highly sophisticated testing procedures, and results of their tests were incontestable. Autoantibodies specifically against each of the body areas involved with yeast infections were detected.

Treatment against *Candida albicans*, using the effective anti-Candida drug ketoconazole, was given to four of these six patients. Retesting showed that all signs of autoantibodies had disappeared.[3]

A research study carried forward by the Institute of Microbiology, Universidad Nacional de Tucuman, Argentina, was designed to detect some soluble immunosuppressor substance in the blood of mice after they were infected with *C. albicans*. The research team reported that a suppression of the immune response was obtained from as early as the second day of yeast innoculation up to the twenty-eighth day. In their 1984 paper published in *Mycopathologia*, the researchers concluded, "Systemic infection by *Candida albicans* induces a nonspecific immunosuppression."[4]

In 1983 *The Journal of Immunology* published a report of *C. albicans*–induced immune response suppression in mice, which confirmed a fear that had been slowly but steadily growing in the minds of medical scientists. The report's authors wrote:

> Human chronic mucocutaneous candidiasis [a severe disease syndrome, where yeast infection can be found on the mucous membranes and skin, around the lips and in the mouth, or on the buttocks and in the anus] has been associated with a depressed cellular immune system. . . . Little evidence exists that might link this disease to a defect in the humoral [body fluids] immune system. It has been assumed in most cases that defects in T-lymphocyte function predispose to the infection by this pathogenic yeast. Recent studies suggest that the infection may contribute to the immunodepressions."[5]

Scientists in the Department of Human Microbiology, Sackler School of Medicine, Tel Aviv University, Tel Aviv, Israel, did a study to determine whether *C. albicans* infection has a suppressive effect on the immune response in mice.

The research findings, published in 1979, were interpreted as showing *C. albicans* does affect the early phase of the immune response.[6]

The Journal of Clinical Investigation published a paper, in 1976, describing function of the thymus-derived lymphocyte (T-cell or T-lymphocyte) in fourteen patients infected with a variety of fungal organisms. The patients' T-cells were weakened possibly as a result of the fungus being present in their bodies. The investigators wrote: "Patients with localized or disseminated fungal infection do manifest deficiencies in T-cell reactivity although it is difficult to decide whether the defect precedes or is secondary to the infection."[7]

As indicated by these and other research citations, candidiasis is a complicating condition as well as a prime suspicious factor in human immunity weakness. Paralysis of the immune response or tolerance to the body's antigen overload could be the mechanisms involved. The exact significance of *C. albicans* in causing any disease process is difficult to establish. Yeast toxins appear to circulate throughout the body and organisms themselves can grow in or on many tissues as well. We are increasingly aware that Candida is a saprophyte turned pathogenic by changes in the internal ecology (balance) of the body.

YEAST TOXIN ATTACKS

Since *C. albicans* may be found on the skin and in the mouth, intestinal tract, vagina, and other body areas of healthy individuals, little diagnostic value can be attached to the finding of a positive skin test. In fact, absence of a positive skin reaction is often considered as evidence of a defect in immune system function. Therefore, in "normal" people, physicians expect to find a positive skin test result for Candida.

Scientific reports indicate that a high percentage of sera (the fluid portion of blood) from "normal" persons contain antibodies to yeast toxins. This means that the organisms are continuously excreting toxic substances. Thus, B-cell immune system defenses (antibodies) must unceasingly counteract them. Nutritional status must be kept optimal in order to avoid deficiencies that may arise due to effects of yeast waste products and toxins. This observation again emphasizes that *the real medical difficulty for a person having the Candida syndrome is with the immune defense system and not simply with yeast overgrowth itself.*

Infections of the lungs, such as bronchitis or pneumonia, often involve fungus as a secondary invader superimposed upon viruses or bacterial germs. As we shall discover in the next chapter, this situation may be partially due to antibiotics used to control bacterial invaders, with a result of encouraging yeast overgrowth. Yeast may also be cultured from lesions of the skin or mucous membranes that originally initiate from dietary deficiencies. Dietary deficiencies invariably compromise the body's overall defensive status.

Using a variety of intricate mechanisms, your immune system neutralizes, conquers, or literally consumes and digests foreign proteins such as enemy micoorganisms that don't belong in the body. The skin, mucous membranes, antibodies, neutrophils, lymphocytes, macrophages, basophils, eosinophils, and a host of other natural barriers comprising the immunological mechanism combine with and defeat invaders. But when yeasts are stimulated to multiply by some alteration of the internal ecology (such as ingesting quantities of antibiotics in the meat supply or during treatment of an infection), the subsequent Candida overgrowth puts out toxins which circulate and weaken your defenses. As time passes, symptoms of illness develop.

The excessive toxins will make membrane linings in the gut leak, for instance, which then allows many abnormal and larger protein molecules to be absorbed. People with multiple food and chemical sensitivities often appear to have developed these reactivities because antibody formation is stimulated by abnormal absorption of antigenic proteins in food, pollens, and their own normal microbiological flora. Candida toxins seem to contribute greatly, then, to the onset and worsening of these allergic sensitivities. Moreover, affected individuals devote a great deal of biochemical energy trying to mount an immune defense response to the Candida as well.

When alive, yeasts seem able to evade the immune system to some degree. But when killed, yeast cell-wall proteins are absorbed through the weakened mucous membrane and cause allergic reactions. Antibodies stimulated by Candida infections can react at sites in the tissues of present or previous Candida infection. "Die-off," sometimes referred to as "Herxheimer reactions," occurs when treatment for infection kills large numbers of yeast germs rather quickly and your membranes absorb toxic products from these dead organisms. The large amount of foreign antigens triggers an increasing immune response, in addition to interfering with usual biochemical processes, and these effects can temporarily worsen your symptoms. Physicians believe that this "die-off reaction" indicates that the treatment is working. "Die-off" suggests that you may have an excellent response to a properly designed treatment program.

Some of the symptoms of the Herxheimer reaction appear to be due to formation of immune complexes (antigens reacting with antibodies) with resulting histamine release, swelling, and pain. Thus, surfaces where *C. albicans* may infect and where histamine reactions can be most distressing are mucous membranes in the mouth, esophagus, stomach, small and large intestines, sexual and urinary organs, sinuses, Eustachian tubes in the ears, bronchi, lymphatics, and possibly other membranes such as the meninges (protective wrappings) of the brain and synovial linings of the joints.

A yeast cell can produce a direct toxic action by penetration of its germ tubes into tissues. Germ tubes, known as "mycelia," are filamentous, threadlike structures that it puts out in search of nutrients for the organism. Tangled masses can develop when local growth conditions change and large numbers of budding yeast suddenly decide to "move out" by forming mycelia. A candidiasis patient's gastrointestinal mucosa (the lining of the digestive tract) can be invaded by these germ tubes in the same way that tree roots push deeply into the ground. Similar invasion has been documented in kidney tissue and in the lining of the vagina.

Sending its protoplasmic threads into the gut's wall, the fungus appears to cause lesions that can contribute to abnormal absorption of large protein molecules in the intestine. This is the plausible explanation for the sometimes severe food allergies seen in patients suffering with the yeast syndrome. Many people don't realize that food sensitivity reactions can show up as muscle or joint pains, headaches, asthma, nose congestion, or a myriad of other symptoms, not just as distressing upset of the digestive tract. Toxins, yeast waste products, and invasive germ tubes can bring about gastrointestinal compromise and, eventually, malabsorption difficulties.

Certain microscopic organisms present as normal flora in your gastrointestinal tract help prevent extension of *C. albicans* mycelia. These bacteria are *Lactobacillus acidophilus, Lactobacillus bifidus,* and other sometimes pathogenic bacteria which will ordinarily be kept under control when your immunological resistance stays at high-level wellness.

The prevention of yeast-related disease by friendly bacteria in the gut was confirmed in 1977 with a published study from the Department of Pathology and Microbiology of the medical college in Rajasthan, India. Formation of germtubes by twelve clinical isolates (cultures of germs grown from specimens obtained from infected patients) of *C. albicans* was studied in human blood containing *Staphylococcus pyogenes, Escherechia coli, Klebsiella pneumoniae, Lactobacillus acidophilus,* and *Proteus vulgaris.* The four Indian researchers concluded,

All of the five bacteria inhibited formation of germtubes by *C. albicans* at all concentrations, and the percentage of germtube formation diminished with increasing concentration of the bacteria. *Lactobacillus acidophilus* [the bacterial culture in yogurt] inhibited the formation of germtubes maximally. . . . Since germtubes of *C. albicans* are invasive, it is suggested that inhibition of blastopore germtube transformation may be significantly responsible for prevention of infection by *C. albicans* by coexisting bacterial flora.[8]

NOTES

1. John W. Rhinehart, "Chronic Metabolic Distress," *Journal of Holistic Medicine*, 1985, 7:38.

2. C. Orian Truss, *The Missing Diagnosis*, Birmingham, Ala.: The Author, 1983, p. 23.

3. Moncef Zouali, Edouard Drouhet, and André Eyquem, "Evaluation of Auto-Antibodies in Chronic Mucocutaneous Can-

didiasis Without Endocrinopathy," *Mycopathologia*, 1983, 1984, 84:87–94.

4. Juan Carlos Valdez, Oscar Enrique Meson, Garciela Aciar de Valdez, and Angel Sirena, "Suppression of Humoral Response During the Course of *Candida albicans* Infection in Mice," *Mycopathologia*, 1984, 88:61–63.

5. Victor Rivas and Thomas J. Rogers, "Studies on the Cellular Nature of *Candida albicans*-Induced Suppression," *Journal of Immunology*, January 1983, 130:376.

6. Nurith Vardinon and Esther Segal, "Suppressive Action of *Candida albicans* on the Immune Response in Mice," *Exploratory Cell Biology*, 1979, 47:275–280.

7. John D. Stobo, Sigrun Paul, Robert E. Van Scoy, and Paul E. Hermans, "Suppressor Thymus-Derived Lymphocytes in Fungal Infection," *Journal of Clinical Investigation*, February 1976, 57:319–328.

8. Bharati C. Purohit, K. R. Joshi, I. N. Ramdeo, and T. P. Bharadwaj, "The Formation of Germtubes by *Candida albicans, When Grown with Staphylococcus pyogenes, Escherichia coli, Klebsiella pneumoniae, Lactobacillus acidophilus,* and *Proteus vulgaris*," *Mycopathologia*, 1977, 62,3:187–189.

4

Antibiotics Encourage Yeast Overgrowth

For twenty-eight years, forty-nine-year-old Norma Meyer, an employee for the Kelly Insurance Agency in Leipsic, Ohio, had problems with her left kidney. X-ray examination showed that it was smaller than the right kidney, and this was thought to come from frequent urinary tract infections. She often suffered with burning on urination and severe pain located toward the back of her left side. Occasionally Mrs. Meyer needed antibiotics prescribed for the chronic recurring condition. Then, starting in 1980, kidney infections hit the woman badly, with an acute attack at least once every month. Antibiotic usage became a regular ritual in her lifestyle. She swallowed the germ-destroying drugs routinely, almost as though they were vitamin pills.

Nutritional supplementation with vitamins and minerals did, indeed, do the patient some good. She began a Shaklee Company nutrient program, and her problem improved somewhat for the next three years. Antibiotic usage could be slacked off and only the nutritional supplements continued.

However, kidney and bladder difficulties returned in late 1983, which again forced Mrs. Meyer to seek aid from a urologist. Several visits to this specialist netted her more kidney X-rays, plus some sophisticated clinical tests, laboratory tests, and an echogram (ultrasound testing, like sonar on a submarine). A fibroid tumor was found to be growing in her uterus. The surgeon suspected the enlarged uterus was pressing on her bladder and possibly causing the urination discomfort and blockages of the kidney drainage tubes leading to repeated kidney infections. A hysterectomy was performed in January 1985. Antibiotics were routinely used postoperatively.

Mrs. Meyer hoped that her problem was solved, but one month later the urinary tract infections began all over again. She experienced renewed monthly acute attacks, despite adopting a healthier way of living, including drinking cranberry juice, taking vitamin C and multivitamins, and exercising.

Once again she required extensive courses of prescribed antibiotics, but still continued to complain of severe burning on urination, and her left kidney area continued to be sore. She felt herself functioning poorly at home, on the job, and in other normal endeavors.

Her eyes smarted. Spots floated in front of them. She had ongoing fatigue, irritability and jitteriness, almost daily headaches, and a persistent sense of pressure that lingered above her ears. She suffered with poor memory, the feeling of being drained of energy, numbness in her extremities, a bad taste in her mouth, and continuous nasal congestion or discharge. The constant urinary urgency, frequency, and burning had Mrs. Meyer distraught. Worse, she was struck with a new bout of troublesome vaginal discharge, accompanied by unrelenting vulvovaginal itching. Although she had no clue about the underlying problem, hers was a classic case of the Candida syndrome.

In April 1985, Norma Meyer consulted family practice specialist L. Terry Chappell, M.D., of Bluffton, Ohio. A number of special diagnostic techniques demonstrated to Dr. Chappell that his patient had urethritis, an inflammation of the bladder tube, the urethra. Her yeast questionnaire susceptibility Y-score (a series of diagnostic questions devised by William G. Crook, M.D.) was 98. When the Y-score is less than 60 for a woman, yeast is not apt to be playing a role in illness; with a score between 61 and 120, yeast is a possible source of difficulty; 121 and over means that yeast probably is causing trouble; over 180 indicates that the patient almost certainly is suffering with the yeast syndrome.

Mrs. Meyer had gone through five pregnancies, and pregnancy encourages yeast growth. She reported a few mild vaginal yeast infections in the past. The only atypical aspect of her suspected candidiasis was that she did not now complain of any digestive disorder.

Dr. Chappell concluded that large and repeated doses of antibiotics and sulfa drugs during nearly three decades of kidney and bladder trouble had lowered Mrs. Meyer's resistance to yeast invasion. She exhibited immunodeficiency denoting that her many chronic complaints were a collection of Candida-connected illnesses.

The environmentally oriented doctor did not again use antibiotics or other Candida-stimulating drugs for the urethritis that plagued his patient. (Before visiting him, in fact, Mrs. Meyer had just completed a course of therapy with Sultrin® triple sulfa cream and vaginal tablets. Sulfa drugs are among the many broad spectrum antibiotics known to stimulate the Candida syndrome. Manufactured by Ortho Pharmaceutical Corporation of Raritan, New Jersey 08869, Sultrin® is indicated for the intravaginal treatment of *Gardnerella vaginalis* vaginitis, a bacterial infection.) In contrast to the traditional drug methods already used, Dr. Chappell cleared up Mrs. Meyer's health problems with nutritional and nontoxic remedies. He advised three natural items: (1) deodorized garlic; (2) elevated doses of vitamin C; and (3) Serodex,™ a homeopathic remedy. (Homeopathic remedies use infinitesimally small doses of drugs.) He placed her daily on three liquid capsules of aged special garlic preparation (SGP), a professional-strength formulation of the over-the-counter Japanese product brand-named Kyolic™. SGP™ is packaged and distributed in the United States by the Wakunaga of America Company, Ltd., of Torrance, California. Her vitamin C dosage was increased to 3,000 mg a day, and she began on Serodex™ at the sixfold dilution (6x) as the initial concentration. Serodex™ is a homeopathic formulation with no known contraindications and no known side effects, intended to help develop immunity against the yeast organism. These and other nontoxic remedies will be discussed in detail in Chapters Eleven and Twelve.

When she entered Dr. Chappell's practice, Norma Meyer

had blood pressure elevated to 146/94. With nontoxic treatment for the Candida syndrome, it soon dropped to 130/78, and has since remained normal. The burning with voiding stopped within three weeks. Then she ran out of Serodex™ just prior to her one-month return consultation and experienced another episode of burning. Starting back on the homeopathic drops, which originally were intended to be continued for three months, her urethritis symptoms disappeared again. There was still some voiding frequency, but fatigue didn't bother her anymore, and plenty of energy was left at the end of her working day to accomplish homemaker tasks.

Today Mrs. Meyer no longer feels drained and anxious. Her vaginal discharge went away quickly, and the absence of burning and itching has helped to restore her usual cheerfulness. Smarting eyes and the spots in front of them have floated away forever; she has discomfort only when discourteous cigarette smokers blow their residue her way. Minimal feelings of irritability or jitteriness remained for just a few months. The bad taste in her mouth left permanently, and her nasal congestion and postnasal drip cleared altogether. The left side where her kidney used to feel tortured hasn't given her pain in months.

By December 10, 1985, the woman reported to us that she is living a happy and trouble-free existence. "It's been really good," said Norma Meyer. "I've not needed any Serodex™ now for at least four months. All I use is special garlic preparation and vitamins." Knowing that antibiotics were the source of her candidiasis, she intends to avoid their use unless she faces a serious or life-threatening bacterial infection. "I won't take antibiotics anymore," she declares.

ANTIBIOTICS

Antibiotics are chemical substances, produced primarily by the growth of molds from plants or animals (some are manufactured synthetically), that are capable in small amounts of destroying or inhibiting the growth of living things such as germs. The antibiotic lincomycin hydrochloride, for instance, can kill the pathogenic bacteria pneumococci, which causes pneumonia. But lincomycin and other antibiotics also kill the friendly Lactobacilli which live synergistically in your intestines and keep down the spread of the Candida organism.

Antibiotics are often combined together and with other drugs, to enhance their killing effects and to minimize undesirable side effects. Typical antibacterial drugs in common use today are penicillin-V, -K, or -G, plus its derivatives, such as ampicillin and amoxicillin; close cousins to penicillin, such as cephalosporins; chlortetracyclin, also known as Aureomycin®; oxytetracycline, also called Terramycin®; tetracycline, such as Achromycin®, Vibramycin®, Minocin; trimethoprim-sulfa combinations such as Septra® or Bactrim®; furadantin as the brand name Macrodantin®; the rarely used chloramphenicol, as the brand name Chloromycetin®; topicals bacitracin, neomycin, and polymyxin; streptomycin (an injection only) and used less often than tobramycin (Nebcin®) or gentamycin (Garramycin®). There are thousands of different antibiotics—so many that literally a dictionary of antibiotics has been published. Different antibiotics act against different microbes. Those that are effective against a great number of microbes are called broad spectrum antibiotics; these are the ones most likely to stimulate the illness-producing overgrowth of *C. albicans*.

The increased incidence of candidiasis in recent years has been clearly shown to be related to the increased use of antibiotics. In particular, the incidence of various systemic disorders and localized visceral candidal infections has been convincingly correlated with the administration of combined antibiotics or broad spectrum antibiotics, with or without corticosteroid (cortisone) treatment. This first review article on the effect of antibiotics on *C. albicans*, written by Mildred S. Seelig, M.D., M.P.H., was researched twenty years ago. Dr. Seelig's perceptive revelations are startlingly more pertinent today.[1]

Oftentimes, the fungus comes about as a result of our own demands for antibiotic prescriptions or from the actions of doctors who are uneducated about the ways of the yeast syndrome. Here the coauthors ask, "Isn't it time to stop gambling with the excessive prescribing of antibiotics?" We're sure that this chapter furnishes an affirmative answer to this question. Read on and be shocked at what's been foisted on consumers of medical services and consumers of meat and poultry.

INCREASED COLONY-FORMING CANDIDA
AFTER ANTIBIOTIC USE

Antibiotic use disrupts the normal competition between the separate members of the resident flora of a human being's gut, as well as between the collective resident flora and any new organisms taken in. Every person ingesting an antibiotic becomes a self-contained factory tending to produce resistant strains of germs. This occurs because antibiotics select for survival any existing or newly emerging resistant organisms. Not every germ is killed by an antibiotic. To get over an infection, you depend on your immune defense system to clean up the remaining microbes that continue to grow because they have developed resistance to the antibiotic you're using.

The wholesale use of antibiotics for every little infection such as mild illnesses in children has negative consequences not immediately obvious. For instance, commonly prescribed broad spectrum antibiotics help to create resistant strains of nonpathogenic bacteria such as *Escherichia coli*. Each surviving *E. coli* bacterium thereby becomes a reservoir of transferable resistance genes.

We have selected *E. coli* as our example because it is one of the aerobic bacteria that naturally lives in your gut, the same place where *C. albicans* is most likely to flourish and begin its destructive work leading to the Candida syndrome. Like this commensal yeast we've been condemning, *E. coli* basically is saprophytic, and its family is widespread throughout your body as normal flora. Under certain conditions, however, the bacterium also may invade and produce devastating disease. *E. coli* is held back from pathological overgrowth by coexisting friendly bacteria such as *Lactobacillus acidophilus* and *Lactobacillus bifidus*. When you use antibiotics systematically instead of topically, your friendly *L. acidophilus* and *L. bifidus* are easily killed. Any antibiotic-resistant and potentially dangerous *E. coli* get left behind along with the unaffected *C. albicans*. Thus remaining are two germs, a bacterium and a fungus, either of which might cause much damage to you, the host organism.

A study on *Escherichia coli* was performed in 1980 at a

renowned microbiological institute in Oslo, Norway. Results indicated that the defensive effects of human white blood cells (WBCs) were reduced when cell preparations were treated with antibiotics. *E. coli* which were exposed to antibiotics and then put in contact with WBCs did not get vigorously attacked by the usually phagocytic (devouring) defense cells. The researchers wrote: "There was a tendency towards depression of the process of phagocytosis in the presence of high concentrations of the various antibiotics."[2]

Another 1980 study was carried out by investigators at the University of Pavia in Italy. They tested the effect of five antibiotics on the candidacidal activity of human white blood cells capable of ingesting and killing bacteria. Each of the antibiotics blocked the action of the WCBs against *Candida albicans*, an organism on which they ordinarily would feast. As mentioned, the antibiotics have no effect on the yeast organism,[3] so Candida overgrowth can proceed uninhibited when an important white blood cell defense action has been stunned.

At the Ohio State University College of Dentistry forty rats were divided into two groups. Group 1 received a tetracycline solution as drinking water. Group 2 received distilled water. Animals in both groups were inoculated in the mouth equally with pathogenic *C. albicans*. After twenty weeks, sixteen group 1 animals and seventeen group 2 animals developed lesions on their tongues. No difference was shown between the lesions in the two groups, except the antibiotic-treated animals had significantly larger fungus lesions than did the untreated ones. The induction of experimental oral candidiasis in the rat has been considerably enhanced by the use of tetracycline. Antibiotics help yeasts grow well in the human host.[4]

Investigators from the University of Wisconsin Medical School in Madison studied the natural killer cells of the alimentary tract of mice. After creating colonization of the alimentary tracts in the animals with pure cultures of *C. albicans*, pathogenic bacillus bacteria were introduced, but they did not stimulate natural killer cell activity. The bacilli grew in the mice without difficulty. Increased quantities of yeast present in their intestinal flora inhibited the usual immune response and presumably aided bacteria to grow.[5]

Among other recent studies, the Mycology Laboratory at the Eastern Michigan University in Ypsilanti conducted a valuable animal experiment in 1985, with important implications for humans. Antibiotic-treated and untreated hamsters were inoculated in the stomach with *C. albicans;* the question was whether the yeast could opportunistically colonize the gastrointestinal tract and then disseminate to the pancreas, liver, spleen, and other vital gut organs.

In their article published in the September 1985 issue of *Infection and Immunity,* the mycologists wrote:

Antibiotic treatment decreased the total population levels of the indigenous bacterial flora and predisposed hamsters to gastrointestinal overgrowth and subsequent systemic dissemination by *C. albicans* in 86 percent of the animals . . . The results indicate that the indigenous microflora reduced the mucosal association of *C. albicans* by forming a dense layer of bacteria in the mucus gel, out-competing yeast cells for adhesion sites, and producing inhibitor substances (possibly fatty acids, secondary bile acids, or both) that reduce *C. albicans* adhesion. It is suggested, therefore, that the indigenous intestinal microflora suppresses *C. albicans* colonization and dissemination from the gut by inhibiting Candida-mucosal association and reducing *C. albicans* population levels in the gut.

The two mycologists went on to confirm what we believe and have ourselves stated. "Systemic Candida infections are important causes of morbidity [illness] and mortality [death] among patients who are compromised immunologically or who are undergoing prolonged antibiotic therapy. The passage of viable *Candida albicans* through the gastrointestinal (GI) mucosa into the host bloodstream is believed to be an important mechanism leading to systemic candidosis."[6]

Disturbingly, polyene antibiotics (such as nystatin, used to treat yeast infections including candidiasis) may induce an increase in the number of colony-forming units of yeast cells of *C. albicans,* according to microbiologists in the Divisions of Infectious Diseases, Dermatology, and Laboratory Medicine at Washington University School of Medicine, St. Louis,

Missouri. Researchers reported that the normally yeast-killing polyene antibiotics were bound to the fatty acids in the cell wall of the fungi, but they produced no toxic effect and actually stimulated the yeasts to increase the number of their colonies.[7] No matter what the intended effect of antibiotics, they all hold the prospect of making our lives more difficult— even the ones we often rely on to help eradicate the yeast syndrome.

ANTIBIOTICS IN ANIMAL FEED AS A STIMULATOR OF CANDIDIASIS

In 1949 antibiotic use was still in its infancy, since only a few of these drugs had recently been discovered. Thomas Jukes, Ph.D., then a research director at American Cyanamid's Lederle Laboratories, stumbled on the curious fact that baby chicks fed mash containing residual amounts of the antibiotic chlortetracycline gained 10–20 percent more weight than other chicks. Dr. Jukes found that piglets did even better on subtherapeutic levels of antibiotic. They grew fat fast![8]

The Jukes discovery was a commercial bonanza, leading to an antibiotics market now worth over $250 million each year to U.S. drug makers. In 1985, more than 11 million pounds of the drugs—about one-third of the approximately 35 million pounds of antibiotics made in the United States—were sold as feed additives for livestock. Drug companies supplying this ever-increasing demand include American Cyanamid, American Hoechst, Eli Lilly, Pfizer, SmithKline Beckman, and a few smaller ones.

Today, subtherapeutic amounts of broad spectrum antibiotics are routinely added to animal feeds to promote more rapid and enhanced meat production in nearly all domestic edible animals.

In promoting this abnormal growth, antibiotic additives also enable farmers to use less feed to produce more meat. The economics of antibiotic use have proved irresistible: almost all the poultry, about 70 percent of the cattle, and 90 percent of the pigs raised commercially in the United States are ingesting subtherapeutic doses of antibiotics at mealtimes. And drug firms continue to invest heavily in research.

The Animal Health Institute (a meat industry lobby) says that its members spend over $200 million each year to develop new growth-promoting feed additives.[9]

The widespread use of antibiotics, for both veterinary and agricultural purposes, has its dark side. Adding such drugs to livestock feed has been accompanied by an increase in the number of drug-resistant microbe strains. A review of salmonella-induced dysentery in America from 1971 to 1983 showed that food animals were the source of 69 percent of the outbreaks caused by resistant salmonella and 46 percent of those caused by antibiotic-sensitive strains of microorganisms.[10] Now it's reported that spread of multiply resistant salmonella from calves to people is definite, including the spread to a hospital nursery.[11]

In England in the 1960s, serious human disease caused by the same multiply-resistant *Salmonella typhimurium* type 29 originally found in cattle led to establishment of the Swann Committee. This committee's report attributed the rise in resistant organisms in humans to low-level (subtherapeutic) use of antibiotics in animals. As a result antibiotics routinely needed for therapy of infections were removed from subtherapeutic use in England. In 1976, all other countries of the European Economic Community followed suit.[12]

Putting the same antibiotics in feed troughs that are found in pharmacies contributes to the rise of even "cross-resistant" strains of bacteria that effectively resist more than one drug. The medical community is concerned about this documented relationship of antibiotics in animal feed and pathogenic cross-resistance.[13] General agreement exists that antibiotic use is responsible for the recent rise in resistant bacteria, but the meat and poultry industries continue, in the face of mounting criticism, to point to excessive use of therapeutic prescriptions for people as the primary culprit.

The arguments back and forth—especially from the profit-minded industrialists—would appear to be irrelevant; the environments of animals and human beings are not separate. Exchange of bacteria occurs between both. Organisms originating in the animal gut can find their way into the human intestinal tract.[14] When pathogenic, they can cause human disease.

The 1984 publication of a book devastatingly condemning

the meat industry, *Modern Meat: Antibiotics, Hormones and the Pharmaceutical Farm,* has stimulated public interest in the use both of antibiotics and of hormones to stimulate animal growth.[15]

The New England Journal of Medicine in 1984 published a scientific paper and an editorial about a study which had been conducted by the Center for Disease Control (CDC) in Atlanta, Georgia. This experiment established a link between the use of antibiotics in feed and the transmission of antibiotic-resistant microorganisms to humans who ate the meat.[16] The article and editorial were picked up by the *New York Times,* the *Washington Post,* and dozens of other newspapers. Representative Jim Weaver (Democrat-Oregon) then wrote to House colleagues urging them to support legislation "to ban the addition to livestock feed of subtherapeutic doses of antibiotics that have been licensed for human use." As you might have guessed, nothing has come from that proposed legislation. In a directive to the U.S. Food and Drug Administration (FDA), the Senate Appropriations Committee asked that no further action be taken on the antibiotic–animal feed question until an FDA report on the issue had been completed and reviewed. What's happened to the report? Have the powerful food industry and drug industry lobbies persuaded our public officials to dispose of it?

On January 13, 1986, the House Government Operations Subcommittee on Intergovernmental Relations and Human Resources, which held hearings on Capitol Hill in the summer of 1985, issued a study, "Human Food Safety and the Regulation of Animal Drugs." It condemned the U.S. Food and Drug Administration for inadequately monitoring the use of toxic drugs and nutrition supplements in raising and fattening livestock. The subcommittee chairman, Representative Ted Weiss, Democrat of New York City, said: "The law requires and consumers deserve far more public health protection than the agency has provided. The FDA has repeatedly put what it perceives are interests of veterinarians and the livestock industry ahead of its legal obligation to protect consumers."[17]

Probably worse than drug-resistant strains of bacteria created by antibiotics in animal feed is the resulting stimulation of yeast overgrowth in people. The agricultural industry, the pharmaceutical industry, the medical industry, and governmental consumer advocates do not yet seem aware of this greater danger to the American public. Perhaps it's because the yeast syndrome has been recognized only recently and is now just emerging as the epidemic of the 1980s. If we as a society fail to take action—or if powerful special interest lobbies block our efforts—then we will have forfeited our birthright of good health.

NOTES

1. Mildred S. Seelig, "Role of Antibiotic in the Pathogenesis of Candida Infections," *American Journal of Medicine*, 1966, 40:887–917.

2. Kjetil Melby and Tore Midtvedt, "Effects of Some Antibacterial Agents on the Phagocytosis of [32] P-Labelled *Escherichia coli* by Human Polymorphonuclear Cells," *Acta Pathology and Microbiology, Scandinavian Section B*, 1980, 88:103–106.

3. Franco A. Ferrari, Ambrogio Pagani, Massimo Marconi, Renzo Stefanoni, and Antonio G. Siccardi, "Inhibition of Candidacidal Activity of Human Neutrophil Leukocytes by Aminoglycoside Antibiotics," *Antimicrobial Agents and Chemotherapy*, January 1980, 17:87–88.

4. Carl M. Allen, Frank M. Beck, Fredrick A. Lurie, and H. Mark Pinsky, "Role of Tetracycline in Pathogenesis of Chronic Candidiasis of Rat Tongues," *Infection and Immunity*, February 1985, 47:480–483.

5. K. F. Bartizal, C. Salkowski, and E. Balish, "The Influence of a Gastrointestinal Microflora on Natural Killer Cell Activity," *RES: Journal of the Reticuloendothelial Society*, 1983, 33:381–390.

6. Michael J. Kennedy and Paul A. Volz, "Ecology of *Candida albicans* Gut Colonization: Inhibition of Candida Adhesion, Colonization, and Dissemination from the Gastrointestinal Tract by Bacterial Antagonism," *Infection and Immunity*, September 1985, 49:654–663.

7. Anina Brajtburg, Svetlana Elberg, Gerald Medoff, and George S. Kobayashi, "Increase in Colony-Forming Units of *Candida albicans* After Treatment with Polyene Antibiotics," *Antimicrobial Agents and Chemotherapy*, January 1981, 19:199–200.

8. E.L.R. Stokstad and T. H. Jukes, "Further Observations on the 'Animal Protein Factor,'" *Proceedings of the Society of Experimental Biology and Medicine*, 1950, 73:523–528.

9. "Antibiotics in Animal Feed," *Chemical Week*, October 10, 1984, pp. 44–48.

10. S. D. Holmberg, J. G. Wells, and M. L. Cohen, "Animal-to-Man Transmission of Antimicrobial-Resistant *Salmonella:* Investigations of U.S. Outbreaks, 1971–1983," *Science*, 1984, 225:833–835.

11. T. F. O'Brien, J. D. Hopkins, B. S. Gilleece, et al., "Molecular Epidemiology of Antibiotic Resistance in *Salmonella* from Animals and Human Beings in the United States," *New England Journal of Medicine*, 1982, 307:1–6; R. W. Lyons, C. L. Samples, H. N. DeSilva, K. A. Ross, E. M. Julian, P. J. Checko, "An Epidemic of Resistant *Salmonella* in a Nursery: Animal-to-Animal Spread," *Journal of the American Medical Association*, 1980, 243:546–547.

12. E. S. Anderson and M. J. Lewis, "Drug Resistance and Its Transfer in *Salmonella typhimurium*," *Nature*, 1965, 206:579–583.

13. S. B. Levy, G. B. FitzGerald, and A. B. Macone, "Spread of Antibiotic-Resistant Plasmids from Chicken to Chicken and from Chicken to Man," *Nature*, 1976, 260:40–42.

14. A. H. Linton, "Animal to Man Transmission of Enterobacteriacea," Royal Society of Health Journal, 1977, 97:115–118.

15. Orville Schell, *Modern Meat: Antibiotics, Hormones, and the Pharmaceutical Farm*, New York: Random House, 1984.

16. Stuart B. Levy, "Playing Antibiotic Pool: Time to Tally the Score," *New England Journal of Medicine*, September 6, 1984, 311:663–664.

17. Keith Schneider, "F.D.A. Faulted in Threat from Animal Drugs," *New York Times*, January 13, 1986, p. 1.

5

Additional Stimulators of the Yeast Syndrome

Until June 1984, a secretary working in the marketing department at the headquarters of a large automotive company, thirty-four-year-old Sally Whiteburn of Detroit, Michigan, thought that she was a normal, healthy person. Thin, small-framed, and athletically inclined, Mrs. Whiteburn exercised several times a week until she began experiencing severe menstrual pain and repeated bladder infections, both of which progressively worsened.

In September 1984, her physician performed a laparoscopy that revealed the presence of a benign tumor plus endometriosis. Laparoscopy, sometimes called "bandaid surgery," is an examination of the internal abdominal structures by means of an illuminated tubular instrument somewhat like a thin telescope and called a laparoscope, which is passed through a small incision in the wall of the abdomen. Endometriosis is the condition in which membranous material of the kind lining the womb is abnormally present at other sites within the cavity of the pelvis. Any fragments of womb lining tissue will show the same periodic changes and cyclical bleeding in response to the female hormone phases, wherever located. Since there was no outlet for the bleeding that occurred from this womb tissue located on the organs of her pelvic cavity, Mrs. Whiteburn suffered severe pain for several days each month. To correct these problems she underwent a total hysterectomy along with extensive bladder repair in January 1985.

"Because of widespread infection, I was again hospitalized two weeks later," Mrs. Whiteburn wrote in a highly literate and detailed letter. "In all, I was given five different types of antibiotics, some of them repeatedly." Three years prior to this she had taken tetracycline for a full year and a half to control a frustrating acne problem. Additionally, she had taken birth control pills for most of the preceding ten years. She also had suffered for four years with a discharge from yeast vaginitis.

The operative experience left her with a bevy of strange symptoms. "I had a pounding in my head (not like a headache, but as if you could hear your heart beating in your brain), clicking noises in my head, spots in front of my eyes, dizziness and uncoordination, headaches, extreme fatigue, and weird visual disturbances like lights flashing when my eyes blinked. I heard another noise in my head every time I moved my eyes. My memory was poor, and I would become confused very easily."

Her gynecologist prescribed estrogen in the form of 2.5 mg of Premarin®, a medical approach which, although standard, is somewhat surprising, since estrogens have been reported to increase the risk of endometrial cancer. Theoretically, any abnormal fragments of endometrial tissue that might have been missed at operation may undergo a cancerous change much later, due to excess estrogen effect. Three case control studies reported that the risk of endometrial cancer in estrogen users was about 4.5 to 13.9 times greater than in nonusers.[1] These studies are further supported by the finding that incidence rates of endometrial cancer have increased sharply since 1969 in eight different areas of the United States with population-based cancer reporting systems. The increase may be related to the rapidly expanding use of estrogens during the last decade.[2]

Estrogen also was among the ingredients in the birth control pills that Mrs. Whiteburn had taken. When handing her his Premarin® prescription, the gynecologist assured the woman that most of her weird head complaints would disappear. But they did not!

"When the pounding in my head did not go away, I decided to consult a neurologist," she said. "In March 1985, the nerve specialist performed a brain CAT scan using a dye injected into my vein. During that procedure, my throat swelled closed and my heart started beating irregularly. It was a severe [and potentially fatal] allergic reaction to the dye. I was given adrenaline and several other medications to counteract the iodine dye, but from that day forward, I was allergic to almost every chemical I would come into contact with. My throat starts to swell, and I develop typically asthmatic symptoms."

Soon after this episode, the patient began developing allergies to many different foods. Mrs. Whiteburn explained, "The brain CAT scan was negative and my neurologist referred me to an ear specialist, who also could find no reason for the pulsating sensations and other symptoms. The ear doctor suggested that an angiogram should be taken, again using more iodine dye into a main artery in my leg. I refused to have this done as the doctors who conducted the brain CAT scan to which I had reacted told me never to have another test using dye. The next time it could produce a fatal allergic reaction."

The frightened woman went to three more doctors trying to find an answer for the subtle but persistent perception of head pounding, worried that it might be a cerebral artery problem or something else quite serious. Searching for a diagnosis and its solution among many different physicians, she could not find any.

THE PATIENT CONFRONTS THE YEAST SYNDROME

"About this time I read Dr. Crook's book, *The Yeast Connection*, and made an appointment with an allergist who works extensively with Candida. He couldn't see me until April 1985, so I went ahead and just put myself on the book's anti-Candida diet," said the patient. "Soon thereafter I came upon Sally Rockwell's Candida cookbook. She recommended that completely cutting out grains and fruits would reduce the yeast at a much faster rate.[3] I did this."

Early in April 1985, Sally Whiteburn did consult allergist and clinical ecologist John Rechsteiner, M.D., of Springfield, Ohio. Dr. Rechsteiner is a former member of the Board of Directors of the American Academy of Environmental Medicine. This academy, previously named the Society of Clinical Ecology, is comprised of health professionals concerned with adverse reactions to environmental insults to people, as modified by individual susceptibility and specific adaptation. These adverse reactions, manifested as a wide variety of physical and mental symptoms, are often chronic in nature and cyclic in occurrence. The conditions they produce are frequently undiagnosed, misdiagnosed, or poorly identified by traditionally practicing, establishment-type physicians. Polysystemic chronic candidiasis—the yeast syndrome—is one such health problem. The science of environmental medicine (clinical ecology) is particularly concerned with impersonal environmental excitants (those to which any of us can be exposed) in air, water, food, drugs, and environmental chemicals in our habitat. For referrals to clinical ecologists who are now known as environmental medicine specialists near your area, contact the academy at P.O. Box 16106, Denver, CO 80216; (303) 622–9755.

Mrs. Whiteburn's environmental medicine specialist, Dr. Rechsteiner, emphasizes treatment of candidiasis, chemical intolerances (especially petrochemicals), food allergies, and inhalant problems. From the patient's description of her symptoms, the Candida syndrome, with associated chemical sensitivities and allergies, was apparently her trouble. Dr. Rechsteiner recorded a thorough health history and sent the patient to a local medical laboratory to have blood specimens drawn.

Research for detecting the presence of candidiasis has resulted in a few accurate laboratory tests now being used (see Chapter Nine). One of them is the "light" blood test developed by the California Allergy Laboratories Hemogenetics Division, which measures the immune response of patients to *Candida albicans*. Dr. Rechsteiner packaged the woman's blood and mailed it for testing to California Allergy Laboratories in San Mateo, California.

"The normal test reading for a healthy person is 8. I had a Candida count of 41.7," Mrs. Whiteburn told us in a subsequent interview.

Sally Whiteburn subsequently conquered her Candida syndrome, but this chapter's focus is another area: additional stimulators of the Candida syndrome, besides the overuse of antibiotic drugs. While antibiotics are the primary factors, there is something else that brings on the Candida syndrome. That something else is the birth control pill.

THE CONTENT OF BIRTH CONTROL PILLS

Synthetic hormones containing both estrogens and progesterones are incorporated into birth control pills. Doctors are uncertain about whether the estrogen fraction encourages the growth of *C. albicans* in a woman's body. The progesterone (also referred to as progestin) component, though, does tend to foster candidiasis. Taking progestin also alters mucous membranes of the mouth, throat, lungs, and vaginal vault, in which yeasts are invariably present. Progesterone-induced membrane changes, for example, occurred among 2,000 birth control pill users studied for candidiasis in 1983 at the University of Southern California School of Medicine in Los Angeles. Results indicated that all of them possessed vaginal yeast invasion and nearly 30 percent suffered with associated local discomfort. They complained of chronic vaginitis with itching, pain from friction (as with sexual intercourse), irritability, fatigue, and depression. These more general complaints suggest that many of them might also be suffering with systemic yeast effects—the Candida syndrome.

Oral contraceptives are comprised of steroid hormones and are divided into three types: combination, sequential, and daily progestin. The most common, often simply called "the Pill," is the combination type and consists of a synthetic estrogen and a synthetic progestin, representing the two female hormones. The amount of estrogen and progestin can vary, but the amount of estrogen is most important. Both the effectiveness and the major dangers of oral contraceptives are related to the quantity of estrogen.

A second type of oral contraceptive, often referred to as the "mini-pill," contains only a progestin. It works in part by preventing release of an egg from the ovary, by keeping sperm from reaching the egg, and by making the womb less receptive to any fertilized egg that might reach it. The mini-pill is about 2 percent less effective than the combination oral contraceptive. In addition, the synthetic progestin-only pill has a tendency to cause irregular bleeding or cessation of bleeding entirely (called amenorrhea, or absence of expected periods). Mini-pills are taken daily and continuously. Use of the mini-pill is sometimes desirable for women who must avoid estrogen-containing medications: women over thirty-five, those who have experienced estrogen-related side effects from the combination type of oral contraceptives, and those with a history of headaches, hypertension, or varicose veins (where inflammation from thrombophlebitis would be more likely).

The third type of oral contraception, no longer allowed for use in the United States, is the sequential pill, which contains much higher doses of estrogen. With the sequential type, estrogen is given alone for two weeks, and then a combination of estrogen and a synthetic progestin is given for one week. This regimen is associated with a relatively high incidence of irregular bleeding and a pregnancy rate of up to 8 percent per year.

HOW ORAL CONTRACEPTIVES STIMULATE SYSTEMIC CANDIDA COLONIES

At the third Yeast–Human Interaction Symposium held in San Francisco, March 29–31, 1985, David Feldman, M.D., Professor of Medicine and Chief in the Division of Endocrinology at the Stanford University School of Medicine, Stanford, California, spoke of steroid receptors which are present in yeast and the production of steroids by yeasts.

"*Candida albicans* has a steroid-binding protein. It binds corticoids [steroids such as cortisone] and progesterones," Dr. Feldman declared. In the same way that a woman transports steroids into the cytoplasm of her body cells, the yeast takes steroids into its own cellular protoplasm.

From his studies, Dr. Feldman found that corticosterone

and progesterone were the yeast's two most favored steroids. He found that the Candida receptor is even better at absorbing steroids and seeking steroid substance than were the animal receptors also studied. "Bidirectional interaction is possible," he concluded, meaning that yeast can potentially participate in, and interfere with, human hormone signal systems. (See Chapter Two for the way Clarissa Candida describes her use of hormones to interfere with a person's metabolic traffic.)

A speculation derived from Dr. Feldman's microbiochemical research is that the attachment of steroids in birth control pills to receptor sites on *C. albicans* might "feed" the yeast a desired molecule. Thus, oral contraceptives probably promote Candida colony growth through a direct and unavoidable mechanism.

At the same 1985 Candida conference, internist Leo Galland, M.D., formerly with the Gesell Institute of New Haven, Connecticut, and now Assistant Medical Director at the World Health Medical Group in New York City, discussed how the Candida organism finds nourishment and spreads its colony. "A yeast that is happy and well fed will grow rapidly and bud," Dr. Galland said. "Candida goes into germtubes or hyphae formation when it is deprived of nutrients. [Hyphae are germtubes, the branching tubular filaments comprising the vegetative portion of fungi.] Human serum contains certain food factors for the yeast, including transferin, which binds iron (another key nutrient for yeast), and the serum may also deprive it of [other] nutrients."

When malnourishment occurs for *C. albicans*, "It goes into this hyphal form in the organism's search for nutrients. One of the changes that occurs is at the tips of the hyphae: an enzyme called phospholipase is elaborated, which is capable of disrupting human cell membranes, allowing the yeast looking for food to penetrate into the cell," said Dr. Galland. "The Candida's phospholipase works by splitting fatty acids from phospholipids present in the human cell membrane. There will then be peroxide generation which accounts for some of the local inflammation [with skin eruptions, gut wall distress, and other disorders]."

A woman swallowing her daily hormone-containing birth

control pill might therefore be helping to meet the metabolic needs of *C. albicans*. Her own cells are absorbing the progesterone from the Pill. In penetrating human cells while searching for nutrients, the fungus is likely also to be stimulated by the steroids found within—resulting in more vigorous symptoms of the yeast syndrome.

CORTICOSTEROIDS FEED YEAST

We have suggested that Candida colonies are stimulated to grow by the taking of oral contraceptives. The same steroid receptor response appears to be true for the utilization of that class of drugs known as corticosteroids, more particularly glucocorticoids such as cortisone. Corticosteroid drugs should be avoided by Candida syndrome victims and those who wish to minimize their chance of becoming a victim. Where possible, the corticosteroids to avoid include hydrocortisone (cortisol), cortisone, desoxycorticosterone, fludrocortisone, prednisolone, prednisone, fluprednisolone, meprednisolone, methylprednisolone, paramethasone, triamcinolone, dexamethasone, and betamethasone. Over fifty corticosteroids have been isolated from the adrenal glands. Some of the pathological conditions in which they are administered include acute allergic reactions, chronic allergic conditions, rheumatoid arthritis, Addison's disease (adrenal insufficiency), cancer chemotherapy, skin eruptions, bronchial asthma, emphysema, hypersensitivity conditions, and various disorders of the adrenal glands.

NUTRITIONAL DEFICIENCIES GIVE RISE TO CANDIDIASIS

Overall observations among clinicians who routinely diagnose and treat candidiasis is that an immunodeficient state due to malnutrition of the patient is probably a precursor to the disease. Even in the midst of plenty among the rich and the middle class of industrialized countries such as Great Britain, Canada, the United States, France, Holland, and Japan, malnourishment is a major and undermining problem for growing numbers of people. Malnourishment is malnutrition in the sense of biochemical *quality* of the food, not the quantity of its consumption.

Patients often are selectively nutrient deficient. The B vitamin biotin, for instance, seems consistently inadequately consumed in daily food supplies. Biotin is lacking in the empty-calorie prepared meals so common in commercial fast food restaurants. Their highly refined white sugar, white flour breads and pastries, French fried potatoes, and other "fake food" depletes a person of nutrients—while at the same time feeding his yeast invader with simple carbohydrates. Supplementation with biotin may help prevent the conversion of the budding yeast form of *C. albicans* to its invasive hyphae or germtube form.

Candida can move rapidly to become invasive if it finds itself unhappy with its present environment. The organism may change its anatomical and physiological state from a rounded yeastlike form to a puncturing mycelial form. As earlier noted, mycelia are those tangled masses of fine branching threads which make up the "moving on" part of a fungus like *C. albicans*. The mycelium is its invasive fungal form, which penetrates human cells, seeking food. Candida organisms are dimorphic, meaning that they can exist in two states. The yeastlike state is sugar-fermenting, actively reproducing, and noninvasive. Eating foods such as brown rice (not white rice, which has been "polished"), soybeans, liver, kidney, egg yolk, and other sources of biotin or even taking vitamins with biotin might help to hold Candida in its yeastlike state and stop its conversion to the invasive fungal form.

How many consumers know this about biotin and other nutrients? Most traditionally trained physicians are completely unaware of the significance of biotin nutrition and its connection to candidiasis. So why should *you* know? The answer is that it's *your* body, *your* health, *your* life that's endangered by the Candida syndrome.

There are many aspects to the anti-Candida diet, which we will be covering in Chapter Eleven. Too many ramifications exist for us to attempt to include them here. To illustrate, a final complication relating to biotin nutrition: *C. albicans* growth is known to be stimulated by the simultaneous presence of carbohydrates, biotin, some other B vitamins, and a few minerals. Biotin and other B vitamins should be taken several hours before or after meals, at which time little or no carbohydrate will be present on the mucous membranes. That's the preferred way to swallow your required daily intake of the B vitamins. (See Chapter Twelve to receive more detailed information on nutritional supplementation for the treatment of the yeast syndrome.)

BACTERIAL INFECTION FOSTERS CANDIDA GROWTH

In a series of three published scientific papers and in her followup lecture at the second Yeast–Human Interaction Symposium, December 9–11, 1983, in Birmingham, Alabama, Eunice Carlson, Ph.D., Associate Professor of Microbiology, Technological University, Houghton, Michigan, advised that bacterial infection fosters the systemic growth of *C. albicans*.

In her first study, published in December 1982, Dr. Carlson showed the synergistic effect on mouse mortality by the combined infection of mice with *C. albicans* and *Staphylococcus aureus* isolated from a patient with toxic shock syndrome (TSS). Mice exhibited very high resistance when inoculated within the peritoneum (abdominal cavity) by either pathogen alone. But when both organisms were injected simultaneously, 100 percent of her test animals died.[5]

In Dr. Carlson's second paper, published in January 1983, she described a study which showed that mice inoculated with *S. aureus* along with a nonlethal dose of *C. albicans* developed widespread staphylococcal infection. Yet *S. aureus* injected alone at the same or considerably higher doses did not establish such an infection. A minimum dose of *C. albicans*, indeed, also enhanced similar bacterial infections with *Serratia marcescens* and *Streptococcus faecalis*,[6] both of which can be as pathogenic for humans, as is *S. aureus*.

The final paper in Dr. Carlson's series was published in October 1983 and absolutely proved the synergism between *S. aureus* and the yeast organism. Bacterial strains isolated from patients with toxic shock syndrome were combined with sublethal doses of *C. albicans*. Mice were inoculated intraperitoneally (into the space surrounding their abdominal organs) with the infectious agents. TSS developed in the animals, but some differences in their signs and symptoms occurred, depending on the mouse strain. The symptoms included conjunctivitis (eye inflammation); gastrointestinal, neurological, and circulatory abnormalities; a rash followed by scaling and then sloughing of the skin; and patchy baldness.

Although Dr. Carlson observed overlap in symptoms between animal treatment groups, certain symptoms (neurological and bleeding) were seen only in animals inoculated with particular strains of *S. aureus* combined with *C. albicans*.[7]

Dr. Carlson's research has major implications for people who suffer with recurrent deep-seated tissue infections such as pyelonephritis (kidney infections), bronchitis/bronchial pneumonia/lobar pneumonia, and perhaps even diverticulitis (infection forming in wall pockets of the large intestine in older people).

New treatment concept: We believe that controlled clinical trials are needed to compare the present treatment regimen of antibiotics alone with programs that combine antibiotics and various anti-Candida medications that are described in Chapter Ten. We anticipate that many patients now suffering with such recurrent infections will likely find permanent relief. (For nearly three years, coauthor Dr. John Trowbridge has been using this combined therapy in his practice and attaining excellent patient success.) If bacterial colonies are remaining in tissues after antibiotics are discontinued, safely shielded inside a colony of surrounding yeast, then only by killing the *C. albicans* at the same time can a physician effectively eradicate all of the patient's bacterial organisms. It's the only way to rid his patient of the bacteria that would remain to seed the next infection in the following weeks or months.

POLLUTANTS AND POISONS
PROMOTE THE YEAST SYNDROME

Toxic and poisonous substances, such as the heavy metals and organic chemicals and pesticides floating in our water and air from industrial pollution, are promoters of the Candida syndrome. Household pollutants do this, too. We can't individually take much action to reduce the total amount of industrial toxins, but we can all improve our own home situation and remove toxic products from surroundings in which we live.

C. albicans growth is aided by suppression of your immune system response from commonly used, unsafe consumer goods that are a preventable stress upon your body. While the listing below primarily applies to the surroundings in your home—which you readily control—several categories also apply to offices and other working environments. By consulting an ecologically minded physician specialist and referring to several excellent personal environmental clean-up guides that he or she can recommend, you're able to do a great deal to minimize the stresses on your immune defense system.

Some of the toxic home-care and self-care substances which turn your internal ecology into one highly favorable for yeast growth are given in the following classifications and listings:[8]

Aerosol Sprays, Personal:
Hair sprays, tints, or dyes
Underarm deodorants
Antiperspirants (especially those containing aluminum)
Shaving cream
Feminine "hygiene deodorants"
Medicines

Building Materials:
Asbestos insulation
Asbestos caulking
Asbestos shingles
Fiberglass

Clothing and Fabric Care Products:
Spot removers and dry cleaning materials
Aerosol fabric finishes
Antistatic agents (fabric softener sheets used in driers)
Aerosol spray starches
Nonflammable clothing

Dust Accumulation:
Ragweed growing near home
Uncleaned fireplace chimneys and ash chute
Collector screen in clothes drier
Full or leaking vacuum cleaner bag

Heating and Cooling Device Emissions:
Coal, natural gas, or heating oil furnace
Gas stove or ranges
Bedroom over attached garage

Idling auto exhaust
Leaking refrigerator or air conditioner coolant
Kerosene stove, lanterns, or camping stove
Wood-burning stove
Smoking fireplace
Glowing charcoal burner
Burning trash

Furniture and Floor Polishes:
Aerosol floor polish, wax, or cleaner
Aerosol furniture polish or wax
Metal polish and cleaners
Rust remover
Tarnish preventers
Aerosol rug cleaner or tack-down material

Garbage and Solid Wastes:
Open garbage bags
Undefrosted refrigerator
Stored rotten vegetables or fruits
Moldy bread, fruits, or vegetables

Hobbies, Arts and Crafts:
Oil-based paint
Photographic and painting supplies
Wood lacquers
Sculpting, welding, or etching supplies
Fast-fixing glues and cements

Insecticides and Other Chemical Pesticides:
Herbicides
Fungicides
Insecticides
No-pest strips
Mothballs
Aerosol insect repellents

Germicides and Disinfectants:
Aerosol air fresheners or room deodorizers
Aerosol disinfectants

Kitchen and Laundry Soaps and Detergents:
Strong soaps
Brighteners
Detergents

Lead and Other Heavy Metals:
Lead-based paint
Lead water pipes
Some copper water pipes

Peeling or cracking paint on walls
Unglazed pottery used for drinking or food service
Mercury (silver) amalgams as dental fillings

Motor Vehicle Products:
Gasoline
Aerosol antirust
Waste oil
Commercial deicing agents
Antifreeze

Noise Pollution:
Typewriter
Hair drier
Vacuum cleaner
Stereo
Radio
Television
Computer printer
Electric mixer
Refrigerator or freezer motor
Forced convection oven
Food processor
Blender
Power drill
Leaf chopper
Children's toys
Power chain saw
Power lawn mower
Power leaf and litter blower/vacuum
Metal garbage cans
Lathe
Vibrator
Motorcycle
Loud pets—yours and your neighbors
Late night telephone calls

Oven and Other Cleaners:
Glass cleaners
Bleaches
Toilet bowl cleaners
Scouring powders
Aerosol oven cleaners
Silver cleaners
Surface disinfectant solutions
Ammonia and bleach or acid cleaners
Aerosol drain cleaners

Plastics and Plasticizers:
Auto plastic fixtures and trim
Auto window plastic film
Burning plastic
Plastic house furnishings
Plastic dishware
Plastic fixtures
Plastic bottles holding beverages
Plastic wraps
PVC furniture

Radiation:
Microwave oven
Microwave transmission towers nearby
Computer terminal
Television set
Personal photocopier machines
Ultraviolet lamps
High-tension electric wires nearby
"Black lights"
Excessive sunbathing
Powerful transmitters or defense electronic equipment

Solvents:
Paint thinners, removers, or solvents
Lighter fluid for charcoal or tobacco
Butane lighter containers
Kerosene
Aerosol paint products
Oily rags
Petroleum-based solvents
Cement solvents

Tobacco:
Cigars, cigarettes, or pipes smoked—sidestream smoke
  from careless co-workers or thoughtless "friends"
Marijuana smoked
Chewing tobacco or "snuff"

Utensil Coatings:
Teflon
Plastic

Vegetation:
Poisonous plants
Plants producing allergic response or sensitization
Fertilizer

Water Contaminants:
Asbestos pipes
Polyvinyl chloride pipes
Dirty gutters or downspouts
Organic chemical contaminants in drinking water
Particulate in drinking water
Contaminated well water
Swimming pool cleaners
Backed-up toilets
Water conditioners

Extra Chemicals:
Lye and other corrosives
Fireworks
Matches
Aerosol medicines (local anesthetics, skin preparations)
Salt and other compounds for melting snow and ice

Yuletide Decorations:
Cut-off Christmas tree
Aerosol decorative materials
Aerosol cocktail chillers

Zoological Waste:
Rat, dog, or other excrement
Cat hair and dander
Cat litter boxes
Fleas and ticks
Bird nests, bird droppings, or bird feathers ("down")
Pet turtles
Parrots and canaries

NOTES

1. H. K. Ziel et al., *New England Journal of Medicine*, 1975, 293:1167–1170; D. C. Smith et al. *New England Journal of Medicine*, 1975, 292:1164–1167; T. M. Mack et al., *New England Journal of Medicine*, 1976, 294:1262–1267.

2. N. S. Weiss et al., *New England Journal of Medicine*, 1976, 294:1259–1262.

3. Sally Rockwell, *Coping with Candida Cook Book*, Seattle: Diet Design by Rockwell, 1984.

4. "The Pill Takes a Bow on Its 25th," *Medical World News*, January 28, 1985, p. 23.

5. Eunice Carlson, "Synergistic Effect of *Candida albicans* and *Staphylococcus aureus* on Mouse Mortality," *Infection and Immunology*, December 1982, 38:921–924.

6. Eunice Carlson, "Enhancement by *Candida albicans* of *Staphylococcus aureus*, *Serratia marcescens*, and *Streptococcus faecalis* in Establishment of Infection in Mice," *Infection and Immunology*, January 1983, 39:193–197.

7. Eunice Carlson, "Effect of Strain of *Staphylococcus aureus* on Synergism with *Candida albicans* Resulting in Mouse Mortality and Morbidity," *Infection and Immunology*, October 1983, 42:285–292.

8. Adapted from Center for Science in the Public Interest, *The Household Pollutants Guide*, Garden City, N.Y.: Anchor Books, 1978, pp. 14–22.

6

Why Many Physicians Miss the Candida Connection

Immunologist Alan S. Levin, M.D., of San Francisco, a member of the American Medical Association, the California Medical Association, and the San Francisco Medical Society, is a maverick even when it comes to accumulating credentials within the modern medical Establishment. He has gathered many more than is usual. Having served in Vietnam as a flight surgeon with the U.S. Marine Corps, Dr. Levin is presently a member of the Medical Quality Assurance Review Committee of the State of California and an Adjunct Associate Professor of Immunology in the Department of Dermatology at the University of California School of Medicine in San Francisco. He is a Certified Diplomate of the Board of Allergy and Immunology and a Certified Diplomate of both the Board of Pathology and the Board of Clinical Pathology, a Fellow of the American College of Pathologists, a Fellow of the American Society of Clinical Pathologists, a Fellow of the American Academy of Allergy and Immunology, a Fellow of the American Association of Clinical Chemists, a Fellow of the American College of Emergency Physicians, and a Fellow of the American Academy of Environmental Medicine. He is also a recipient of the American Cancer

Society Faculty Research Award. You might correctly conclude from these credentials and honors that Dr. Levin is no wild-eyed kook with "off-the-wall" ideas about current medical practices.

At the 1983 Yeast–Human Interaction Symposium in Birmingham, and again at the 1985 symposium in San Francisco, Dr. Levin repeatedly referred to the "bible" of medical practice, *The New England Journal of Medicine* (*NEJM*). He showed slides to illustrate that it is the main medical source to which members of the American electronic and press media turn for dramatic headline news. To be published in the *NEJM*'s pages is even more prestigious for research physicians than in the *Journal of the American Medical Association* (*JAMA*).

Dr. Levin emphasized that this "is a peer-reviewed journal, publishing very august material, which sets the standard of practice in the United States." Then he described his content study on the September 8, 1983, issue of the *NEJM*: it contained fifty-one pages of scientific editorial matter and ninety-nine pages of pharmaceutical advertising. By weight three-fifths and by volume two-thirds of the *NEJM* was filled with drug ads.

"What's happening in the United States today is that the drug industry is setting the standard of medical practice. Drug companies have invaded the academic institutions. As much as two-thirds of the research funding in most major institutions comes directly or indirectly from drug industry interests; therefore, chemotherapy is dominant," declared Dr. Levin. "Immunotherapy is secondary. The market for immunotherapy in the U.S. is in the range of $50 million. In contrast, the market for just one drug, antihistamines, is about $2 billion. The sale of drugs is more profitable than any other industrial product. There's little wonder why health industrialists have taken over the practice of medicine. . . .

"The *NEJM* helps to create and sustain an environment in which our medical science is dictated by the interests of the drug industry that is promoting its financial welfare. We see this with its published articles advocating cancer chemotherapy, Inderal® [a drug that lowers blood pressure by decreasing heart output, manufactured by Ayerst Laboratories, New York City] for delaying second heart attacks, and other items," said the acclaimed immunologist. His point is simple: Since treatment of the Candida syndrome requires fewer drugs but more immune system buildup and better nutritional support, prestigious journals such as the *NEJM* would not have much interest in the condition as a disease entity. You aren't likely to see articles on polysystemic chronic candidiasis published in its pages. The ordinary physician who depends on journals like the *NEJM* will, most likely, miss the Candida connection.

THE SMEAR CAMPAIGN
AGAINST IMMUNOTHERAPY

As you learned from prior chapters, treatment for the Candida syndrome is largely dependent on your resistance to the yeast's growth through a healthy immune system. Physicians trained to minister to candidiasis patients attempt to provide them with the best possible support for the immune defense system. For that reason, it was extremely alarming when, at the 1983 Yeast–Human Interaction Conference, Dr. Levin went on to announce, "The American Academy of Allergy and Immunology [AAAI] is in a big smear campaign. I have heard from high-ranking officials in the Academy that 'immunotherapy will be dead within ten years.'

"Roughly one-third of the population suffers from allergy. If immunotherapy is removed from the marketplace, what happens to the [$2 billion annual] market for antihistamines?" he asked.

Antihistamines are drugs which tend to counteract allergic symptoms. If all that's left to treat allergy is antihistamines, drug product sales will spring upward, product prices will skyrocket, and profits for the antihistamine manufacturers could quadruple their current returns.

"My point is that this is no laughing matter," Dr. Levin continued. "We are being taken over by the drug industry. It is using the academic institutions to do this. If you don't think so, read any of the so-called peer-review journals, and you will realize that they are dominated by the drug industry."

THE MEDICRATS

Dr. Levin's December 1983 and March 1985 warnings to his candidiasis-treating colleagues were well placed. Just four months after the third Yeast–Human Interaction Symposium, in the summer of 1985, the AAAI piously declared that the Candida syndrome—giving it their own label, the "candidiasis hypersensitivity syndrome"—was both speculative and unproven. (See Chapter Seven for the AAAI's complete rebuff and our full response.)

Such medicrats have lots of tools to keep would-be medical mavericks in line. For instance, they use a demand for double-blind controlled studies to slow the rate of acceptance of new observations made by clinicians. Primary care physicians are on the front lines of patient care. Facing patients across the desk or in treatment rooms, they minister directly to people's needs. In the minds of medicrats, a lack of controlled experiments means invalidity of even the most well-founded observations based on the clinicians' firsthand findings. Yet, candidiasis is a clinical disease. Few laboratory tests can substantiate its existence; diagnosis and therapeutic result are established by observations of planned medical treatment programs, adapting to changes that occur in the patient's condition.

We have spoken with leading authorities who regularly diagnose and treat the yeast syndrome. They believe that the principles of medical ethics, properly applied in the best interests of the patient, prevent them from carrying out double-blind, controlled clinical studies. Such crossover, placebo-controlled, double-blind trials would mean that half their patients would receive appropriate anti-Candida therapy and the other half must get only the poorly effective, conventional remedies, including drugs for their complaints, but nothing to eliminate the generalized condition. In effect, nearly every patient who finally seeks out a candidiasis-conscious physician has already completed this ineffective phase of medical "treatment"—because if the standard approaches had worked for the yeast syndrome problems, the patient would never have needed to look for a different method.

DISEASE IS A FUNCTION OF THE HOST

Establishment types in medicine are following a belief system
that blames disease formation on causative agents that affect
humans—the germ theory of disease advanced by Louis Pasteur over 120 years ago. Dr. Levin disavows this general type
of traditional thinking as erroneous for many current health
difficulties. He said:

All disease is the function of the host response and not
necessarily the etiological [causative] agent. Every host
is different; individuals are unique. Therefore, the
[present] concept of diagnosis is obsolete [because it is
inadequate], inasmuch as we can't really say that a person has some disease simply because it fits into a particular classification.

We are studying disorders of biological regulation or
disruptions of biological response modifying systems. It
is no longer feasible to say that diabetes is an endocrine
disease or that schizophrenia is neurological; rather they
fit into similar patterns. Each germ layer from the embryo has its system to recognize specific antigens—sights,
sounds, pressures, temperatures, and other stressors.
The mechanisms by which germ layers recognize these
changes are the same—enzyme systems. We are beginning to see interactions between, for instance, the neurologic, the endocrine, and the immunologic systems.
Each system has control over the other.

People may share signs and symptoms that are similar
so that we pigeon-hole them, but there is no way that
two persons can have the same disease. Even identical
twins are different. Therefore, when we speak of candidiasis we mean a generalized concept and not specific
moieties [characteristics] which are reproducible from
individual to individual. This is important since no human being can be an adequate control [in a medical trial]
for another human being.

He is confirming that double-blind controlled trials disallow
clinical observation and patients' subjective feelings, which
are the foundations for determining the presence of—and

monitoring the treatment for—the Candida syndrome. He continued:

> We merely have normal ranges, but a range does not fit one person. For example, the measles virus in the appropriately susceptible host is associated with a symptom complex that in a young Caucasian we call measles; in a Samoan, the same virus would cause a devastating vasculitis [patchy inflammation of small blood vessels with potential kidney failure, arthritis, and other serious problems]. So the disease measles is really a function of the host and not the etiologic agent. This was widely known until the advent of antibiotics. But the antibiotic mentality changed medical thinking to looking for the magic bullet to cure every disease.

Conclusion? Establishment-type doctors still looking for the magic bullet invariably miss the target with the Candida connection.

BEING OUTSIDE THE PATIENT

The common causes of most diseases are assumed by the traditionally trained medical doctor to be "outside the patient." Indeed, the yeast problem does represent a situation in which the patient is affected by an outside agent, a saprophytic organism turned pathogenic. In this instance, however, symptoms of yeast-related illness are considerably different from other infections. The patient carries the disease around inside him—within the gut most often—which is actually "outside" the patient. The gut is an open organ, a hollow tube opened to the outside at both ends, and the body literally surrounds it. Therefore, what is in the gut actually lies outside the body.

Yet, because of its coiled location within the abdominal cavity, the gut is considered to be "internal." The patient is therefore carrying around—inside, but really outside—a disease-manufacturing system consisting of yeast cells making poison, the Candida toxin. This toxin is absorbed and distributed throughout the body, able to cause widely variable effects in every body system of the victim.

Medical traditionalists miss the Candida connection because they focus their treatment efforts on the patient's presenting complaints and urgent problems. Typically, they concentrate on the results of the problem, rather than on locating and treating the root cause. Each symptom or sign is like an individual branch of a tree far removed from the roots. Laboratory diagnostic findings—abnormalities—are other individual branches or smaller twigs, reflecting changes occurring in the cells and body systems. A patient's basic biochemical processes, common to cells in all nine body systems, could be compared to the tree's trunk and roots.

Physicians practicing orthodox medicine prescribe medications and other therapies for "correcting" the smaller branches—trying to push the laboratory tests toward normal and to resolve (or cover up) symptoms and signs of illness—while difficulties continue to rise from the root cause.

In candidiasis, local disorders such as vaginitis deserve local treatment. But the more troublesome symptomatic problems of the full Candida syndrome manifest themselves as a reflection of dysfunctions from a more basic level. Persistent chemical damages created by the Candida toxin interfere with individual cells throughout the body. This toxin has been shown in various studies to disrupt vitamin B_6 metabolism, sugar metabolism, magnesium metabolism, protein metabolism, and multiple other aspects of hormone and biochemical function. Consequently, the fundamental disturbances of biochemical activity are gradually reflected at the smaller branch level, either as laboratory test abnormalities or as varied and numerous disease discomforts. For example, toxin effects may show themselves as psoriaform lesions (noncontagious, chronic, reddish silvery patches collectively labeled psoriasis) on the skin. Or the body's response to yeast toxin might be bloating from indigestion changes in the gut. Or, as we have seen in Chapter Two, drunkenness.

When a traditionally trained doctor directs medications and other treatments at the smaller branches of the patient-tree, the therapy must be unremittingly applied: chemical insult for the patient continues unabated from that individual's source of chemical events. Administering only to the twigs or small branches representing a patient's deeper health difficulty— candidiasis—is bound to fail.

The basic difference here is between the wholistic concept of health care versus orthodoxy's crisis or emergency approach to drug-oriented disease care. The conflict is real: proper use of medications, diet, nutrition, and advice for the whole person as opposed to fancy bandaids that cover but don't cure disorders seen in isolated body parts. Wholistic physicians view the body as a harmony of interacting processes, quite unlike conventional specialists who after medical school graduation take a body part—skin, brain, endocrine glands—or class of person—babies, elderly, women—and "run with it."

DESCRIPTION OF A WHOLISTIC PHYSICIAN

Any doctor who achieves lasting therapeutic success with the yeast syndrome is practicing wholistic medicine. The wholistic physician dispenses humanistic medicine that is more person-oriented than disease-oriented. Treatment programs arise from the idea that health care should take full consideration of human needs and be humane in attitude, ethic, and behavior. The wholistic physician does not confine his thinking to traditional methods alone. Recognized, studied, and put into service are other kinds of activities, instruments, and healers to accomplish therapeutic goals. Any technique is allowed that provides valuable treatment, aids prevention of disease, and safeguards the maintenance of good health. His approach is based on the realization that merely the absence of disease does not itself equal the presence of health. He makes use of the best that modern Western medicine has to offer as well as ancient wisdoms and the most successful of health practices from the East.

More than that, the wholistic practitioner does not consider himself finished with his patient after providing technical services. He is a counselor who brings in other aspects of the individual's life such as his family and his community. They are a part of the larger whole, and each needs to be seen as interacting on that basis. The doctor helps to stimulate healthy interactions. In wholistic medicine, there is no "active doctor–passive patient" role; the patient participates all the way as an equal-but-different partner.

Finally, the wholistic physician actively informs his patients of issues they need to know related to their bodies and minds. The wholistic doctor is a health educator, a facilitator of the healing processes. He recognizes that his function is not merely that of clinician and scientist but also that of physician-teacher. At the very least, teaching might be by example. Indeed, health education of patients and the public at large may be the most important function of the wholistic physician.[1]

NOTES

1. Morton Walker, *Total Health: The Holistic Alternative to Traditional Medicine That Stresses Preventative Care, Nutrition, and Treatment of the Whole Person*, New York: Everest House, 1979, pp. 22, 23.

7

The Yeast
Syndrome Controversy

Kathryn Lazarou of Brooklyn, a budding actress in her early 30's, enjoyed a successful career in theatre and a carefree lifestyle until, as she described it, "I began feeling just awful all the time. I started to have all kinds of health problems."

A neighborhood doctor, the grandfather of Kathryn's closest girlfriend, became her primary care physician. This kindly, establishment-type of family practice specialist put her through numerous diagnostic procedures but couldn't pin a label on Kathryn's problem. He therefore decided to remedy her individual complaints with referrals to medical experts in the different body systems and organ parts that troubled her.

Because Kathryn was experiencing vaginal discharge, premenstrual tension, abdominal pain, fluid retention, and other menstrual difficulties, she first was referred to a gynecologist for medical attention. He gave her relief with some local treatment.

Accompanying the patient's gynecological symptoms were headaches, and when they became almost unbearable, her primary care physician then referred the actress to a neurologist.

The nerve specialist performed a variety of tests on Kathryn, including a full neurological examination, a brain scan, and electroencephalographic (EEG) studies. All of her neurological tests were reported back as being "normal."

For her continuing troubles with abdominal pain, gas, bloating, and other complaints connected with her digestive system, the referring doctor sent Kathryn to see a gastroenterologist. After upper (UGI) and lower gastrointestinal tract (barium enema) X-ray films were taken, the patient also went through a series of gall bladder X-ray studies. A week later, the gastroenterologist told her, "Your G.I. and gall bladder studies are just fine. There's nothing wrong."

But her abdominal distress did not let up; occasionally it was complicated by a urinary tract infection, as well. Consequently, her girlfriend's grandfather, who continued to treat Kathryn at little cost, sent her to a urologist for a cystoscopic examination and kidney X-rays. Nothing unusual showed for her urinary tract either.

No "disease" could be identified—but Kathryn felt anxious, tired, depressed, and her many physical signs and symptoms lingered. The older doctor, as he had done previously, questioned the young woman about her Midwestern background, if her family life had been happy, was she feeling fulfilled now. He frankly wondered if the patient's problems were "all in her head." To find out, he suggested that psychiatry might hold some answers.

Following six months of reduced-rate, twice-weekly visits to a psychiatrist, Kathryn concluded that she felt no better— worse, if anything—and decided to take matters into her own hands.

Searching for a series of symptoms similar to her own, the woman purchased or borrowed every health book and magazine that she could acquire. Furthermore, Kathryn attended medical consumer lectures or films at hospitals, natural healing seminars, health fairs, and even some physician conferences. It was during this investigation that she came upon the pattern of disorders described as candidiasis. Her signs and symptoms exactly matched its syndrome, except that oral thrush had not yet affected her.

She brought these suspicions about her health problem to the physician who had taken such an interest in helping, but his mind was absolutely closed to the concept. Polysystemic chronic candidiasis was not a condition that he recognized, and their visit ended with his saying outright that Kathryn's troubles were partly psychosomatic. He thought that the physical difficulties might actually be created by her mind.

That's when Kathryn went looking for another doctor who might be open to this relatively new disease entity—generalized, chronic candidiasis. Eventually she found her way to a physician regularly applying alternative techniques of healing—Warren M. Levin, M.D., Medical Director of the World Health Medical Group in New York City. Dr. Levin's type of wholistic medicine is complementary to traditional methods. He determined that the patient was, indeed, ensnared by the Candida syndrome.

Before her correct diagnosis was finally made and appropriate treatment administered, however, Kathryn Lazarou had been the victim of another problem associated with the social changes occurring in medicine today—a medical revolution. She was the unwitting pawn in an ongoing medical tug-of-war. Heretofore kept at low profile, the battle between the traditionalists and mavericks in medicine finally broke into the open during the summer of 1985.

CONTROVERSY SURROUNDING CANDIDIASIS

Traditionalists in medicine tag the Candida syndrome with another name—the "candidiasis hypersensitivity syndrome."

In the summer of 1985, the Practice Standards Committee of the American Academy of Allergy and Immunology (AAAI) declared that it not only found multiple problems with the proposed treatments of candidiasis hypersensitivity syndrome, but it also even questioned the existence of the condition as a clinical entity. A declarative statement from that committee said the medical maverick's concept of polysystemic chronic candidiasis is speculative and unproven, for several reasons:

1. It would apply to almost all sick patients at some time.
2. The complaints are essentially universal.
3. The broad treatment program would produce remission in most illnesses regardless of cause.
4. There is no published proof that *Candida albicans* is responsible for the syndrome.

5. There is no published proof that treatment of *C. albicans* infection with specific antifungal agents benefits the syndrome.

6. There is no proof that neutralization with *C. albicans* allergenic extracts benefits the syndrome.

7. There is no proof that the special studies used to track down Candida are effective diagnostic tests.

8. Resistant species of yeast and other pathogenic fungi may arise from use of antifungal agents.

9. Untoward effects from oral antifungal agents are rare, but some inevitably will occur.

In conclusion, the AAAI committee's official proclamation to its members was that "the concept of the candidiasis hypersensitivity syndrome is unproven. The diagnosis, the special laboratory tests, and the special aspects of treatment should be considered experimental and reserved for use with informed consent in appropriate controlled trials which have been approved for scientific merit and safety by competent institutional review boards."

Such erroneous arguments put forth by the AAAI for *non*-recognition of any chronic and generalized candidiasis condition as a disease entity are poorly considered. The yeast syndrome is real, should be recognized, must be diagnosed, and demands to be appropriately treated with the therapies shown to work. This narrow-minded committee of a major medical-specialty academy is typically falling into the trap of defending its own form of allopathic practice at the expense of the medical consumer's welfare.

In the summer 1985 issue of the AAAI newsletter, *News and Notes*, the Chairman of this Practice Standards Committee, I. Leonard Bernstein, M.D., of Milwaukee, Wisconsin, delivered a direct attack on the precepts of William G. Crook, M.D., as set forth in *The Yeast Connection*.[1] Dr. Crook answered Dr. Bernstein with patience, gentleness, and full documentation. He even offered to send complimentary copies of the book to any AAAI members who requested them. We wish to add our response to offset harm done to the millions of *C. albicans* victims around the world by the arguments of the American Academy of Allergy and Immunology.

OUR RESPONSE TO THE AAAI
PRACTICE STANDARDS COMMITTEE

Our reply is stated below in accordance with the Practice
Standards Committee numbered arguments.

1. That the disease symptoms might apply to almost all sick
patients at some time is exactly the point made by those
informed pioneers—the medical mavericks—who have educated themselves about the condition and regularly treat the
Candida syndrome. Indications of ill health from this yeast
syndrome are wide ranging. They involve multiple body systems and include fatigue, lethargy, depression, inability to
concentrate, hyperactivity, headache, skin problems such as
hives and psoriasis, gastrointestinal disorders of constipation,
abdominal pain, diarrhea, gas, and bloating, respiratory tract
troubles, and other health problems affecting the urinary
tract and reproductive organs.

2. Yes, the complaints truly do affect people universally
and worldwide. That's part of the reason Dr. Truss's discovery is such a medical breakthrough. Acting on the information presented in this book will improve the quality of life,
literally, for millions. People are functioning at extremely low
levels of wellness or with the outright signs of illness because
the Candida syndrome is sapping their strength and removing normal health faculties.

3. The mere remission of illness symptoms is quite acceptable to those unhappy patients beset by chronic disorders.
Indeed, if people have wandered from doctor to doctor looking for the cause and cure of their discomforts and nothing
brings them relief, isn't it logical for empathetic and aware
physicians to try them on a program that reduces the growth
of *C. albicans*? Like chicken soup, a little anti-Candida treatment can't hurt. Treating candidiasis is correct procedure,
especially if the patient's medical history, test scores, and
symptomatology are typical of yeast-connected health troubles.

4. It's false to state, as does the AAAI committee, that no
published proof is available showing *C. albicans* causes the
yeast syndrome. Just look at the footnotes at the end of
this and other chapters and at the bibliography for reliable
published medical sources. Furthermore, Dr. Crook points

out that the Japanese mycologist, Dr. Kazuo Iwata, had published a series of 1977 journal articles reporting on the organism's potent, lethal toxin, *canditoxin*.[2] The Iwata work was also cited in a brief 1985 report printed in the *Journal of the American Medical Association*.[3]

The committee's fourth argument against recognizing the Candida syndrome is answered, as well, by four scientific papers published by Dr. Truss.[4] Next read Dr. Truss's trailblazing book, *The Missing Diagnosis*. Much of his two dozen years of study on candidiasis are laid out in that one comprehensive text.[5]

5. Published proof that *C. albicans* treatment with specific antifungal agents benefits the Candida syndrome is immediately furnished by two articles currently presented in prestigious medical journals. Writing in the *New England Journal of Medicine*, William Rosenberg, M.D., Professor and Chairman, Division of Dermatology, University of Tennessee Center for the Health Sciences in Memphis, said: "We have become aware . . . of improvement of both psoriasis and inflammatory bowel disease in patients treated with oral nystatin, an agent that was expected to work only on yeast in the gut lumen. . . . We suspect that gut yeast may have a role in some instances of psoriasis."[6] Dr. Rosenberg's statement answers both the Committee's fourth and fifth condemnations of the Candida syndrome concept.

Argument five is also rebuffed by Dr. Rosenberg and Sidney M. Baker, M.D., a member of the clinical faculty at Yale University School of Medicine and Medical Director of the Gesell Institute of Human Development, New Haven, Connecticut. In the April 1984 *Archives of Dermatology*, they and their colleagues describe the response of four patients with longstanding psoriasis and inflammatory bowel disease to oral nystatin therapy. All four patients showed remarkable recovery from psoriasis when *C. albicans* was treated. One of their patients, a sixty-three-year-old man whose psoriasis began at the age of twenty-two, showed remarkable improvement after just four months on 500,000 units of oral nystatin four times a day for three months, and 1,000,000 units four times a day for one month. Remaining were only some pale redness and fine scale where before large thick plaques had been present.

Rosenberg and Baker reported on another man, age sixty-five, who had suffered with thick scaling psoriasis on his hands and multiple lesions on his trunk and legs. On 1,000,000 units of oral nystatin four times a day, after six months, "He was without any lesions except for some pale redness on his legs," they wrote.[7]

6. Chapter Three is a response to the AAAI committee's refusal to accept that "immunotherapy or provocation and/or neutralization with *Candida albicans* allergenic extracts benefit the syndrome." We also describe immunotherapy's role in Chapter Twelve. Dr. Crook's own response cited an editorial written by James S. Goodwin, M.D., of the Department of Medicine and Jean M. Goodwin, M.D., M.P.H., of the Department of Psychiatry at the University of New Mexico School of Medicine. Entitled "The Tomato Effect . . . Rejection of Highly Efficacious Therapies," it was published in a 1984 issue of the *Journal of the American Medical Association*.[8]

Tomatoes were rejected as a food by North Americans almost until the twentieth century because "everyone knew they were poisonous." In the same way, said the Drs. Goodwin, "The tomato effect in medicine occurs when an efficacious treatment for a certain disease is ignored or rejected because it does not 'make sense' in the light of accepted theories of disease mechanism and drug action." They name several instances where "the tomato effect has retarded the use of effective therapies, including the use of gold, colchicine, and aspirin for the treatment of various types of arthritic joint dysfunction." The Goodwins conclude:

> Modern medicine is particularly vulnerable to the tomato effect. What gets lost are the only three issues that matter in picking a therapy: Does it work? How toxic is it? How much does it cost? We are at risk for rejecting a safe, inexpensive therapy in favor of an alternative treatment perhaps less efficacious and more toxic. . . . Before we accept a treatment we should ask, "Is this a placebo?" and before we reject a treatment we should ask, "Is this a tomato?"

Has the AAAI Practice Standards Committee turned neutralization, provocation testing, and immunotherapy with *Candida albicans* allergenic extracts into . . . tomatoes?!

7. Plenty of proof exists for effective diagnostic tests for the Candida syndrome. Edward Winger, M.D., a pathologist and faculty member of the University of California San Francisco School of Public Health at Berkeley, has perfected a test for candidiasis of which the AAAI committee seemingly has no knowledge. We describe it in the next chapter. Studies by Dr. Winger show that patients with the "candidiasis hypersensitivity syndrome" exhibit higher levels of anti-Candida antibodies than do patients who don't have this problem. Similar studies have been carried out by F. T. Guilford, M.D., of San Mateo, California.

Howard E. Hagglund, M.D., of Norman, Oklahoma, author of the yeast treatment booklet, *Why Do I Feel So Bad (When the Doctor Says I'm O.K.)?*[9] and David S. Bauman, Ph.D., Adjunct Professor of Microbiology at the University of Oklahoma College of Medicine, have studied control groups of patients as well as patients with the typical history of candidiasis. They have identified and corroborated the presence of yeast-related health disorders with a reliable test, the candida enzyme immuno assay in conjunction with a history/symptom worksheet. In the next chapter, we also describe the way their test works.

Steven S. Witkin, Ph.D., of Cornell University Medical College, carried out studies illustrating that membrane infections with *C. albicans* produce changes in the immune system and in the endocrine system. His studies were published in the May-June 1985 medical journal, *Infections in Medicine*[10] and are discussed by us in Chapter Sixteen.

8. As with the use of any medication, a resistant species of Candida may be produced by the long-term oral use of the antifungal agents. That's immunologically true with most medicines, including antibiotics against bacteria, the chemotherapies for various cancers, and other drug items. Conscious of the possibility that Candida can grow resistant, the physician tries quickly to rid the patient of the entire Candida syndrome so that antifungal medication becomes unnecessary in the long term.

Better yet, the conscientious wholistic doctor will rely heavily on nontoxic therapies, diagnostics, and lifestyle improvement for candidiasis: regular exercise; mental health programming; avoidance of chemical pollutants; the taking of antioxidant nutrients; continuing observation so that concomitant diseases can be detected and accurately diagnosed; special laboratory tests—blood vitamin studies, mineral studies of the hair, blood, and urine, amino acid studies in urine, essential fatty acid profiles; a special dietary program with diversity and fresh foods from a variety of sources, avoidance of refined and fabricated foods, avoidance of fruits and milk, complete elimination of all yeast- and mold-containing foods, routine intake of sugar-free yogurt, daily nutritional supplementation, and only incidental use of antifungal agents and allergenic extracts of *C. albicans* for immunotherapy and provocation/-neutralization.

9. Just one of the contentions made by the AAAI Practice Standards Committee has any validity. Although extremely rare, untoward effects from oral antifungal agents could conceivably occur.

In conclusion, as medical consumer advocates and journalists, we confirm the role of *Candida albicans* toxins in making people sick. We are backed up by " 'Think Yeast' . . . the Expanding Spectrum of Candidiasis," an article published in *The Journal of the South Carolina Medical Association*, one of the most conservative medical journals published in the United States. Martin H. Zwerling, M.D., Kenneth N. Owens, M.D., and Nancy H. Ruth, R.N., B.S., who appear to be former traditionalists newly converted to the medical maverick cause, write:

> Consider the following "incurable" patient who is being treated by several specialists. Her gynecologist is treating her recurrent vaginitis and irregular menstrual periods, while an otolaryngologist is trying to control her external otitis and chronic rhinitis. At the same time, her internist is unsuccessfully attempting to manage symptoms of bloating, indigestion, and abdominal pain, and her dermatologist is struggling with bizarre skin rashes, hives, and psoriasis. Lastly, her psychiatrist has been unable to convince the patient that her "nerves" are the cause of her extreme irritability, inability to concentrate, and depression. We have all been guilty of

labeling such patients as "psychosomatic" and, since there is "nothing physically wrong," conclude we cannot cure them. Incurable? Not if you *Think yeast*.

This patient and thousands like her are suffering from chronic candidiasis.[11]

NOTES

1. William G. Crook, *The Yeast Connection*, 2nd ed., Jackson, Tenn.: Professional Books, 1984, pp. 5–7.

2. K. Iwata and Y. Yamamoto, "Glycoprotein Toxins Produced by *Candida albicans*," Proceedings of the Fourth International Conference on the Mycoses, PAHO Scientific Publication no. 356, June 1977; K. Iwata, *Recent Advances in Medical and Veterinary Mycology*, Tokyo: University of Tokyo Press, 1977; K. Iwata and K. Uchida, "Cellular Immunity in Experimental Fungus Infections in Mice," *Medical Mycology*, January 1977.

3. D. A. Edwards, "Depression and Candida," *Journal of the American Medical Association*, 1985, 253:3400.

4. C. Orian Truss, "Tissue Injury Induced by *Candida albicans*," *Journal of Orthomolecular Medicine*, 1978, 7:17–21; C. Orian Truss, "Restoration of Immunologic Competence to *Candida albicans*," *Journal of Orthomolecular Medicine*, 1980, 9:287–301; C. Orian Truss, "The Role of *Candida albicans* in Human Illness," *Journal of Orthomolecular Medicine*, 1981, 10:228–238; C. Orian Truss, "Metabolic Abnormalities in Patients with Chronic Candidiasis: The Acetaldehyde Hypothesis," *Journal of Orthomolecular Medicine*, 1984, 13:66–93.

5. C. Orian Truss, *The Missing Diagnosis*, Birmingham, Ala.: The Author, 1983.

6. F. William Rosenberg et al., "Crohn's Disease and Psoriasis," *New England Journal of Medicine*, 1983, 308:101.

7. F. William Rosenberg, Sidney M. Baker, et al., "Oral Nystatin in the Treatment of Psoriasis," *Archives of Dermatology*, 1984, 120:435.

8. James S. Goodwin and Jean M. Goodwin, "The Tomato Effect . . . Rejection of Highly Efficacious Therapies," *Journal of the American Medical Association*, 1984, 251:2387–2390.

9. Howard E. Hagglund, *Why Do I Feel So Bad (When the Doctor Says I'm OK)?* 2nd ed., Oklahoma City: IED Press, 1984.

10. Steven S. Witkin, "Defective Immune Responses in Patients with Recurrent Candidiasis," *Infections in Medicine*, May-June 1985.

11. M. H. Zwerling, K. N. Owens, and N. H. Ruth, " 'Think Yeast' . . . The Expanding Spectrum of Candidiasis," *Journal of the South Carolina Medical Association*, 1984, 80:454–456.

Diagnosis and Treatment of the Yeast Syndrome

8

How To Recognize
When You Have Candidiasis

My name is Martha Etta Mansell, and today is August 16, 1984. I live in Pasadena, Texas. I am aware that numbers of disorders from which I've suffered over time are typical of some clinical complaints people have when they endure generalized, chronic candidiasis. I've decided to write this letter so that Dr. Trowbridge can paste it into his clinic's exhibit book. That way, others may benefit from reading of my experiences. They could recognize their own signs and symptoms.

I am thirty-four years old and have had hay fever–type allergies all of my life. I have taken various prescription drugs for the hay fever but would have to change them frequently, as they only remained effective for a short time. I mainly learned to live with the stuffy nose, sinus drainage, sore throats, and dark circles under my eyes.

I also have had severe headaches since about age seventeen. These frequently felt especially bad for about one week before I menstruated and during the first two or three days of my period. I went to a doctor about the headaches in 1975. He took an EEG [a brain wave recording] and told me the headaches were caused by stress and tension. I was given a prescription drug for the headaches, but it was not any more effective than plain old aspirin. I was told that I just had to learn to live with the headaches.

When I was twenty-four years old I became aware of my body's fluid retention, as much as five to eight pounds, if I ate something like pizza or Mexican food. I assumed that it was salt that was causing the problem and completely cut out salt from the food I prepared. However, I still retained fluid and especially felt bloated prior to my period. I usually became irritable and depressed before my period and decided that this was due to the fluid retention.

For a number of years, I have also had a problem with fatigue. I envied people who were always cheerful and energetic as I barely had enough energy to get to work. I needed more physical exercise but just did not have the strength to do it, and gradually my weight increased by an extra thirty pounds.

I have a stressful job and some days would notice that I had no coping skills. The least little thing out of the ordinary would bring on my severe mood swings. On one occasion, I was able to notice a definite correlation between my mood and what I had eaten. I had chili dogs, baked beans, pickles, potato chips, and cookies for lunch and then was wild all afternoon. At other times I would be so drowsy that I could barely work. I even fell asleep once at a restaurant during lunch.

I felt crummy and drained all the time but never said anything to a doctor about it. Since I had always been this way, I just assumed that feeling awful was normal. I then heard about the cytotoxic food testing program and thought I could possibly benefit from it. I was tested in September 1983 and reacted to forty-two foods. Among these were baker's yeast, brewer's yeast, malt, and mushrooms. I eliminated all forty-two items from my diet and immediately started feeling better and also lost ten pounds. I soon discovered that the yeasts and related items were my main food allergy problems. I learned to also eliminate enriched flour, vinegar, fruit juices, and cheeses. My disposition also improved and people commented that I was a different, nicer person.

Then I attended a lecture on the yeast syndrome. Since my symptoms exactly matched the condition described, I started the antiyeast treatment in February 1984. I continued my anticytotoxic diet and also started taking one-quarter teaspoonful of nystatin four times a day for my yeast trouble. After a couple of days I felt just terrible. [She was having a "die-off" of *Candida albicans* known as the Herxheimer reaction, which we discuss at length in Chapter Ten.] I was bloated; my legs ached; I felt depressed, exhausted, and had headaches again. I felt like every symptom I had ever experienced was magnified ten times. I increased the nystatin to one-half teaspoon four times a day and started feeling normal again after just a couple of days.

In March 1984, I went on the Candida control diet, started losing my excess weight, and saw a gradual improvement in my energy level. In July 1984, I was able to reintroduce fruit and grains into my eating program while still taking the nystatin. I no longer have headaches as long as I stay on this diet. My overall health continues to improve. I certainly believe that the antiyeast treatment has made a significant difference in my life.

MARTHA MANSELL FIGHTS HER YEAST INVADER

Mrs. Mansell was begun on a therapeutic program designed both to help her fight against the yeast syndrome and to restore her health. Today, while response to yeast syndrome therapy is still diagnostic, questionnaires and new laboratory tests provide more exacting indicators of the condition's presence.

Martha Mansell began her fight against the Candida syndrome in February 1984, nine months before the introduction of any currently accurate special laboratory tests for the condition. Even though several of Mrs. Mansell's body systems were obviously malfunctioning, her clinical examination and laboratory test readings were mostly in the normal ranges—a common disguise of the Candida syndrome. For making the diagnosis, Dr. Trowbridge had only his patient's history, her answers to the yeast questionnaire from Dr. William G. Crook's book, *The Yeast Connection*, and the notes from her physical examination. He told the patient, "You might well have a yeast-related problem. Your yeast Y-score was 190 before you eliminated the forty-two foods to which your cytotoxic testing showed you are allergic, but today it's down to 140. Your Y-score is still on the high side of normal."

A SUMMARY OF CANDIDIASIS SIGNS AND SYMPTOMS

The typical clinical picture of Candida-connected health problems occurs in people of all ages and both sexes. Women have been most likely to exhibit candidiasis, but men now manifest almost as many difficulties. The invasion of *Candida albicans* shows no major preference for one individual over another, as long as the physiological conditions for yeast overgrowth are ripe.

You may recognize symptoms and signs of having the Candida syndrome by matching your state of health to the following brief description of yeast-related problems:

1. You feel lousy—"bad all over"—even having had many types of treatment.

2. The cause of your feeling rotten can't be identified.

3. Courses of broad spectrum antibiotic drugs, including the tetracyclines (Achromycin®, Sumycin®, Panmycin®, Vibramycin®, Minocin®), ampicillin (Amcill®, Omnipen®, Polycillin®, Principen®), amoxicillin (Amoxil®, Larotid®, Polymox®), the cephalosporins (Keflex®, Ceclor®, Velosef®, Anspor®, Duricef®), or sulfa combinations (Septra®, Bactrim®), that you may have taken for the present problem or for others present or past haven't helped much—or even have made you feel worse.

4. You have a subconscious preference for foods made with yeast—bread, beer, wine, alcohol, and certain cheeses.

5. You crave sweets and other sugar-containing edibles.

6. You have an insistent desire for refined carbohydrates—candy, chocolate, cake, cookies, soda pop, "junk foods."

7. You find that eating sweets or refined carbohydrates gives you a quick pickup soon followed by a letdown, so that the uncomfortable feelings become worse.

8. Although tests may fail to confirm hypoglycemia, you still suspect that low blood sugar is one of your problems because some of the characteristic symptoms—fatigue, sudden hunger, weakness, trembling, lethargy, a drowsy mental state, headache, cold sweats, dizziness, rapid heartbeat, numbness, irritability, hostility, blurred vision—are often present.

9. You like to imbibe alcoholic beverages more than do other people.

10. You routinely take birth control pills.

11. You have regularly utilized corticosteroids (such as cortisone, prednisone, Decadron®, Medrol®, Aristopak®), or other such anti-inflammatory or immunosuppressive drugs.

12. You have gone through multiple pregnancies.

13. You recently or chronically are troubled by abdominal pain, vaginal infection, premenstrual tension, menstrual irregularities, menstrual pain, discomfort during sexual intercourse, a loss of interest in having sex, prostatitis, impotence, or other reproductive organ difficulties.

14. You are troubled by persistent athlete's foot, jock itch, fungus infection of the toenails or fingernails (thickening, discoloration, or splitting), or fungus infection of the skin (blisters, peeling, dry scaling, or color changes).

15. You feel tired or dragged out on damp days or when you find yourself around moldy places such as basements, root cellars, and turned over soil in gardens.

16. You experience discomfort in the presence of tobacco smoke, household chemicals, petrochemicals, or perfumed toiletries.

Because all human beings are colonized in a benign fashion by yeasts, skin tests and other tests of the immune system are almost useless for diagnosing the Candida syndrome. For this reason, if you suspect you're infected with *C. albicans*, seeing how well you fit this description of signs and symptoms is vital. Candida organisms are usually present on everyone's mucous membranes, including the mouth, other areas of the digestive tract, and the vagina. Smears and cultures which show—or don't show—the microbe are of little help in making a diagnosis. Accordingly, the clinical diagnosis of the Candida syndrome is based on the rating you give your own health, your personal clinical history, your physical examination, perhaps a laboratory test or two, and your response to a therapeutic trial of the anti-Candida treatment programs discussed in this book.

"RATE YOUR HEALTH QUIZ" FOR THE YEAST SYNDROME

There are several ways you can privately determine at home whether you have been affected by *C. albicans*. The most important question that you might ask yourself or that you may be asked by your doctor is: "When was the last time that I (you) really felt well?" Added to that very basic piece of information should be responses to Dr. Trowbridge's Rate Your Health Quiz. Take the quiz and learn if you may need treatment for Candida illness.

Circle the number of a question to which you must answer "yes." If you have four or five yes answers, you may suffer with yeast-related illness; if you have six or seven yes answers, you probably are a Candida infection victim; if you have eight or more yes answers, you almost certainly need medical treatment for chronic, generalized candidiasis or for unusual illnesses that occasionally mimic the condition and for which proper medical diagnosis and care should be sought.

Questions for Adults and Teenagers

Have you suffered with . . .

1. Frequent infections, constant skin problems—or taken antibiotics (or cortisone medications) often or for long periods?
2. Feelings of fatigue, being drained of energy, drowsiness—or the same symptoms on damp, muggy days or in moldy places such as a basement?
3. Feelings of anxiety, irritability, insomnia—or cravings for sugary foods, breads, alcoholic beverages?
4. Food sensitivities, allergy reactions—or digestion problems, bloating, heartburn, constipation, bad breath?

5. Feeling "spacy" or "unreal," difficulty in concentrating, or being bothered by perfumes, chemical fumes, tobacco smoke?

6. Poor coordination, muscle weakness, or joints painful or swollen?

7. Mood swings, depression, or loss of sexual feelings?

8. Dry mouth or throat, nose congestion or drainage, pressure above or behind the eyes or ears, or frequent headaches?

9. Pains in the chest, shortness of breath, dizziness, or easy bruising?

10. Frustration at going from doctor to doctor, never getting your health completely well—or being told that your symptoms are "mental" or "psychological" or "psychosomatic"?

For Women Only

Have you suffered with . . .

1. Vaginal burning or itching, discharge, infections—or urinary problems?

2. A difficult time getting pregnant—or been pregnant two or more times—or taken birth control pills?

3. Premenstrual symptoms: moodiness, fluid loading, tension—or irregular cycles, other menstrual or sexual problems?

Especially for Children

Do you suffer with . . .

1. Frequent infections, particularly of the ears, tonsils, bronchitis, history of frequent diaper rash?

2. Continuous nasal congestion or drainage?

3. Dark circles under the eyes—or periods of hyperactivity, poor attention span?

DR. CROOK'S YEAST QUESTIONNAIRE AND SCORE SHEET

Dr. Trowbridge has also utilized the Candida Questionnaire and Score Sheet (the Y-score) as developed and described by William G. Crook, M.D., of Jackson, Tennessee, in his book, *The Yeast Connection.*[1] This questionnaire is often provided as a diagnostic tool by Candida-conscious physicians as part of recording the patient's health history. An inquiring doctor then is able quickly to evaluate the likely role of *C. albicans* in contributing to illness.

Dr. Crook's yeast questionnaire gives additional scoring emphasis to a patient's answers in the following categories that are the source of, or are often found associated with, yeast-related illness:

1. taking antibiotics such as tetracyclines, sulfas and sulfa combinations, synthetic penicillins, and other "broad spectrum" antibiotics

2. taking birth control pills or having been pregnant

3. taking cortisone or other steroid medications

4. having "chemical sensitivities" or other significant allergy problems

5. reacting to molds, fungi, yeasts, and other parasites

6. craving sweets, alcohol, or breads

7. frequently feeling the wide variety of symptoms noted at the beginning of this chapter.

The patient's scores are totalled to determine whether there is a symptomatic relationship to yeast disease. A yeast questionnaire also exists for children, which Dr. Crook has made a part of another small book that he published in 1984.[2]

REVIEW OF PERSONAL
HEALTH PROBLEMS AND CONCERNS

A full review of your own clinical history is a critical part in the correct approach to ascertaining whether you are the unwilling host for expanding colonies of yeast organisms. Your present feelings and observations about yourself are every bit as valuable as any laboratory or physical examination. Your physician will want to know what you sense about your own body's functions and how your mind and emotions are working. Review of Personal Health Problems and Concerns supplied below can be an important tool for you and your health professional. It was adapted by Dr. Trowbridge from an earlier symptom survey form distributed by Standard Process Laboratories, Milwaukee, Wisconsin.

Although extensively used by doctors for diagnostic purposes, this evaluation form is not necessarily a physician's patient history document. Rather, it's a patient self-testing technique. You are creating a diagnostic tool in your own home when you have the time and opportunity to reflect on your discomforts. Seeing, for instance, that you have thyroid stress or adrenal stress, a health professional trained in wholistic approaches to healing illness will be more efficiently able to counsel you. This will save you time, discomfort, and money. You will need less testing from the beginning because fewer areas will have to be examined.

Do the following:

1. Use a pen and mark in the space provided your numbered point score to the question asked, if the question fits what you have been experiencing.

2. Mark only the signs, symptoms, or complaints that apply specifically to you—leave all others *unmarked*.

3. Use the number codes of 1, 2, or 3 for scoring your answers, placing your assessment score on the line between the question and the question's number:

- 3 for problems you notice *every day* or at least *once a week*
- 2 for problems you notice about *once* or *twice a month*
- 1 for problems you notice *irregularly* or only *every so often*.

Leave blank the space for any problem *not* bothering you.

1—Sympathetic Nervous System Function

1 _____ "Lump" in throat
2 _____ Dry mouth, eyes, nose
3 _____ Strong light irritates eyes
4 _____ Gag easily
5 _____ Body temperature easily raised
6 _____ Arms, legs cold, clammy
7 _____ "Goosebumps" common
8 _____ Staring, blink little
9 _____ Pulse speeds up after meals
10 _____ Heart pounds after retiring
11 _____ "Keyed up"—can't relax
12 _____ Jumpy, mind overly active
13 _____ Burning, tingling, sharp pains felt
14 _____ Cuts heal slowly
15 _____ Urine amount reduced
16 _____ Cold sweats often
17 _____ Appetite reduced
18 _____ Acid foods upset stomach
19 _____ "Nervous" stomach
20 _____ Sour stomach often

Related problems not mentioned above:_____

_____

2—Parasympathetic Nervous System Function

1 _____ Joint stiffness after arising
2 _____ Muscle-leg-toe cramps at night
3 _____ Perspire easily
4 _____ Eyes or nose watery
5 _____ Eyes blink often
6 _____ Eyelids swollen or puffy
7 _____ Hoarseness
8 _____ Breathing irregular
9 _____ Pulse slow, maybe irregular
10 _____ Difficulty swallowing
11 _____ Need to eat often or feel hunger pains, faintness
12 _____ Indigestion soon after meals
13 _____ Stomach growling, churning
14 _____ Vomit easily or frequently
15 _____ "Butterfly" stomach, cramps
16 _____ Alternating constipation/diarrhea
17 _____ Circulation poor, hands or feet sensitive to cold
18 _____ Slow reflexes
19 _____ Easily get colds, bronchitis, asthma

Related problems not mentioned above:_____

_____

3—Adrenal System Function

1 ____ Pounding headaches
2 ____ Tendency to higher blood pressure
3 ____ "Hot flashes"
4 ____ Dizziness sensations
5 ____ Exhaustion, can't cope
6 ____ Constant fatigue
7 ____ Tend to have lower blood pressure
8 ____ Circulation poor in hands or feet
9 ____ Abnormal sweating
10 ____ History of kidney trouble or swelling ankles
11 ____ Crave salt, salty foods
12 ____ Brown spots or bronzing of skin
13 ____ Nails weak or have ridges
14 ____ (Women) Masculine body traits
15 ____ (Women) Hair growth on face or body
16 ____ History of sugar in urine but not told to have diabetes
17 ____ Weakness, dizziness
18 ____ Joint or arthritislike pains
19 ____ Tend to have hives or welts
20 ____ Tend to have allergies or asthma
21 ____ Frequent or continuing colds or infections
22 ____ Weakness prolonged after colds or flu

Related problems not mentioned above:_____

_____

4—Cardiovascular/Respiratory System Functions

1 ____ Aware of "breathing heavily"
2 ____ Want to open windows when in closed rooms
3 ____ Sigh often, "hunger for air"
4 ____ High altitude causes discomfort
5 ____ Shortness of breath with increased activity
6 ____ Dull pressure or pain in chest or left arm, worse with increased activity
7 ____ "Tightness" in chest, worse with increased activity
8 ____ Muscle cramps, worse with exercise—"charley horses"
9 ____ Hands-feet "go to sleep" or feel tingling or numbness
10 ____ Swollen ankles, worse in the evening
11 ____ Bruise easily, "black and blue" spots
12 ____ Nose bleeds easily
13 ____ History of anemia, low blood count
14 ____ Noises or "ringing" in ears
15 ____ Easily get colds or fevers
16 ____ Afternoon "yawner"
17 ____ Get drowsy during day or early evening

Related problems not mentioned above:_____

_____

5—Thyroid Gland Function

1 ____ Insomnia or too easily awakened
2 ____ Nervousness, anxiety
3 ____ Highly emotional
4 ____ Inward trembling
5 ____ Irritable and restless
6 ____ Heart pounds or skips
7 ____ Pulse fast at rest
8 ____ Increase in weight
9 ____ Decreased appetite
10 ____ Sleepy during day
11 ____ Mental sluggishness
12 ____ Fatigue easily
13 ____ Headaches upon arising, wear off during day
14 ____ "Get up and go" has "got up and gone"
15 ____ Night sweats
16 ____ Flush easily
17 ____ Feel drained in heat
18 ____ Thin (unpadded), moist skin
19 ____ Eyelids and face twitch
20 ____ Can't work under pressure
21 ____ Increased appetite
22 ____ Can't gain weight
23 ____ Slow pulse
24 ____ Poor hearing
25 ____ Noises or "ringing" in ears
26 ____ Frequent urination
27 ____ Hair coarse, falls out easily
28 ____ Dry or scaly skin
29 ____ Constipation or hard stools
30 ____ Sensitive to cold

Related problems not mentioned above:_____

_____

6—Sugar-Handling Ability

1 ____ Hungry between meals
2 ____ Irritable or moody before meals
3 ____ Get "shaky" when hungry
4 ____ Faintness when meals delayed
5 ____ Fatigue relieved by food
6 ____ Heart pounds or skips when meals missed or delayed
7 ____ Afternoon or late morning headaches
8 ____ Awaken after few hours of sleep—hard to return to sleep
9 ____ Abnormal craving for sweets, snacks between meals, at bedtime
10 ____ Crave candy or coffee, tea, cola in afternoon
11 ____ Overeating sweets upsets body or mind
12 ____ Appetite excessive
13 ____ Eat when nervous or upset
14 ____ Moods of depression, "blues," or melancholy

Related problems not mentioned above:_____

_____

7—Pituitary Gland Function

1 _____ Failing memory
2 _____ "Splitting" headaches, forehead or temples
3 _____ Excessive thirst
4 _____ Weight gain around hips or waist
5 _____ Feel better after eating sweets
6 _____ Have lower blood pressure
7 _____ Increased sexual desire
8 _____ Sexual desire reduced or lacking
9 _____ Sugar-handling problems
10 _____ Tend to have ulcers or bowel problems
11 _____ Bloating of intestines

Related problems not mentioned above:_____

_____

8A—Liver and Gall Bladder Function

1 _____ Bitter, metallic taste in mouth in the morning
2 _____ Stools that float, or an "oil slick" on water in toilet
3 _____ Stools light brown, tan, or gray
4 _____ Greasy foods cause digestive upset
5 _____ Pains in upper right belly after eating
6 _____ Pains behind right shoulder or right shoulder blade
7 _____ Bowel movements painful or difficult
8 _____ Laxatives needed for regularity
9 _____ Stools alternate from formed to watery
10 _____ Blurred vision
11 _____ Burning feet
12 _____ Skin peels on soles of feet
13 _____ History of gall bladder attacks or gall stones
14 _____ Dry skin
15 _____ Skin rashes
16 _____ Itching skin and itchy feet
17 _____ Hair falling out excessively

8B—Allergy Interrelated with Liver System Function

18 _____ Dizziness
19 _____ Nightmares
20 _____ Sneezing attacks
21 _____ Bad breath, "halitosis"
22 _____ Milk, milk products, or cheese cause distress

23 _____ Crave sweets
24 _____ Feel drained in hot weather
25 _____ Burning or itching anus
26 _____ Hemorrhoid problems

Related problems not mentioned in Groups Eight A and B above:

_____

9—Gastrointestinal Function From Stomach to Anus

1 _____ Feel burning stomach, relieved by eating
2 _____ Dark tarlike color to stools
3 _____ Indigestion one-half to one hour after eating (or may occur in three or four hours)
4 _____ Gas or rumbling shortly after eating
5 _____ Stomach "bloating" after eating
6 _____ Loss of taste for meat

7 _____ Coated tongue
8 _____ Lower bowel gas several hours after eating
9 _____ Stools have foul odor
10 _____ Stools lumpy or hard, constipation
11 _____ Stools runny or watery, diarrhea
12 _____ Mucus mixed with stools
13 _____ Blood mixed with stools

Related problems not mentioned above:_____

_____

10A—For Women Only

1 _____ Premenstrual tension

2 _____ Premenstrual swelling or "puffiness"

3 _____ Depressed feelings before menses

4 _____ Very easily fatigued

5 _____ Painful menses

6 _____ Menses excessive and prolonged

7 _____ Menses usually closer than twenty-six days

8 _____ Painful breasts

9 _____ Sexual desire reduced or lacking

10 _____ Vaginal discharge

11 _____ Had hysterectomy with both ovaries removed

12 _____ Menopause "hot flashes" or mood changes

13 _____ Menses scanty or missed

14 _____ Acne worse at menses

15 _____ Melancholy, sadness, or depression

16 _____ History of kidney or urine infections or blood in urine

Related problems not mentioned above:_____

_____

10B—For Men Only

1 _____ Feeling of incomplete emptying of bowel

2 _____ Urination two or more times per night

3 _____ Urination difficult or with dribbling

4 _____ Prostate trouble history

5 _____ Pain on inside of legs or heels

6 _____ Legs jerking or restless in bed at night

7 _____ History of kidney or urine infections or blood in urine

8 _____ Tire too easily

9 _____ Lack of energy

10 _____ Avoid physical activity

11 _____ Melancholy, sadness, or depression

12 _____ Aches and pains that seem to move about the body

13 _____ Sexual desire reduced or gone

Related problems not mentioned above:_____

_____

Score yourself for the yeast syndrome. Here is what your numbered scorings mean:

Any group in which you score fifteen points or more, you must consider that candidiasis might be causing problems in that body system.

Any group in which you score ten to fourteen points, you should consider that candidiasis possibly contributes to problems in that body system.

Any group in which you score less than ten points but you've marked several answers with the number 3 or 2, consider that candidiasis may be weakening that body system.

In fact, pay attention to any individual 3 response. This higher number will alert your physician to check more closely that particular body tissue, part, organ, or system for effects of yeast infestation or other disturbance to healthy function.

A total score for the entire questionnaire is not relevant. The Review of Personal Health Problems and Concerns does not work that way. You may be exceedingly affected in one area and not at all in another. These are actually ten small health history tests, which together indicate a pattern of illness for evaluation by your wholistic physician. Traditionally practicing physicians could also find your information valuable, directing them to look more closely at areas of health problems for you that previously had been ignored or simply skipped over in earlier evaluations.

NOTES

1. William G. Crook, *The Yeast Connection*, Jackson, Tenn.: Professional Books, 1984.

2. William G. Crook, *Yeasts and How They Can Make You Sick*, Jackson, Tenn.: Professional Books, 1984.

9

New Laboratory Tests for Yeast-Related Illness

Barbara Lynn Herrington, age thirty-four, now lives with her five-year-old son in Joliet, Illinois. No longer married, Mrs. Herrington has returned to the profession for which she had trained—teaching occupational therapy in a school for handicapped children. She sustained much stress as a result of her divorce, and emotional difficulties at that time were complicated by some physical symptoms: headaches, frequent colds, aches and pains in the joints, backache, anxiety, and mental depression.

Mrs. Herrington was no stranger to subclinical illness (chronic unwellness). From the time she was a youngster in the sixth grade, she had a history of spastic colon discomforts, terrible intestinal gas, and a lack of energy. She suffered with three or four severe colds each year, was on prolonged antibiotic therapy, painkillers, and muscle relaxers, and underwent much chiropractic treatment. While married, she took birth control pills for two years. During her second year in college, Mrs. Herrington changed her diet radically, eating much more carbohydrates not only out of convenience but also because of her cravings.

She had simply been feeding a fungus, she later realized,

for in October 1984 the woman learned that the yeast syndrome was the source of her physical disorders. The doctors Mrs. Herrington consulted in Joliet then put her on various antiyeast diets and prescribed different strengths of Candida-combating medications. Seeking relief for her health problems, the patient received from one doctor a prescription for 50,000 units of Mycostatin™ tablets; from another she got quantities of nystatin; a third physician tried her on Nizoral™. She attempted to stay on the prescribed medications but soon found herself so sick with apparent side effects from each that she was forced to discontinue them.

Finally, during an extended visit to her sister in Emmaus, Pennsylvania, Mrs. Herrington made her way to the preventive medicine office of Conrad G. Maulfair, Jr., D.O., of Mertztown, Pennsylvania. Dr. Maulfair is an wholistic osteopathic physician who specializes in testing for allergy and utilizes nutrition for the treatment of hypoglycemia and other conditions. He also administers chelation therapy. At her first visit, the patient told him about her chronic unwellness, noting that her headaches, depression, and fatigue were all worsening.

In furnishing us with the health history of Barbara Lynn Herrington, Dr. Maulfair wrote:

> She felt fatigue both in the morning and all day. (I am specifically interested in morning fatigue, as it can be a sign of adrenal gland malfunction.) At this juncture, in addition to the patient's provisional diagnosis of systemic candidiasis, I was suspicious that she might have bio-ecologic illness. Bio-ecologic illness refers to the condition that occurs when someone becomes sensitive to, or allergic to, or even addicted to something in the environment. That "something" is often a food or foods, but it can also be any of the thousands of chemicals that we are exposed to. These sensitizing foods or chemicals can contribute to, if not cause, multiple symptoms over and above the typical "allergic" symptoms such as sneezing, runny nose, and rash. Symptoms such as tiredness, headache, fatigue, blurred vision, decreased concentration, decreased memory, joint pain, abdominal pain, and many

others can be caused by these often hidden food or chemical sensitivities.

I consequently asked Mrs. Herrington to complete an allergy questionnaire and also to keep a diary of all foods or fluids that she ate or drank. This information allows me to select those foods or chemicals that are suspicious, thereby decreasing the number of items to be tested. The patient was then scheduled to have sublingual provocative testing. This sublingual testing entails placing drops of different strengths of the particular test item under the patient's tongue. The test drop is allowed to remain there for ten minutes, while it is absorbed into the circulation. The patient then relates to the testing personnel what symptoms he or she is feeling. This particular environmental medicine procedure often allows a wholistic physician to reproduce many of the symptoms that the patient has had for years.

I was unable to complete the testing procedure as the patient reacted to the first item tested, which is phenol. Phenol is the preservative used in all of the test antigens. The patient therefore was unable to be tested as she would have reacted to all substances, since they were preserved with phenol. I decided at this point to bypass any additional testing procedure and commence treatments . . . with a natural antifungal agent called Capristatin™ [see Chapter Twelve] and a nutrition program [see Section Three]. I use a number of nutrients guided by a computer-derived nutritional evaluation and hair analysis examination. In addition, I taught the patient how to "listen to her own body" to determine what foods or chemicals she may be exposed to.

Dr. Maulfair would have preferred to utilize the full extent of his sublingual provocative testing procedure, plus other new laboratory tests for Candida-connected illness. Laboratory tests help to pinpoint for the physician the extent of his patient's allergic response and *C. albicans* infestation. Thus a doctor could help achieve for the patient a quicker and finer-tuned result with appropriate treatment. As it is, on January 28, 1986, Dr. Maulfair told us, "The combination of the natural antifungal preparation plus intravenous and oral nutrition support with adrenal support has allowed Barbara Lynn Herrington to restore her internal biochemical balance, to improve to the point where virtually all of her symptoms are improved and, to date, many have been totally eliminated."

CHRONIC UNWELLNESS DIAGNOSED BY THE ANTI-CANDIDA ANTIBODY TEST

Board-certified clinical pathologist and immunopathology specialist Edward Winger, M.D., on the faculty of the School of Public Health, University of California at Berkeley, has perfected and was among the first to announce a laboratory method for diagnosing chronic unwellness created by the Candida syndrome. His is an elegant and accurate testing procedure. At his ImmunoDiagnostic Laboratories in Oakland, California, Dr. Winger reports on a patient's blood test results as measured levels of activity of several antibody immunoglobulins produced by your body and directed against Candida antigens.

The anti-Candida antibody test is performed on a sample of the patient's serum, obtained by a venipuncture and then processed and mailed to the medical mycology laboratory by the physician. Skilled technicians perform sophisticated tests to separate various immunoglobulins and to test them against antigens from *C. albicans*. Although your body usually makes an immune response against the yeast, the antigens "seen" by the body in an infestation are different than those reacted against in the usual benign yeast–human interaction. Elevated levels of immunoglobulins against these specific Candida antigens are suggestive of the Candida syndrome.

The ImmunoDiagnostic Laboratories report summarizes the levels of three major immunoglobulins: IgM (frontline), IgG (second-line), and IgA (antibody usually associated with body surfaces—mouth, gut, bladder, vagina). Understanding the result is made simpler for physicians who are not immunologists by Dr. Winger's development of a unique reporting system called "MONA" units. "MONA" means "multiples of normal activity," and normal is from 0 to 100 for each of the immunoglobulin classes. A report of 200 is "twice normal activity"; 350 would mean "three and one-half times normal activity." When levels of all three immunoglobulins are elevated two or more times above the expected "normal activity," a diagnosis of the Candida syndrome is difficult to refute. The physician should then seriously consider treatment for his candidiasis-involved patient.

Because of his special research interests, Dr. Winger was asked by Phyllis L. Saifer, M.D., M.P.H., a Professor at the School of Medicine at San Francisco, the University of California, to develop a test for antiovarian antibodies. Dr. Saifer's and Dr. Winger's correct suspicion was that human antibodies directed against the human ovary were present in *C. albicans* infections, contributing to infertility, premenstrual syndrome, and other menstrual irregularities often found in patients with the Candida syndrome.

Dr. Winger's antiovarian antibody test demonstrates the cross-reaction of a patient's antibodies: the very same ones reacting with Candida antigens also react with ovary tissue as well. Patients who are successfully treated for the yeast syndrome will show a decrease in the level of both reactions. Demonstration of cross-reactions to both Candida and ovary confirms the immunological process that seems to injure the ovaries and contribute to "female" symptoms.

In performing the antiovarian antibody test, Dr. Winger's laboratory is looking for an aberrant immune response. This situation results in actually creating symptoms of candidiasis instead of accomplishing the intended neutralization of Candida infection. When a patient suffers with "female organ" symptoms, an improper cross-reaction attack by body defenses (accidentally striking at its own ovary glands) must be considered. Dr. Winger declares that a triad develops in the patient involved with yeast overgrowth. The triad results in candidiasis, autoimmune antibody production (body defenses turned against itself), and endocrinopathy (dysfunction of one or more of the hormone glands). He adds that ovarian disorders can be seen in as many as 75 percent of women with chronic vaginal candidiasis. Resulting or associated hormone dysfunctions might include fertility problems (perhaps including spontaneous or threatened abortions or difficulty carrying an infant to term), possible endometriosis, reduced libido, and diminished or absent sexual activity.

Physicians interested in technical details of the anti-Candida antibody test, the antiovarian antibody test, and several other comprehensive immunology tests and profiles available under Dr. Winger's direction are invited to telephone the Immuno-Diagnostic Laboratories at (415) 839-6477.

THE CANDIDA ANTIGEN PROFILE

At the Antibody Assay Laboratories, pathologist Alan Broughton, M.D., also offers laboratory-assisted diagnosis of the Candida syndrome. Dr. Broughton suggests that the testing should include (1) an immunonutritional profile to give a precise indication of the nutritional state of the patient; (2) an immunoglobulin food hypersensitivity profile to measure IgG antibodies to fifty different foods; (3) a fungal hypersensitivity profile to screen for IgG and IgE antibodies to nineteen fungi; (4) a chronic fungal disease profile, specifically focusing on antibodies to Candida antigen as well as IgG, IgA, and IgM antibodies to trichophyton and epidermophyton; and (5) a chronic viral disease profile, seeking evidence of past, present, or chronic EBV, CMV, and herpes virus infections.

Of these profiles, the laboratory testing we are most concerned with is the fourth, the Candida antigen profile. Establishing the presence of yeast in stool cultures does not prove Candida overgrowth, since many normal people have this microorganism present in small amounts in their bowel. Quantitative stool cultures can be a valuable diagnostic procedure, but they are expensive, time consuming, and not always readily available. Serum antibody determinations have proven useful, but high antibody levels do not invariably indicate active overgrowth with yeast. Rather, serum antibody determinations may merely reflect recent past involvement. Dr. Broughton suggests that the detection of Candida-specific immune complexes and circulating free Candida antigens are consistent with acute Candida overload, with active replication of the yeast.

The origin of immune complexes and the course leading up to their full development is easy to understand. The presence of foreign antigen inside an organism initiates an immune response, with the resultant production of antibodies. These antibodies are present in high levels (high titers) only for days or weeks, but even after the antigen has been removed, specific antibodies can often be detected for months or years, steadily falling in concentration. A second appearance of the antigen results in prompt formation of an immune complex in which the already present antibody combines with the antigen and with fractions of complement. (Complement is a heat-sensitive, complicated protein system in fresh human blood serum. When activated in combination with antibodies, it is an integral part of the host defense mechanism against invading microorganisms.) Antigen in the blood may be transient. After you eat eggs, for example, egg albumin is absorbed from the gut and specific immune complexes can form. These albumin-immune complexes last only a matter of hours, often being removed by the spleen. When antigen persists in the blood for a prolonged period, on the other hand, such as from a heavy colonization with *C. albicans*, then the immune complexes are continually produced.

The detection of free circulating antigen is unusual in human blood samples. This indicates one of two situations: either antibody production has not yet commenced, or more antigen is present than antibody is being produced. Such insufficient production means that not all of the antigen is complexed or bound and some of it is floating freely in the blood.

When the candidiasis-conscious physician performs a chronic fungal disease profile on his patient's blood sample, four possibilities can arise:

1. When there are no immune complexes or circulating antigen, active Candida infestation is less likely in the patient.

2. When Candida-specific immune complexes are present without circulating antigen, the patient probably has active Candida overgrowth with a satisfactory (or even aggressive) immune response underway, completely tying up the antigen into immune complexes.

3. When Candida-specific immune complexes are present along with circulating free antigen, the patient most likely has active candidiasis to which the immune response is insufficient, so the laboratory test detects an excess amount of antigen compared to antibody.

4. When circulating antigen alone is detected with no

immune complexes present, the patient probably has active candidiasis to which he is not mounting an effective immune response, so that virtually no antibody is available for immune complex formation.

In addition to the symptoms discussed in the last chapter and the laboratory diagnostic tests described here, Candida syndrome patients may have a reduction in total numbers of T-cell lymphocytes. These immune system changes can be seen as a reduction of T-helper cells or T-suppressor cells or both. Such changes appear to depend at least partially on the nutritional status of the patient.

Physicians who desire more detailed discussion of technical aspects on the laboratory testing available from Antibody Assay Laboratories are invited to contact pathologist Alan Broughton, M.D., at (714) 538-3255.

THE CANDI-SPHERE SERODIAGNOSTIC ANALYSIS

Howard E. Hagglund, M.D., board-certified in family practice and Medical Director of the Hagglund Clinic, Inc., of Norman, Oklahoma, together with David S. Bauman, Ph.D., Adjunct Professor of Microbiology at the University of Oklahoma and President of Immuno-Mycologics, Inc., of Norman, Oklahoma, developed the Candi-sphere serodiagnostic analysis (a test). Working under the commercial name of Cerodex Laboratories, Inc., of Norman, Oklahoma, Drs. Hagglund and Bauman have evolved a somewhat different method to evaluate the overgrowth of yeast.

The Candi-sphere serodiagnostic analysis, more commonly referred to as the Candida enzyme immuno assay (CEIA) is a test with a claimed 95 percent accuracy when results are interpreted in concert with results of a patient questionnaire. The physician takes a blood sample from his patient by the finger-stick method or from a venipuncture (venous needle stick) specimen. The blood can be drawn into capillary tubes provided in the test kit. This blood is sent in a prepaid mailer to Cerodex Laboratories for their enzyme immunoassay. Testing supplies are distributed under Cerodex Laboratories license by a marketing company, Meditrend, Inc., of Albuquerque, New Mexico, (800) 545-9800, or in New Mexico, (505) 292-0700.

Your blood immunoassay is carried out using an unusual detection device, a small plastic sphere, invented by Drs. Bauman and Hagglund. The technician coats the sphere with a carrier protein called cytoplasmic protein antigen (which acts like a binder or glue) to which is chemically coupled a Candida antigen. The antigen bristles all over this plastic sphere, like metal filings on a magnet. The sphere is incubated with your serum, then processed so that a technician can identify spheres bristling with Candida antigens that also have your antibodies attached to them. This evidence that you have antibodies against Candida in your blood is reported to your doctor.

A patient with characteristic Candida syndrome symptoms (as documented on the history questionnaire and by physical examination) who also has a positive color change on the CEIA test is considered to have a confirmed diagnosis of candidiasis. Only in a few unusual situations will the test be positive while the patient does not, in fact, respond to treatment for the Candida syndrome.

For the patient having a negative CEIA but having clearly positive symptoms, diagnoses to consider include a prediabetic condition, a previous infection (such as with *Aspergillus*), infectious mononucleosis, or other unusual conditions that mimic the Candida syndrome. When the Candi-sphere serodiagnostic analysis was originally developed, Drs. Hagglund and Bauman incorporated the patient's answers on his candidiasis questionnaire into the total scoring. This practice does not appear to be essential and is no longer followed. Questionnaires are still furnished to physicians as part of the test kit and are used in screening patients to help determine who should be evaluated further with the CEIA test. Low-scoring responses on the questionnaire suggest that a patient is less likely to have a positive result on the CEIA test.

Meditrend, Inc., supplies an overlay-type scoring system, which is used by the doctor or his assistant to quickly grade the answers. A weighted Candida score is thus assigned to the patient. This score, combined with serological testing, helps to establish a positive or negative diagnosis for the Candida syndrome.

Physicians who want additional technical information about the Candi-sphere serodiagnostic analysis should contact Cerodex Laboratories at (800) 654-3639; in Oklahoma, (405) 288-2458.

THE CANDIDA ALBICANS ANTIBODY TITER TEST

J. Alexander Bralley, Ph.D., Director of the MetaMetrix Medical Research Laboratory in Norcross, Georgia, provides an antibody titer test for *C. albicans* similar to those already reported.

The MetaMetrix test has three components: a questionnaire and two specific antibody titers (IgE and IgG) to the fungal organism. The laboratory uses a small disc, on which are mixed a sample of the patient's blood, antigen from the fungus, and a radioactive tracer. The disc is run through a gamma ray counter, which measures radioactivity. The amount of radioactivity is proportional to the yeast-specific IgE and IgG antibodies present in the patient's blood.

In an interview Dr. Bralley stated,

We at MetaMetrix have found that any [high] score of IgG indicates an active overgrowth of Candida, hence the patient's elevation of the IgG level in an attempt to control it. The antigen is critical. It is important to test for both cytoplasmic as well as cell wall fragments, as we do. High IgE levels indicate an allergic reaction occurring in the patient to his own Candida. I view this as a more serious case of long-term Candida overgrowth, with drastic effects on the immune system. IgG levels will often be low [immune suppression] plus an allergic reaction [IgE levels elevated] to the normally resident Candida, which in a sense is like an autoimmune reaction going on in the gut. These patients will often have rampant food and chemical allergies.

MetaMetrix Medical Research Laboratory staff work under the supervision of pathologist Robert S. Waite, M.D., Ph.D.

The laboratory makes available *C. albicans* antibody titer diagnostic test kits, questionnaires, and support services. Physicians wanting technical information are asked to contact Dr. Bralley at (800) 221-4640; in Georgia, (404) 446-5483

THE CONTROVERSIAL CANDIDA ALBICANS LIVE BLOOD CELL ANALYSIS

Live blood cell analysis is a new and unproven method of viewing human blood elements under the microscope. Even among open-minded medical mavericks who routinely minister to yeast-related illness, this search technique for *C. albicans* is highly controversial and not widely accepted.

Live blood cell analysis involves assessment of a blood sample taken by a finger-stick and is reported as a composite of over twenty-five "measurements" of this freshly drawn blood. "Darkfield" microscopy technique is used. Developers of the method claim that observation of blood cells and other elements can give immediate information on multiple vitamin and mineral deficiencies, "toxicity," relative degree of oxygenation, tendencies toward "liver weakness," allergies, excess fat in the bloodstream, clotting, arteriosclerosis, and plaque. The technique's endorsers say that tendencies toward pathology may be detected and treated before complications to the patient arise.

Combining darkfield microscopy with television monitors and photomicrography, proponents suggest that they are advancing the fields of both hematology (the science of blood) and metabolic (body chemistry processes) research. They describe live blood cell analysis as an effective tool for the early detection of disease, identifying individual needs and effective dosage levels of nutrients. Malabsorption disorders and oversupplementation with too many (or too high a dosage of) nutritional supplements are also claimed to be eligible for detection, along with assessment of the degree of immunity that a person possesses. Live blood cell analysis equipment is employed in the office setting within twenty to thirty minutes.

Philip Hoekstra, III, Ph.D., has adapted high resolution optical microscopic techniques to demonstrate what he declares to be the consistent presence of significantly increased numbers of *Candida albicans* in the peripheral blood of candidiasis patients. These findings have high correlation with symptomatology and known risk factors of personal history. The majority of these organisms have been found to exist as cell wall–deficient aggregates termed "spheroplasts." These organisms have been consistently observed to undergo a rapid reversion to the parent, classical form in the *in vitro* microenvironment of a thin wet-mount slide.

Dr. Hoekstra says that fungi have a variant state so small that they can attain viruslike pervasiveness. This variant state he terms "cell wall deficiency" (CWD), and he asserts that it results in a less aggressive and less osmotically vulnerable organism, with altered nutritional requirements. Dr. Hoekstra states that his discovery of CWD yeast organisms in the individual suggests that these variant forms might be induced by taking antifungal antibiotics such as nystatin or ketoconizole. He claims that the CWD state is difficult to culture in the test tube and that CWDs are frequently killed or are not recognized because of their slow, altered growth. Thus, he maintains, standard microbiologic laboratory techniques fail to demonstrate their existence.

The failure of common laboratory methods to demonstrate CWD forms has been a source of much controversy in the medical community, including among candidiasis-conscious practitioners. Expert technicians, board-certified research pathologists, medical mycologists, and immunologists have not been able to substantiate the existence of the CWD yeast forms as claimed by Dr. Hoekstra. They have declared to us that they do not use or recommend live blood analysis to detect Candida organisms in a person who might be afflicted with candidiasis.

We feel a responsibility to report Dr. Hoekstra's work, but we must also point out that not only other microbiologists but also other live cell analysis experts have decried Dr. Hoekstra's findings. For instance, James R. Privitera, M.D., Medical Advisor and Founder of a live blood analysis laboratory, NutriScreen™ of Covina, California, says: "We've consulted with immunologists, pathologists, and university microbiologists who soundly denounce the claims that Candida is commonly seen in the blood of ambulatory patients. Until such iconoclastic claims are published and confirmed by independent investigators, we caution all health professionals to use only effective and proven tests to confirm your clinical impressions of *Candida albicans*."[1]

NOTES

1. James R. Privitera, "Enough Is Too Much," *Townsend Letter for Doctors*, January 1986, 34:26.

10

The Antiyeast
Drug Therapy Program

In late 1982, a little more than a year following the birth of her third child and while she was still nursing, Roberta Dominguez, age thirty-five, noticed that she was experiencing a great amount of gastrointestinal gas, stomach cramps, and other alimentary tract symptoms. Mrs. Dominguez, who resides in the Los Angeles suburb of North Ridge, California, suffered with the distress for a number of weeks before finally deciding to seek medical help.

Luckily, the woman chose a doctor well versed in the human body's reactions to our technologically altered internal and external environments, clinical ecologist Harvey Ross, M.D., an allergist and wholistic physician located in Hollywood, California. Dr. Ross, Vice President of the American Schizophrenic Association and the author of two popular books on physical and mental illnesses stemming from changes in the ecology, advised his patient that she had spontaneously acquired a yeast sensitivity. To help remedy her candidiasis, he prescribed the drug nystatin, four daily oral tablets of 500,000 units each.

Mrs. Dominguez improved dramatically on the nystatin and got rid of her alimentary tract symptoms rather quickly.

Consequently, she gave that first bout of candidiasis hardly any additional thought and continued with her life as a wife and mother of three children. But then, after traveling through Mexico on a vacation trip, Mrs. Dominguez had a relapse.

When we got home I sort of collapsed. I didn't know what it was. However, suspecting that my yeast problem had returned, I started building myself up slowly with good nutrition and the resumption of my nystatin prescription. When I stopped taking nystatin in September 1983, the disease hit me hard. My weight dropped to ninety-six pounds; I felt weak, had anemia, and worse. My husband got worried at the state of my condition and insisted that I go to an internist. But that specialist didn't believe in any systemic clinical entity caused by *Candida albicans*. He refused to treat what he considered to be an imaginary disease. So again I started to treat myself with what I knew to be excellent nutrition, acidophilus cultures, and a special anti-Candida diet that Dr. Ross had originally put me on.

In January 1984, following a visit out of town when I cheated on my antiyeast diet, I got candidiasis a third time. This recurrent attack was really severe and laid me low with more intestinal symptoms, vaginal symptoms [itching and discharge], and thrush all striking me at once. [Thrush is a Candida fungus infection of the mouth diagnosed by white patches on the tongue and oral mucous membranes.] My cotton-coated-like tongue was so stiff that I could hardly talk, plus I felt an insatiable thirst; I thought I had the thirst of diabetes. Not water nor any other liquid would quench it. My lips dried up and looked like prunes. I knew that I had to get back to Dr. Ross, and when I did, he represcribed nystatin.

I eventually doubled the nystatin dose but none of the pills helped to relieve my Candida symptoms. I was really sick. And nursing the baby was wearing me out. Yes, I was still nursing my two-year-old, so my mother advised me to stop and to eat quantities of garlic cloves. From a friend who is knowledgeable about herbs, my mother learned that garlic is a fine remedy for yeast infections. She had heard of its use for migraine headaches, too. I ate a lot of garlic, but my breath smelled awful.

Then another friend said I could buy deodorized garlic from the health food store as aged liquid extract produced as capsules and tablets. The brand name is Kyolic® [distributed by Wakunaga of America Company, Ltd., Torrance, California]. I used a bottle of the liquid every day. It worked! I started to feel alive again. I began to resume doing my housework and take care of the kids properly. My weight, which had dropped to just ninety pounds, started increasing. My strength came back. Of course, I continued with the nystatin too.

Taking so much of the garlic food supplement got expensive, but as soon as I let it go, thrush came back strongly. I kept my tongue clean with the liquid, and I brought in other remedies such as acidophilus in yogurt, a resumption of my low carbohydrate, anti-Candida diet, and swallowing more of the nystatin tablets. I kept improving month by month, even with going on a really hard vacation trip to Alaska. It took a year but the combination of ingredients has helped me control candidiasis. Around the time of my menstrual period I must hit the garlic hard, because menstruation seems to stimulate Candida symptoms. I take the garlic and the nystatin together as pills—many of them.

THE BABY HAS YEAST-RELATED ILLNESS

Mrs. Dominguez's baby daughter, three-year-old Jon Marie, had candidiasis manifested by severe symptoms of bronchial asthma. The condition came on as a result of too much antibiotic usage, prescribed by the pediatrician for repeated infections. In January 1984, Jon Marie came down with an acutely painful earache and another oral broad spectrum antibiotic was prescribed. She was first exposed to yeast possibly through contact with it in her mother's birth canal or through kissing or suckling at her mother's breast. The invasion remained quiescent until antibiotics for the earache also killed off friendly bacteria in the child's gut. With no counteracting bacteria remaining to keep down yeast overgrowth, the child had asthma symptoms arise as well. She experienced double discomforts of ear and lung problems.

Simultaneously the baby's bottom broke out in severe diaper rash, irritated by loose black stools. The stools resulted from the reduction of normal gut bacteria by the antibiotic. So Jon Marie's Candida syndrome now involved diarrhea. She was grouchy and cried all the time. Mrs. Dominguez really worried about the toddler.

As they had for her mother, nystatin and aged garlic extract turned out to be lifesavers for the daughter. They aided in ridding her of Candida symptoms and currently control the condition effectively. By putting Jon Marie on a low carbohydrate diet and daily giving her a formula of three-quarters teaspoonful of megadose ascorbic acid (vitamin C) plus one and a half teaspoonsful of liquid aged garlic extract, Mrs. Dominguez keeps her child's bronchial asthma from coming back. The nystatin dosage is scaled down to match the baby's body weight.

MALE CANDIDIASIS TREATMENT WITH NYSTATIN

As we know, men are not immune to the Candida syndrome. But the effects for men usually aren't as devastating as for women. The vastly more complex hormone system of women possibly predisposes them to more potential trouble. Furthermore, men suffer less frequently from candidiasis, probably because they generally are not treated by doctors as often as are women, so they are exposed less often to the wonders— and resulting difficulties—associated with modern medical technology.

In the fall of 1981, Joseph Friedlander of Atlanta, Georgia, a thirty-year-old, previously healthy aircraft mechanic, developed food poisoning—with the typical "both ends" symptoms of vomiting and diarrhea. Two of his co-workers, apparently exposed to the same food contamination, experienced similar symptoms of infection. They recovered in a few days without being seen by physicians and with no drug treatment. Joe Friedlander, on the other hand, chose to consult his airline company's medical department. The clinic was supervised by a traditionally practicing physician who prescribed a tetracycline antibiotic. The drug promptly initiated a long course of illness and misery for the mechanic.

Within days Friedlander developed a severe prostatitis that recurred intermittently for three years. Prostatitis is inflammation of the prostate, a donut-shaped male sexual organ about the size of a chestnut, located at the neck of the bladder, and through the center of which (donut hole) passes the bladder tube to the outside. Inflammation of this muscular and glandular tissue yields pain or a feeling of urgency in the bladder region, frequency of urination, blood in the urine, elevated body temperature, and occasional shivering chills. The man showed all the symptoms of a serious urinary tract infection. More antibiotics cleared up this new acute bacterial infection.

Six months following his prostatitis, Friedlander started to suffer severe constipation, abdominal distention, anxiety, depression, and annoying nervous tension, none of which had ever before been a problem. The discomforts lingered for another whole year until his sister referred him to the Marietta, Georgia, wholistic physician, William Campbell Douglass, M.D., an expert in administering to yeast-related illnesses. Sure enough, Friedlander's Review of Personal Health Problems and Concerns, his background information, and his results on one of the new specialized laboratory tests indicated to Dr. Douglass that his patient had polysystemic chronic candidiasis, the yeast syndrome.

Consulted by Friedlander in March 1985, Dr. Douglass prescribed oral nystatin. To the patient's grateful amazement, his symptoms completely resolved in only ten days. The chronic swelling in his scrotum (from residual inflammation of the prostate) disappeared. Annoying and continuous gastrointestinal distress stopped. His spirits lifted considerably as a result of his newly found freedom from pain and discomfort.

Friedlander then discontinued the nystatin treatment and within two days all of his symptoms returned. He went back to Dr. Douglass with his repeat tale of woe. Resumption of the nystatin prescription cleared the mechanic again, and he has remained well since, thanks in part to continued small daily doses of nystatin.

NYSTATIN

A generic product, nystatin is an antifungal antibiotic which kills or stops the growth of a wide variety of yeasts and yeastlike fungi. The drug is thought to bind with the fungus cell membrane, resulting in changes in membrane permeability. Such changes allow leakage of surrounding fluids into the germ, with subsequent swelling, bursting, and spilling of the organism's intracellular components. Nystatin is the first relatively fast-acting, well-tolerated pharmaceutical of dependable efficacy for the treatment of intestinal, oral, vaginal, skin, and other organ infections caused by *C. albicans* and its sister Candida species. While this medicine provides specific therapy for all localized forms of candidiasis that it can reach directly, it has no known effect on bacteria.

Nystatin is virtually nontoxic and nonsensitizing. All age groups—including debilitated infants—accept the drug without demonstrating major side effects, even on prolonged administration. The generic product, distributed by several companies, was first manufactured by the Lederle Laboratories division of American Cyanamid Company, Wayne, New Jersey. Several other drug houses make brand-name products from the generic ingredients. Nystatin is administered for skin conditions as creams, ointments, and powders; for internal use it is prepared as suppositories, suspensions, tablets, powder, and capsules.

Nystatin has been demonstrated to be safe during more than twenty-six years of medical application. It is available only by a doctor's prescription, mostly and traditionally as a tablet, oral suspension, or suppository. Candida-conscious physicians prefer to prescribe the product as a pure powder. It is less expensive and seemingly more effective that way. The powder, while it has a somewhat unpleasant taste, can be dissolved easily in water and swished around in the mouth to fight the yeast (oral thrush) located there. Some physicians advise women to obtain clear gelatin "medicine" capsules and fill them with the powder (occasionally accompanied by acidophilus powder too) for use as an inexpensive and effective vaginal treatment, rather than the nystatin suppositories that are available. Powder and cream forms are used to treat yeast infections on the skin, such as baby's diaper rash.

Nystatin is still the mainstay for candidiasis therapy, even though new and more powerful products have come along. Some of the new ones have potentially toxic side effects, while nystatin has virtually none or only very minor ones.

Nystatin administration must be prolonged because reducing the number of infecting yeast organisms is only a part of the total treatment program. Nutritional efforts must be concurrently directed at improving the function of the immune defense system, so that it can control future challenges without the need for further anti-Candida medications. Most patients make the greatest progress after taking the medication for three months or more. The drug's broad anti-Candida spectrum, low cost, easy tolerability, and lack of absorption from the gut has made it the most frequently prescribed oral antifungal agent.

Hospitalized patients were evaluated in 1973 before and after nystatin use. When they did not receive the drug, 56 percent of patients were found to have *C. albicans* infestation of the rectum. When taking oral nystatin, only 4 percent of patients were found to have cultures positive for rectal yeast after three weeks of hospitalization. The ability of nystatin to suppress alimentary-tract yeast continued, even for patients who were receiving systemic antibiotics.[1]

The drug appears effective in decreasing major fungal infections even in the diminished dosage of 400,000 units.[2] Administered in the stronger dosage of 1,200,000 units per day, nystatin has been shown to act prophylactically against the Candida syndrome.[3]

NYSTATIN DOSAGES

A pure form of the drug is available as nystatin powder. The usual adult maintenance dose often is one-quarter or one-half teaspoonful (tsp) of powder four times a day. Strictly following your own physician's individual instructions, you will probably start your nystatin powder dosage at ⅛ tsp four times a day and increase it at one- or two-week intervals to ¼ tsp or ½ tsp four times daily. Some patients briefly require dosages of 1 tsp four, five, or more times a day. The powder may be dissolved in the mouth and gradually swallowed. It has a tart taste, reminiscent of stale cardboard. (Some patients have compared nystatin's taste to nibbling on potting soil.) You may choose to dissolve the powder in two to four ounces of purified water.

If juice must be used as a dissolving solution for the nystatin powder, make sure it comes from a non-yeast-contaminated source. For instance, microbiologic culturing performed at the University of Maryland Cancer Center has found species of Candida in the following processed juices: apple, pineapple, orange, tomato, grape, apricot, and lemonade. The presence of fungal contamination was not related to the type of fruit juice but rather to the type of packaging and processing. All fruit juices packaged and sealed with foil wraps were contaminated, while those canned or bottled juices tested were free of fungi. As a general rule, freshly squeezed citrus juices do not contain yeast. (Be sure to check with your physician to see whether you are allowed to drink juices on your particular anti-Candida dietary program. Ice cubes made from ice makers in the cancer center's kitchen were also contaminated with Candida organisms.[4]

A proper dosage of nystatin powder is individualized for you by the prescribing physician. The above dosage schedule is only a guideline. Your doctor will establish your appropriate dose in two ways: by your body weight and by the control and/or disappearance of symptomatic disorders. If you have had irregular bowel movements, indigestion, or heartburn prior to therapy, for example, and such symptoms subside with a specific dosage of nystatin, this amount will likely become your maintenance prescription. Your dosage needs will change over time and as your health and diet vary; regular followup appointments with your physician are essential.

Nystatin in the form of Nilstat® oral tablets are film-coated and produced in 500,000 units per tablet in bottles of 100 by Lederle Laboratories, a Division of American Cyanamid Company, Wayne, New Jersey. The company also manufactures Nilstat® oral suspension, vaginal tablets, topical cream, and topical ointment.

As mentioned earlier, other pharmaceutical companies also make nystatin for oral administration. One of them is E.R. Squibb & Sons, Inc., of Princeton, New Jersey, which produces Mycostatin® oral suspension as well as coated tablets at

500,000 units with yellow dye no. 5 as coloring. The company also produces Mycostatin® vaginal tablets, cream, ointment, and topical powder. Another packager is Premo Pharmaceutical Laboratories, Inc., of South Hackensack, New Jersey. This drug company also offers nystatin oral tablets, vaginal tablets, and cream. Many physicians are reluctant to use oral tablet preparations because they seem to be less effective than the powder form. Incidentally, ⅛ tsp of the powder is supposed to equal about one oral tablet, in terms of potency.

Orally administered nystatin is only partially successful in suppressing gastrointestinal tract yeast. To obtain the most consistent results, you should combine medications with wholistic methods, which will be discussed at length in Chapters Eleven and Twelve.

HERXHEIMER'S REACTION

Named after the German dermatologist, Karl Herxheimer, M.D., the Herxheimer reaction is more correctly given the double-crediting name, "Jarisch-Herxheimer reaction," since Dr. Herxheimer described this body response in association with another German dermatologist, Adolf Jarisch, M.D. The Herxheimer reaction is said to have occurred if a certain quantity of C. albicans "die-off" from the use of nystatin or other antifungal antibiotics causes your body to respond with a series of violent symptoms. Most physicians who treat candidiasis don't consider Herxheimer's reaction to be a side effect but rather anticipate its occurrence as a possible good sign. The definition of a drug side effect is an unwanted harmful effect in addition to the drug's desired therapeutic effect. Except that you may feel unwell for a few days, "die-off" of C. albicans is not necessarily unwanted and not harmful. No serious threat to health or delay of eventual recovery has been noted. The distressing symptoms can be usually treated appropriately by the patient's physician.

Sidney Baker, M.D., Medical Director of the Gesell Institute, explained that patients may have to endure the Herxheimer reaction during the first days (on rare occasions, weeks) of treatment because nystatin kills yeast cells quite brutally: they suddenly release substances that produce a temporary toxic or allergylike reaction in the host. This reaction is not an allergy to the nystatin itself, because it clears up as the nystatin is continued. Some patients have so much discomfort, such as aching, bloating, headache, stuffiness, or worsening of the problem for which they are being treated, that they have to radically modify dosages or even discontinue drug treatment altogether and choose among other options for managing the yeast problem.[5]

ORAL AMPHOTERICIN B

Also called fungilin, fungizone, and amphomoronal, amphotericin B is an antifungal antibiotic formulated into creams, ointments, lotions, lozenges, suspensions, tablets, pessaries (medicated vaginal suppositories), an orabase (medication dentists use to keep some contact between medicine and the gums), and an intravenous preparation. Amphotericin B is extensively utilized in Europe. Because of concern with the preparation's potential side effects, the U.S. Food and Drug Administration disallows its importation and use in the United States.

Amphotericin B was discovered six years after nystatin. A polyene like nystatin, amphotericin B acts on fungi by a similar mechanism. Polyenes bind to the sterol components of the cell membranes of susceptible fungi and alter the permeability functions; an influx of surrounding fluids leads to metabolic disruptions and cell death. Clinically, amphotericin B has been applied as topical applications with success to nearly every form of oral, vaginal, and other superficial candidiasis. Since it is not absorbed from the gut, it has to be administered by intravenous injection in order to have a direct effect on Candida invasion in deeper tissues.

But amphotericin B can be highly toxic, easily causing kidney damage, uremia, and other troubles. In serious infections, however, a person is presumably better off alive with some kidney damage than dead with untreated rampant fungal disease. In hospital usage, amphotericin B is administered intravenously. Since this is a book for the medical consumer, and since the U.S. FDA objects to its use, no information on its acquisition or dosage or description of administration will be given.[6,7,8,9]

MICONAZOLE

Miconazole was made available by prescription in the United States first as a cream for the treatment of vulvovaginal candidiasis in April 1974. It affects both the yeast (active growth) form of *C. albicans* and the mycelial (invasive) form. Miconazole is believed to start a chain reaction of molecular damage resulting in the cell death of the fungus. Under the microscope, Candida cells incubated with an appropriate dose of miconazole appear to collapse twenty-four hours after the drug is introduced. How the cream, lotion, and suppositories (manufactured by Ortho Pharmaceutical Corporation, Raritan, New Jersey) are used and work will be discussed in Chapter Sixteen.

Miconazole for internal administration has been marketed in the United States as an intravenous preparation by Janssen Pharmaceutica, Inc., of New Brunswick, New Jersey. In Denmark, it has been given orally in a double-blind trial for preventive purposes to patients highly predisposed to fungal infections. Thirty people were in the study and were given either 500 mg of miconazole or a placebo four times daily. The antifungal antibiotic worked as a preventive, apparently through its systemic effect.[10]

KETOCONAZOLE

A synthetic broad spectrum antifungal agent, ketoconazole is marketed for internal use in the United States as scored white tablets under the brand name, Nizoral®, by Janssen Pharmaceutica, Inc., New Brunswick, New Jersey. Its activity against *C. albicans* seems to be from impairment of the organism's synthesis of ergosterol, a vital component of fungal cell membranes. Ketoconazole therapy has been compared to "punching holes in the cell wall and letting the yeast slowly bleed to death."

In some cases (especially of deeper-seated infections), Nizoral® is more effective than nystatin in eliminating yeast. However, as with all oral drugs, ketoconazole can produce some uncomfortable side effects, nausea being the most common one. In rare cases, it can result in "chemical hepatitis." A prescribing physician must monitor the drug's administration by means of monthly liver-testing panels (blood tests) performed on the patient. The drug is also more expensive than bacterial antibiotics, costing approximately one dollar per tablet, but it sometimes achieves symptomatic response somewhat faster than other remedies.

The usual dose of ketoconazole is one or two tablets daily. Some patients and physicians report effective control of the Candida syndrome with a dosage regimen of one-quarter tablet twice a week or doses administered only premenstrually for five or six days. Others use three or four tablets daily—sometimes for many months—to achieve the desired result. As with all details of the anti-yeast program (including nutritional supplementation and dietary changes), you must rely on your physician's constant guidance. There is some worry among mycologists (fungus specialists) that ketoconazole could give rise to a resistant fungal superinfection if it is used clinically for prevention rather than as specific therapy.[11] This concern, while valid, has not been substantiated in clinical experience.

Prophylactic antifungal agents injected intravenously to discourage the development of the Candida syndrome are promising and on the horizon, but new methods need to be developed and more experimentation must be carried out. The number of patients studied to date is small. Antifungal prevention by injection might emerge as a practical technique for restoring the balance between host humans and the Candida organisms that they harbor.

GRISEOFULVIN

The orally administered antibiotic antifungal agent griseofulvin was first discovered in England in 1939. Numerous scientific papers were published about it between 1949 and 1959. Dermatologist Leon Goldman, M.D., said about griseofulvin, "A good way to make something secret is to publish it in the scientific, not medical, literature."[12] Indeed, it went unnoticed on the shelves of biologists and in the journals of allied biological science for nineteen years before it was recognized as an invaluable tool in the fight against fungal disease.

In August 1960, at the Chicago annual meeting of the American Podiatry Association (APA), this book's coauthor, Morton Walker, D.P.M., received the APA's William J. Stickle Annual Award for Research and Writing in Podiatry, for his presentation, "A Study of Griseofulvin as Related to Tinea Pedis." Under an investigational grant-in-aid from Schering Corporation of Kenilworth, New Jersey, and with unprecedented approval from the U.S. Food and Drug Administration (the first time the FDA had approved internal drug research by a podiatrist), Dr. Walker described how griseofulvin is specifically active against fungal organisms, including *C. albicans* occasionally associated with other fungi, which infect the skin of the feet and toenails.[13]

Dr. Walker explained that from infection with yeast organisms, a certain amount of inflammatory reaction occurs in the skin. The inflammation causes dilatation of skin blood vessels and an overgrowth of cellular elements.[14] When you ingest griseofulvin, the drug is absorbed into your bloodstream and is incorporated later in a cellular exudate (fluid) occurring under the tiny blisters created as signs of fungus disease.[15] As skin cells infiltrated with yeast and other fungal organisms grow outwardly from the skin's germ layer—either by the wearing out process or by the actual infiltration of immune defenders—these cells absorb griseofulvin by osmosis in sufficient quantity to stop fungus spread.

The time course of griseofulvin concentration in blood depends on its route of administration and dosage level. When given orally, a slow rise of blood griseofulvin concentration can be detected in the next five to eight hours. Griseofulvin has a "curling factor" action, which causes an actual curling and stunting of the hyphae of the yeast and other fungi, including *C. albicans*.[16] The hyphae coalesce into themselves, forming a tight knot of multibranches. As further griseofulvin-containing skin cells reach the skin's outer surface, the disease process is arrested. The outer skin sloughs off, and eventually noninfected cells replace infected ones. Thus, griseofulvin attacks the invading organisms by bathing the hard keratinous structures in the skin in sufficient concentration to be lethal to the organisms.[17]

Today griseofulvin is FDA-approved and manufactured by several drug companies: Schering Corporation of Kenilworth,

New Jersey, provides Fulvicin® P/G ultramicrosize griseo-fulvin, USP tablets of 125 mg and 250 mg. The adult daily dosage is 375 mg as a single dose or, in divided doses, a maximum of 750 mg daily. It is not recommended for children under age two. Children weighing thirty-five to sixty pounds can take 125–187.5 mg daily. A child over sixty pounds in weight can have from 187.5 mg to 375 mg a day. Fulvicin® also comes in 165 mg, 330 mg, and 500 mg dosages.

Ayerst Laboratories division of American Home Products Corporation of New York City, supplies Grisactin® and Grisactin Ultra®. The Ultra tablets contain griseofulvin ultra-microsize in dosage strengths of 125 mg, 250 mg, and 330 mg. The efficiency of gastrointestinal absorption of ultra-microcrystalline griseofulvin is approximately one and one half times that of the microsized griseofulvin. This factor permits oral intake of two-thirds as much ultramicrocrystalline griseofulvin to be as active as a larger dose of the microsize form.

Ortho Pharmaceutical Corporation of Raritan, New Jersey, manufactures and distributes Grifulvin V® Ortho in 250 mg and 500 mg microsize tablets and Grifulvin V® suspension of 125 mg per 5 cc. The Ortho tablets have a similar dosage schedule.

Herbert Laboratories, Dermatology Division of Allergan Pharmaceuticals, Inc., of Irvine, California, packages an ultra-microsize tablet in 125 mg and 250 mg dosage named Gris-Peg®. The Gris-Peg® adult dose is 375 mg daily as one or more divided doses to a maximum of 750 mg daily, as with the other brands of griseofulvin.

The side effects of griseofulvin usually occur as a result of hypersensitivity of the patient. These include skin rashes, hives, swelling, and numbness or tingling of the hands and feet. There may also be nausea, vomiting, epigastric (in the pit of the stomach) distress, diarrhea, headache, fatigue, dizziness, insomnia, mental confusion, and impairment of performance of routine activities. Although the 1986 *Physicians' Desk Reference* says that griseofulvin is not effective in candidiasis and may also bring on oral thrush as a side effect,[18] numerous physicians have reported its effectiveness when fungus infections are mixed.

CANDICIDIN

Candicidin is presently used only topically in vulvovaginal infections, although previously it was taken orally for systemic candidiasis.

CLOTRIMAZOLE

Also formerly administered by mouth for the Candida syndrome, clotrimazole is now used only topically. When given orally, it can produce serious side effects such as gastrointestinal bleeding, nausea, vomiting, diarrhea, itching, swelling, hives, blistering of the skin, and mental disturbances with hallucinations and disorientation in up to 25 percent of the patients. Clotrimazole will also be discussed in Chapter Nineteen as a topical medication.

FLUCYTOSINE

Manufactured by Roche Laboratories, Inc., a Division of Hoffman-La Roche, Inc., of Nutley, New Jersey, flucytosine was described, in part, in connection with the case of Charlie Swaart, "the drinkless drunk," in Chapter Two. The Roche brand name for flucytosine is Ancobon®.

When given by mouth, flucytosine is distributed widely through body tissues and cerebrospinal fluid. About 50 percent of Candida species are inhibited by flucytosine. Although larger doses are given in Europe, the currently recommended dosage in the United States is 150 mg per kg per day, in four equally divided doses given at six-hour intervals. Flucytosine has potentially serious side effects, such as bowel perforation, rashes, gastrointestinal distress with nausea, vomiting, diarrhea, anemia, lowering of the number of white blood cells, deficiency of blood platelets, liver toxicity, headaches, hallucinations, sleepwalking, and dizziness. Few American physicians have need to prescribe medications with such toxic side effects, in part owing to their success in coordinating drug therapy with the wholistic approaches to be described next.[19,20,21,22,23,24]

NOTES

1. F. R. Stark, N. Ninos, J. Hutton, R. Katz, and M. Butler, "Candida Peritonitis and Cimetidine," *Lancet,* 1978, 2:744.

2. U. Carpenteri, M. E. Haggard, L. H. Lockhart, L. P. Gustavson, Q. T. Box, and E. F. West, "Clinical Experience in Prevention of Candidiasis by Nystatin in Children with Acute Lymphocytic Leukemia," *Journal of Pediatrics,* 1978, 92:593–595.

3. J. Pizzuto, G. Conte, A. Aviles, R. Ambriz, M. Morales, and Centro Medico National Hospital General, "Nystatin Prophylaxis in Leukemia and Lymphoma," *New England Journal of Medicine,* 1978, 299:661–662.

4. James C. Wade and Stephen C. Schimpff, "Epidemiology and Prevention of Candida Infections," in G. P. Bodey and V. Fainstein, eds., *Candidiasis,* New York: Raven Press, 1985, p. 113.

5. Sidney M. Baker, *Notes on the Yeast Problem,* New Haven: Gessell Institute of Human Development, 1985, p. 8.

6. J. Alban and J. T. Groel, "Amphotericin B Oral Suspension in the Treatment of Thrush," *Current Therapeutic Research,* 1970, 12:479–484.

7. M. B. Corkill and N. J. McCarthy, "Comparative Trial of Fungilin (Amphotericin B) and Pimafucin (Natamycin) Pessaries in the Treatment of Vaginal Candidiasis," *Medical Journal of Australia,* 1972, 2:33–44.

8. J. J. Gayford, "The Treatment of Oral Candidosis in Extensively Burned Patients," *British Journal of Plastic Surgery,* 1969, 22:86.

9. W. S. Symmers, "Amphotericin Pharmacophobia," *British Medical Journal,* 1973, 4:460–463.

10. H. Brincker, "Prophylactic Treatment with Miconazole in Patients Highly Predisposed to Fungal Infection," *Acta Medicina of Scandinavia,* 1978, 204:123–128.

11. G. Acuna, D. J. Winston, and L. S. Young, "Ketoconazole Prophylaxis of Fungal Infections in the Granulocytopenic Patient: A Double-Blind, Randomized Controlled Trial," *Programs and Abstracts of the 21st Interscience Conference of Antimicrobial Agents and Chemotherapy,* Chicago, November 1981, abstract 852.

12. Leon Goldman, "Doctor to Doctor, No. 5," *A Round-Table Discussion on Griseofulvin by a Group of Physicians at the AMA Meeting,* June 1959.

13. Morton Walker, "A Study of Griseofulvin as Related to Tinea Pedis," *Journal of the American Podiatry Association,* February 1961, 51:12–14.

14. Oliver S. Ormsby, *Diseases of the Skin*, Philadelphia: Lea & Febiger, 1937.

15. A. Peck, "Epidermophytosis of the Feet and Epidermophytids of the Hands," *Archives of Dermatology and Syphilology*, 1930.

16. Morton Walker, "Report on Griseofulvin," *Journal of the American Podiatry Association*, April 1960, 50:297–303.

17. Marion B. Sulzberger and Rudolph L. Baer, "Griseofulvin, an Oral Antibiotic for the Treatment of Many Common Fungous Infections of the Skin, Hair and Nails," *Excerpta Medica, Dermatology and Venereology*, 13, no. 3, March 1959.

18. *Physicians' Desk Reference*, 40th ed., Oradell, N.J.: Medical Economics, 1986.

19. P. L. Steer, M. I. Marks, P. D. Klite, and T. C. Eickhoff, "5-Fluorocytosine: An Oral Antifungal Compound," *Annals of Internal Medicine*, 1972, 76:15–22.

20. R. Meyer and J. L. Axelrod, "Fatal Aplastic Anemia Resulting from Flucytosine," *Journal of the American Medical Association*, 1974, 228:1573.

21. R. J. Schlegal, G. M. Bernier, J. A. Bellanti, D. A. Maybee, B. S. Osborne, J. L. Stewart, D. S. Pearlman, J. Ouelett, and F. C. Biehusen, "Severe Candidiasis Associated with Thymic Dysplasia, IgA Deficiency, and Plasma Antilymphocyte Effects," *Pediatrics*, 1970, 45:926–936.

22. R. B. Diasio, D. E. Lakings, and J. E. Bennett, "Evidence for Conversion of 5-Fluorocytosine to 5-Fluoroucil in Humans; Possible Factor in 5-Fluorocytosine Clinical Toxicity," *Antimicrobiology Agents and Chemotherapy*, 1978, 14:903–908.

23. G. A. Pankey, W. R. Lockwood, and J. M. Montalvo, "5-Fluorocytosine: A Replacement for Amphotericin B in the Treatment of *Candida* and *Cryptococcus neoformans* Infections," *Journal of the Louisiana State Medical Society*, 1970, 122:365–369.

24. E. J. Harder and P. E. Hermans, "Treatment of Fungal Infections with Flucytosine," *Archives of Internal Medicine*, 1975, 135: 231–237.

11

The Antiyeast Wholistic
Therapy Program—Part One

Nystatin and various other antifungal antibiotic products are merely drug tools in a much larger, full treatment program against the yeast syndrome. Therapy for polysystemic chronic candidiasis has two main goals: (1) to kill the yeast invader (or at least reduce its growth); and (2) to stimulate and repair the patient's immunity so that in the future his body may come to its own defense. The antiyeast wholistic therapeutic program attempts to accomplish the latter.

Immune system stimulation and repair won't entirely eliminate yeast from a patient's body; rather, wholistic therapies are aimed at restoring the original and natural commensal balance between the human host and the Candida parasite. Thus, the "healthy" condition is restored to where an individual and Candida organisms usually live together without harm or prejudice to either.

Candida albicans wait patiently for our death, ever available to recycle you and me as reusable organic matter in nature's synoptic scheme. Yeast organisms are parasites of virtually all warm-blooded animals, especially man. We humans have evolved an ecological balance with the yeast. But when major or even minor changes occur in our physiology, yeast are poised to take advantage of the imbalance and proceed to veritably digest us. In the view of fungi, we are convenient piles of edible material that sooner or later become ripe for recycling. Our human need, in turn, is to hold on to the proper yeast–human interaction balance as long as possible.

Concepts of the antiyeast wholistic therapy program take into account new medical data which are far in advance of therapeutic approaches currently in vogue for traditionally practiced allopathic medicine. The advanced concepts suggest that many diverse diseases, such as migraine headache, ulcerative colitis, asthma, multiple sclerosis, systemic lupus erythematosis, rheumatoid arthritis, and attention-deficit disorders, are all interrelated. These diseases appear to result, at least partially, from environmental, nutritional, biochemical, and other influences that affect the victims' immune systems. By recognizing these correlative causes, and by taking steps to alter them, wholistic physicians are able to help victims of candidiasis without resorting to hospitalization, surgery, radiation, chemotherapy, or other forms of poorly successful and potentially toxic drug treatment.[1]

WHOLISTIC ANTIYEAST THERAPY IN PENNSYLVANIA

Mrs. Cynthia Farris, a sixty-four-year-old homemaker residing outside of Trenton, New Jersey, hosted a widespread chronic candidiasis condition. Her health disorders included nausea, vomiting, severe constipation, great discomfort in the abdomen related to indigestion, persistent vaginal discharge, and severe allergies. These symptoms had been with her intermittently throughout the prior twenty years. She was unable to move her bowels without assistance from either laxatives or enemas. She also suffered with severe headaches and found herself becoming increasingly fatigued—to the point where she could barely take care of herself, let alone perform her housewifely duties.

Eventually it became impossible for Mrs. Farris to fulfill the speaking engagements in which she discusses her victory over cancer by the use of certain nutritional practices. (About ten years ago the woman was diagnosed with melanoma of the skin with metastasis to the liver. After having the skin malignancy surgically removed, her successful treatment was achieved with the help of a wholistic physician who utilizes immune-supportive alternative cancer therapies. He put her on a metabolic program of raw foods, wheat grass, and nutritional supplements. Without undergoing any other traditional treatment, she was informed that her liver biopsy was reported negative for cancer four years after her first being diagnosed— and it has remained negative when biopsy has been repeated periodically during the past five years.)

But Cynthia Farris had discomfort from the other chronic complaints related to yeast infestation. She brought these other troubles to the attention of a second wholistic physician, Pannathpur Jayalakshmi, M.D. In practice with her husband, Kakkadasam R. Sampathachar, M.D., Dr. Jayalakshmi is Medical Director of the New Life Center of Philadelphia, Pennsylvania, where she specializes in the treatment of allergy, arthritis, atherosclerosis, and obesity. She uses a variety of wholistic medical techniques including acupuncture, chelation therapy, and nutrition.

When Mrs. Farris first visited Dr. Jayalakshmi on October 13, 1983, the patient was quite emaciated and obviously malnourished, weighing only eighty-three pounds on a five-foot, two-inch frame. As is common with candidiasis, her physical examination was essentially "noncontributory" or "nondiagnostic," except for her malnourished appearance. When she completed the candidiasis questionnaire, the patient's Y-score (on Dr. Crook's questionnaire) was very high, over 300. The Heidelberg capsule gastrogram test (acid-base evaluation of the stomach and first part of the small intestine, sometimes called a "tubeless gastric analysis") revealed that she produced an insufficient amount of hydrochloric acid (hypochlorhydria).

"We treated her with the antiyeast wholistic therapy program using parenteral [injected] vitamins and minerals; high dosage, orally administered vitamins, minerals, and digestive supplements; yogurt and lactozyme normal flora [*Lactobacillus acidophilus*]; deodorized aged liquid garlic [Kyolic™ and SGP™]; excellent nutrition; and advised her on how to rotate her foods in order to control allergy symptoms," said Dr. Jayalakshmi. "We also approached her multiple allergies (the patient was allergic to more than seventy foods and inhalants) by doing provocative skin testing and neutralization therapy with the injection method developed by Joseph Miller, M.D."

Dr. Miller, of Mobile, Alabama, is a pediatrician specializing in allergy. His testing method is somewhat different from the techniques of skin testing employed by traditionally practicing allergists. Symptoms are provoked by into-the-skin injections of different dilutions (strengths) of antigens, with subsequent neutralization of reactions by further injections. This is an extremely safe method that can provide patients with excellent symptom control despite continuing exposure to environmental allergens. The Miller provocative skin-testing technique enabled Drs. Jayalakshmi and Sampathachar to determine the correct neutralizing dose concentrations for each major allergen causing a reaction in Cynthia Farris.

Wherever possible, the philosophy of medical practice at the New Life Center, as at other wholistic medical centers, is to reduce the amount of drug therapy that a patient must take. Toward this end, the husband and wife medical team employs the wholistic technique of encouraging natural food nutrition. Their recommended eating program includes the elimination of alcoholic beverages, cola drinks, soda pop, tap water, coffee, white flour products, sugar, and processed foods sold in supermarkets, groceries, and other food stores. Of course, smoking and other abusive body and mind practices are discouraged.

Already a prior victim of cancer, Mrs. Farris was devoted to the many good health practices that had helped her to remain free of the life-threatening disease. To this healthful lifestyle, Dr. Jayalakshmi added more approaches for the specific treatment of candidiasis. She prescribed the nutritional supplement evening primrose oil (Efamol™, an English product containing gamma-linolenic acid) distributed by Health from the Sun Products, Inc., of Dover, Massachusetts, plain water retention enemas, freshly brewed caffeinated coffee enemas, nystatin enemas, yogurt douches, inhalant solutions, and other items.

Mrs. Farris was also taught how to relax by applying the Simonton method of visualization. Stephanie Matthews-Simonton and her husband, O. Carl Simonton, M.D., are recognized experts on psychological factors in the treatment of cancer. At their Cancer Counseling and Research Center in Dallas, Texas, the Simontons employ mind dynamics for improved longevity, quality of life, and quality of death. Dr. Sampathachar is a certified medical hypnotist who incorporates relaxation techniques as part of the overall treatment program at the New Life Center.

Cynthia Farris also began a course of nystatin powder. She took the nystatin orally, rectally, and vaginally. Her dosage was gradually increased from one-sixteenth teaspoonful administered orally twice a day to one level teaspoonful three times daily.

Over the course of several months, Dr. Jayalakshmi saw that her patient eventually could tolerate more foods without feeling nauseated or vomiting. Her weight slowly increased to her normal 100 pounds. Most dramatically, Mrs. Farris's energy level became the best it has been for many years. She again became a tireless worker at home and an exciting, invigorated health topic speaker, sharing her stories with large audiences. She has since discontinued the use of nystatin but continues with other alternative nondrug remedies.

Constipation persists some two and a half years later, but Mrs. Farris has no more vaginal discharge or any of her other listed difficulties. She states that employment of the wholistic approach to candidiasis has given her at least a 90 percent improvement.

PHILOSOPHY OF WHOLISTIC DOCTORS
TREATING CANDIDIASIS

When a potential Candida syndrome patient presents her or his litany of discomforts to the candidiasis-conscious doctor, such a physician takes the patient's series of complaints quite seriously. The doctor sees these same health difficulties in his medical practice every day. They are likely to affect the majority of patients. Special training and much experience has almost made candidiasis treatment into a new medical specialty. A yeast-treating doctor's reassuring response to the new patient's multiple complaints might go something like this:

You don't have anything seriously complicating about your presenting symptoms. These are disorders that I routinely handle. What you should understand is that I might not pay close attention today to each and every one of the many disorders causing you discomfort. Why not? Because treatment for the Candida syndrome isn't localized; instead, treatment is generalized, and the condition's variable manifestations will disappear over time. You and I mustn't focus on your separate discomforts; you need to concentrate on exactly what I tell you to do—nothing more, nothing less. Between office visits, you can write down what is of concern or what you think I am not concentrating on enough or what I might be missing and discuss these observations with me at your next consultation.

Take note, Ms. Patient, you've been going to different medical specialists over the past several months or years, reciting all of these newly appearing additional complaints and concerns. Each time the list rolled off your tongue, did it lead to successful diagnosis and treatment being offered by the doctor? No! Now you're presenting me with a new list of more troubles. I understand that these are bothering you. But your symptom list, after you tell it to me the first time, is not so relevant to your treatment. Don't focus on how sick you are but rather on how much better you're going to be—since these symptoms will be disappearing over your treatment period—as long as it takes to get you as completely well as possible.

The physician who treats the Candida syndrome wants to know details about the progress of the few major discomforts troubling his new patient, especially the speed with which they are getting better. Still, visit after visit, he does not need to hear a litany of disorders. Besides, the list starts getting shorter fairly quickly after the start of proper treatment. Knowledge of symptom improvements is essential for the wholistic doctor to be able to discern which chemical systems are being affected in the patient under treatment. The physician who knows about the Candida syndrome possesses a broad nutritional armamentarium to help bring about improvements in symptoms that persist.

In summary, physicians who regularly minister to candidiasis patients approach this health problem with a philosophy that is unique to wholism. Wholistic doctors are aware of how fragile and delicate is our human host balance with organisms in the outside world. All of us depend upon bacterial colonization that serves a protective purpose. Indeed, such colonization is part of our natural defensive mantle. Some bacterial organisms are intensely happy living where they are, on our surface and inside of us. They do a great deal to offset and prevent effects of some other invaders which might be unhappily destructive. Consequently, no one should attempt to become so "sterilized" with disinfectants that all organisms are eliminated. A situation of total disinfection would be downright dangerous.

In the case of *C. albicans* overgrowth, the balance of host–organism commensalism has been tipped too much in favor of the fungus. A treatment philosophy of wholistic doctors therefore involves, in part, restoring the good germs that live all over us. These good germs function for you or me in the same way that the wild water buffalo benefits from tick birds often seen nesting in the animal's fur, eating insect parasites. There is a fine symbiotic relationship between the bird and the buffalo. Similarly, a victim of the yeast syndrome must return to symbiotic balance with friendly bacteria, so that they discourage the invasion of excess *C. albicans* parasites. That's one of the reasons *Lactobacillus acidophilus* and *Lactobacillus bifidus* act as gut-restoring bulwarks in the antiyeast wholistic therapy program.

LACTOBACILLI AS ANTIYEAST THERAPY

The great Russian bacteriologist Elie Metchnikoff succeeded Louis Pasteur as the director of the Pasteur Institute in Paris. This 1908 Nobel Laureate believed that yogurt was the elixir of life. In his study of longevity, Metchnikoff concluded that people should commonly live to the age of 150 years. He found every indication that the basic human mechanism was capable of lasting far longer than it does. One way to last longer, he was convinced, is to eat yogurt containing lactobacilli. [2]

Writing in the December 1985 *Townsend Letter for Doctors*, Carl S. Hangee-Bauer, M.A., N.D., a naturopathic doctor and teacher at the John Bastyr College of Naturopathic Medicine in Seattle, Washington, explained that Professor Metchnikoff's trailblazing yogurt concept is now proving to be correct. Dr. Hangee-Bauer wrote:

> His theory was that putrefactive bacteria in the large intestine produce toxins which invite disease and shorten life. He believed that the eating of yogurt would cause the lactobacilli to become dominant in the colon and displace the putrefactive bacteria. For years these claims of healthful effects from fermented foods were considered unscientific folklore. However, a substantial and growing body of scientific evidence has demonstrated that lactobacilli and fermented foods play a significant role in human health. . . . Foods fermented with lactobacilli have been, and still are, of great importance to the diets of most of the world's people. Most cultures use some form of fermented food in their diet, ranging from cheese and yogurt to miso and other fermented products. The symbiotic relationship between human kind and this genus of bacteria has a long history of important nutritional benefits for humans.[3]

Lactobacillus bifidus is first introduced to the sterile intestines of the infant as a result of breastfeeding. Large numbers can soon be observed in the baby's feces.[4] *L. bulgaricus* is commonly used as a yogurt culture, but it is incapable of proliferating in the human gut. Other friendly bacteria can proliferate and thrive, unless they are attacked by broad spectrum antibiotic drugs (administered for the treatment of infection or already added in the food supply, as discussed in Chapter Four). Additional beneficial lactobacillus strains include *L. acidophilus*, *L. fermentum*, *L. casea*, *L. salivores*, *L. brevis*, and *L. plantarum*. Approximately 200 strains of lactobacilli exist.

Lactobacilli are known to produce natural antibiotics of their own. For instance, *L. acidophilus* manufactures the antibioticlike enzymate agents acidolin, acidophilin, and lactocidin; *L. brevis* makes lactobacillin and lactobrevin; *L.*

bulgaricus produces bulgarican.[5] Of these, the antimicrobial enzymes acidophilin and bulgarican are most effective against food-borne pathogens.[6]

Within a test tube culture (*in vitro*, meaning, literally, "in glass"), *L. acidophilus* has been shown to retard the growth of the yeast *C. albicans*. The fungus grows more slowly, and the maximal population is lessened when grown in broth filtered after this friendly bacterium has grown in it. Clinical studies indicate that the addition of lactobacilli milk products to the vagina assists in the treatment and prevention of recurrent vaginal candidiasis.[7] Yogurt, in fact, has long been a folk remedy for most forms of vaginitis (see Chapter Sixteen for preparing a yogurt douche and other vaginal remedies). *L. acidophilus* is a normal constituent of the vaginal flora, where it contributes to the maintenance of the normal acid reaction (pH) by fermenting glycogen to lactic acid.

Low-fat nonfermented milk products show effects close to those of yogurt; the probable explanation is the presence of lactose, which favors the growth of lactobacilli. Sugar-free (no glucose or lactose) yogurt should be used by people with candidiasis, since high dietary intake of any form of sugar appears to increase the incidence of vaginal yeast infections, and sugar is a known promoter of fungal growth in the genus *Candida*.[8]

Yogurt contains higher levels of free amino acids than milk, mainly due to the heating needed to grow the bacteria and then to the proteolytic (protein-splitting) action of lactobacilli. Lactic acid, produced by fermentation reactions in the friendly bacteria, improves digestibility of the proteins found in acidophilus milk, bifidus milk, yogurt, and buttermilk.[9] The gross protein value of yogurt is 94.5 percent; skim milk (from which yogurt is made) has only 85 percent. The gross measure of protein quality is therefore 9.5 percent greater in yogurt than in skim milk.

Using lactobacilli cultures, the wholistic method of treatment advised by Dr. Hangee-Bauer involves the following:

For infant thrush, treat the mother (especially if she is breastfeeding) with oral supplements of *L. bifidus*. "Paint" the nipples before each infant feeding with a concentrated culture of *L. bifidus*.

For vaginitis, use implants of fresh (sugar-free) yogurt in the vagina—or water plus yogurt douches.

For intestinal infections, eat one or more cups of yogurt three or four times daily or take *L. acidophilus* concentrates that are high in acidophilin, the naturally occurring antibiotic/anticarcinogenic (against cancer) substance produced when acidophilus organisms are cultured and living in a milk base.

For milk-intolerant patients or those with outright milk allergies, an acceptable way to avoid adverse reactions is to introduce potent amounts of the *L. acidophilus* organisms in small increments, beginning with one-quarter teaspoonful of powder or liquid—or one acidophilus capsule—two or three times daily into the gastrointestinal system. This technique will help to establish the production of necessary enzymes that aid in the digestion of milk or milk products, among other foodstuffs. People with lactose intolerance (due to a lack of the digestive enzymes lactase and beta-galactosidase on cells of the small intestine) appear to tolerate cultured dairy products better than milk itself. In one study of lactose-intolerant subjects who reported abdominal symptoms after ingestion of dairy products, no similar symptoms were found when they ate yogurt. Low hydrogen levels in expired breath confirmed their subjective reports.[10]

In addition to their usefulness in antiyeast therapy, lactobacilli strains have advantageous nutritional effects on vitamin and nutrient synthesis, anticholesteremic (lowering blood cholesterol) and antilipidemic (lowering blood fats) benefits, antiviral activity, destructive effects on antinutritional compounds, effects apparently inhibiting to carcinogenesis (the startup of cancer), possible advantages against liver disease, and anti-anxiety and other psychological benefits. Lactobacillus supplementation or yogurt intake should always follow the use of broad spectrum antibiotics to replace the friendly bacteria killed by the nonspecific action of the drug. Attacks of gastroenteritis or diarrhea from any cause also are best treated by including lactobacilli in the medical approach to management.

INGESTING GARLIC TO REDUCE YEAST OVERGROWTH

The School of Health Sciences at the University of Massachusetts at Worcester, Massachusetts, reports that garlic is highly successful in killing *C. albicans*—or at least in reducing Candida overgrowth. Garlic can be taken as fresh whole cloves or in an odorless aged extract form. Both show broad spectrum antifungal and antibacterial activity at concentrations nontoxic to human cells and tissues, but the aged garlic extract appears to be better tolerated in terms of digestive comfort—and sociability. Onion, clove, and horseradish also seem to have similar antifungal properties.

Much of the scientific research on garlic concerns its antimicrobial activity against many genera of bacteria and against opportunistic and infectious fungi, including *C. albicans*. Further, concentrated extract of garlic was more effective than nystatin in several studies of pathogenic yeasts, particularly in complications from candidiasis.[11] Oral administration of garlic extract cured yeast infections after ten days in chicks inoculated with *C. albicans*.[12] Dermatophytic (skin fungus) lesions in rabbits and guinea pigs were treated with topical application of garlic extract. They showed disappearance of skin scales after seven days and complete healing and regrowth of skin after seventeen days.[13]

A major chemical constituent of whole garlic is alliin (allylsulfinyl alanine), which is rapidly converted to allicin (allyl allylthiosulfinate) by the enzymatic action of alliinase when garlic is crushed or eaten. Allicin and resultant sulfide-containing by-products are responsible for the characteristic garlic odor. When garlic is allowed to age for an extended period, the odor disappears and a more socially acceptable, deodorized garlic results with the same properties claimed as for the fresh garlic clove.

The modified, deodorized garlic in extract form—a special garlic preparation, called SGP™—produced as liquid, capsules, and tablets for dispensing by wholistic physicians—is manufactured in Japan by Wakunaga Pharmaceutical Company, Ltd., and is imported into the United States and other Western nations by Wakunaga of America Company, Ltd., of Torrance, California. The product is sold in health food stores as liquid, capsules, and tablets under the brand name, Kyolic™.

The natural oxidizing compound, allicin, exerts suppressive effects on pathogenic fungi.[14] Allicin is primarily fungistatic (slowing or stopping growth of fungi). At concentrations four times higher than that required to inhibit growth, it is fungicidal against *C. albicans*.[15] The substance inhibits fungal growth by inactivating thiol-containing (sulfur-containing) proteins and enzymes. It also decreases the virulence of *C. albicans* by decreasing the yeast-to-mycelial conversion.[16] No clinical strains of *C. albicans* have been shown to develop significant resistance to garlic. Data from published scientific research prove that garlic may play a role in the nutritional enhancement of the body's natural defenses and in the prevention of illness from a variety of causes.

Wakunaga Central Research Laboratory lists more than thirty compounds isolated from garlic. The main medicinally active constituents include, as mentioned, the amino acid alliin, the antifungal active ingredient allicin, and a natural enzyme alliinase.[17] Studies show that effectiveness requires that human dose levels be adequate and that garlic be taken daily. A usual daily dosage for antiyeast therapy is three capsules filled with Kyolic™ or SGP™ liquid at each meal. The liquid comes with a bottle of sixty-two gelatin capsules. Directions are provided to fill each capsule with 1 ml of aged garlic extract. Capsules should not be prefilled, but rather filled and swallowed as needed. Filled capsules (one or two) may also be applied within the vagina (see Chapter Sixteen). The liquid is also appropriate topical medication for treating thrush and acne. Encapsulated powder and tablet preparations of Kyolic™ and SGP™ appear useful but with slightly decreased potency compared to the liquid forms. Some people use the aged garlic liquid as the "oil" in an oil and lemon juice salad dressing each day.

CANDIDIASIS TREATMENT WITH CAPRYLIC ACID

Nutritional supplementation with naturally occurring short-chain fatty acids, such as caprylic acid, has been found to help restore and maintain a normal balance of yeast, bacteria, and other microorganisms in the colon. Such a candidiasis treatment approach fits well with the philosophy of the wholistic physician. When combined with other natural antifungal substances, such as garlic and yogurt, caprylic acid may achieve a broader spectrum of antiyeast activity than can many prescription drugs now used against established yeast infections.

Caprylic acid has been found to exert strong antimycotic effects. *In vitro* tests with this fatty acid demonstrate an almost complete inhibition of *C. albicans* cultures. Successful relief of severe intestinal candidiasis using caprylic acid has been reported for years in the medical literature. Disappearance of Candida from stool specimens of all patients studied occurred within several days. No adverse side effects have been observed from a fatty acid ion-exchange complex (the form used as a nutritional antiyeast supplement) either in patients with known Candida infections or in individuals with a normal gastrointestinal condition.[18]

Ingestion of complexed caprylic acid seems to have a time-release action, allowing the fatty acid to undergo slow hydrolysis (release) throughout the intestinal tract. The finely powdered resin complex tends to coat the walls of the stomach and intestines without upsetting the normal balance of gastrointestinal flora.[19]

Buffered caprylic acid treatment of slowly progressing oral and vaginal thrush that had been resistant to standard therapy produced a prompt and dramatic response in both children and adults.[20]

Vaginal itching and burning were relieved with caprylic acid treatment in a study of 104 patients. Later examination with laboratory methods showed that 92 women (88 percent) were considered clinically cured and free of the organism. Of these, 53 were reexamined four months following completion of therapy and were found to have no recurrence of the infection.[21]

Rapid relief of yeast vaginitis has also been observed with the use of a buffered sorbic acid solution. Commercial products containing sorbic acid as a douche and mouthwash will be described in Chapter Sixteen. Patients with longstanding yeast infections in which standard medications such as nystatin and caprylic acid had been ineffective were treated with sorbic acid. Prompt relief from discomfort occurred with marked soothing effect. Healing was rapid with repeated applications.[22]

Caprylic acid is an antifungal, eight-carbon, short-chain

fatty acid with a white color and a slight soapy odor. The exact mechanism of its fungicidal action is not understood. Scientists speculate that caprylic acid partially dissolves the cell membrane of yeast, causing changes in fluidity and permeability that lead to membrane disaggregation (falling apart). Candida organisms tend to migrate to the mucosal wall of the gut tube. A uniform dispersion of caprylic acid on the gut wall along the length of the intestine probably ensures contact with the organism. Caprylic acid appears to be effective against all Candida species and strains and is recommended in the prophylactic treatment of candidiasis during any long-term bacterial antibiotic drug therapy.

At recommended dosages, caprylic acid is nontoxic and nonsensitizing. Very large doses can cause mucosal irritation and produce diarrhea and nausea. Some patients may suffer with fatigue and flu-like symptoms during the first two to five days of use. This reaction is thought to be a yeast "die-off" and reabsorption phenomenon that we have described as the Herxheimer reaction (see Chapter Ten).

Several manufacturers provide candidiasis-treating physicians with caprylic acid. Brand-name products and their suppliers are the following:

Caprystatin™ consists of enterically coated caprylic acid adsorbed to a nonresinous ion-exchange moiety, designed for slow release of caprylic acid throughout the intestines. The finely powdered complex coats the walls of the stomach and intestinal tract without upsetting the delicate balance of the gut flora. Clinical studies with this complex were performed at the University of Illinois College of Medicine in Chicago, and all patients showed complete disappearance of Candida from stool specimens in several days. Moreover, these patients experienced a remission of symptoms associated with the Candida syndrome. Caprystatin™ exhibits fungistatic and fungicidal properties and is manufactured and distributed by Ecological Formulas, a division of Cardiovascular Research, Ltd., of Concord, California.

Caprystatin™ tablets must be swallowed intact to protect their enteric coating. The product is best taken at least one hour before or two hours after meals. If gastrointestinal discomfort is noted, Caprystatin™ may be taken with meals. A usual dosage regimen is: first week, one tablet two times daily; second week, two tablets two times daily; third week, three tablets two times daily.

For a maintenance regimen, the minimal effective dosage is determined by a titration schedule under the direction of your physician. Caprystatin™ is sold only to health professionals. Jonathan Rothchild, President of Cardiovascular Research, Ltd., advises that the product has a high fiber content, and usage should be monitored in patients who have a history of fiber intolerance. An average duration of treatment with Caprystatin™ is two or three months at a therapeutic dose, followed by four to six or more months at a maintenance dose. Therapeutic response is highly individualized and may be checked by a physician at monthly intervals. Clinical progress may be measured by subjective changes reported by patients, by elimination of symptoms, by reduced fecal yeast count, and by laboratory findings such as reduced antibody titers.

Also available from Cardiovascular Research, Ltd., is *Orithrush™* douche concentrate, containing sorbic acid for the treatment of vaginitis, fungus infection of the toenails, and athlete's foot. Orithrush™ gargle and mouthwash are provided for nasopharyngeal and esophageal candidiasis.

Caprylate Plus™ is a 100 mg caprylic acid compound also containing the minerals selenium (10 mcg), iodine (30 mcg), and magnesium (200 mg); the amino acid L-taurine (125 mg); the vitamins pyridoxine (50 mg) as prydioxine-5'-phosphate, riboflavin (5 mg) as riboflavin-5'-phosphate, and biotin (200 mcg). These additional components were selected, in their specific chemical forms and dosages, because of published reports demonstrating their effects in aiding the body to defend against candidiasis. Nutritional deficiencies are known to contribute to decreased immune system function, the underlying problem that allows for the persistence of candidiasis and the major explanation for the prolonged treatment required to rid your body of the condition. Combination products such as Caprylate Plus™ include several of the nutritional supplements often prescribed individually by wholistic physicians. This therapeutic approach predictably represents the future direction to be taken in product development for treating the Candida syndrome. Caprylate Plus™ is manufactured and distributed by Allergy Research Group of San Leandro, California.

Candistat™ provides a specially complexed form of caprylic acid (70 mg) for slow release throughout the small and large intestine. Also supplied are buffered sorbic acid (50 mg) and *pau d'arco* herb (50 mg), discussed in the section to follow. These items are incorporated into an herbal base containing horseradish and clove extract. The combination of ingredients used in Candistat™ are intended to deter the development of resistant yeast organisms and to increase product effectiveness. Advanced Medical Nutrition, Inc., of Hayward, California, manufactures and distributes the product exclusively to health professionals.

Capricin™ nutritional supplement, broad spectrum fungicide for Candida, is produced by pharmaceutical biochemist Torbin E. Neesby, Ph.D., of Fresno, California. It is distributed nationally by Professional Specialties, Inc., of Bellevue, Washington. The therapeutic dosage of Capricin™ is advised by Dr. Neesby to be 12 capsules per day—4 capsules three times a day, or 6 capsules two times a day—with meals to maximize fungicidal effect and minimize belching. High dosage is continued for sixteen days—two bottles of 100 capsules—then a maintenance dosage of 2 capsules twice daily with meals is begun for the next several weeks. If symptoms of the Herxheimer reaction become intolerable, the therapeutic dose is reduced to 6 capsules per day until the die-off symptoms subside, then gradually increased to 12 capsules daily for a full sixteen-day period.

Professional Specialties, Inc., suggests that Capricin™ should be used in conjunction with a high-yield *L. acidophilus* (some physicians advise *L. bifidus* for children under the age of seven) to aid in the treatment of postantibiotic Candida superinfection by repopulating the normal intestinal flora. The company suggests that any kind of dietary fat such as milk, butter, or salad oil should be included at meals when the product is taken. People who have difficulty in swallowing capsules can simply open the Capricin™ capsules and pour their contents into apple sauce or other palatable foods for eating.

Note: With all of this book's information on therapeutic

programs, food, nutrition, diet, detoxification, and other items of interest, we recommend that you check with your doctor regarding his or her specific guidelines. They may differ from ours and take precedence over what is published here.

TABEBUIA/LA PACHO/TAHEEBO/PAU D'ARCO TEA

Although not touted as a cure for Candida overgrowth, the bark of the tabebuia/la pacho/taheebo tree appears to be helping people whose health is affected by the yeast. Taheebo tea is being used by thousands of Candida syndrome patients across the United States and in other industrialized Western countries. The la pacho trees grow in South American rain forests, especially in Brazil and Argentina. Legends about the curative powers of *pau d'arco* reach back to the time of the ancient Incas. The South American medical press has carried reports for about two decades and North American publications have mentioned it for the past six years. This tea drink is claimed to aid the body's defensive posture to resist candidiasis.

When first drinking *pau d'arco* (the herbal name for the remedy; also designated by Brazilian Indians as "taheebo") tea, many people report experiencing a Herxheimer effect. They have a mild to moderate worsening of symptoms before their discomforts lessen in a few days.

Pau d'arco herbal tea is probably best used as a synergistic remedy combined with other therapeutic agents. When used alone, the effects may be too subtle to be appreciated, although some patients do report that they are less sensitive to molds, chemicals, and foods. Many state that local symptoms persist but their general feeling of physical and mental well-being is enhanced.

When utilized as a douche, *pau d'arco* is sometimes effective for relieving vaginitis. Applied topically, the herbal tea has relieved stubborn cases of athlete's foot, aided skin rashes on the head, face, and hands, and reduced detritus for fungus-ridden toenails and fingernails.

The variety of *pau d'arco* known as *Tecoma curialis* is said to be better tolerated by the chemically sensitive individual than is *Tecoma conspicua*, which can be poorly tolerated in the first months of drinking the tea. The diuretic effect of taheebo tea makes consultation with your wholistic physician advisable, to minimize any possible imbalance in major minerals such as sodium, potassium, calcium, or magnesium, as well as trace minerals.[23]

Taheebo tea is brewed by adding one tablespoonful to eight cups of boiling water for about five minutes. It must then sit for twenty minutes before drinking. It is distributed in tea bags by Alta Health Products of Pasadena, California, and by Nutri-Cology, Inc. of San Leandro, California. It is also available in capsules or as an herbal extract.

A COORDINATED CANDIDA DIAGNOSIS AND TREATMENT SYSTEM

A definite advance in the fight against the yeast syndrome was introduced at the May 1985 semi-annual meeting of the American Academy of Medical Preventics, held in Washington, D.C. During that meeting, Seroyal Brands, Inc., of Concord, California, revealed a coordinated series of techniques for diagnosing and treating candidiasis.

The Candida System™ from Seroyal starts with an initial diagnosis established by the use of a questionnaire and the support of the Candi-sphere serodiagnostic analysis, using the Candida enzyme immuno assay (CEIA test) developed by Drs. Hagglund and Bauman. Seroyal's integrated kit offers information for the physician's initial review, assisting him to determine the likely seriousness of the patient's affliction. If an intensive treatment program seems to be warranted, the physician can consider a full anti-Candida therapy from Seroyal. The coordinated program can be monitored even by the physician who might understand very little about the essential role that nutrition plays in human illness and health.

The Seroyal Candida System™ kit contains the main approaches to candidiasis diagnosis and treatment, with the exception of the prescription medications, which may be prescribed by any licensed physician and obtained from pharmacies. The kit also furnishes patient education materials to aid in understanding the total program. This system and others to follow probably will force establishment-type allopaths and osteopaths to acknowledge that the practice of wholistic medicine has increasingly sound scientific basis.

The Seroyal kit contains:

A. CandiTrak™ diagnostics, based on two researched items: (1) the CandiTrak™ history/symptom worksheet; and (2) the CandiTrak™ serodiagnostic analysis. The Seroyal national polysystemic chronic candidiasis (PSCC) data base, a third element, is in development.

The CandiTrak™ history/symptom worksheet is an inventory of patient symptoms and exposure to the yeast syndrome's causative factors. Patients with symptoms suggesting candidiasis can be screened with this worksheet to determine the advisability of a blood test.

The CandiTrak™ serodiagnostic analysis detects the changes found in the blood with the yeast syndrome. The service includes a computerized analysis of the history/symptom worksheet and performance of the CEIA blood test.

The company is accumulating test results and developing a national PSCC data base to which all physicians are invited to contribute statistics.

B. CandiTrol™ therapy which integrates a broad complement of nutritional products for the abatement of Candida, for the restoration of beneficial bacteria, for intestinal cleansing and detoxification, for oral and vaginal hygiene, and a yeast-free hypoallergenic multiple vitamin and mineral supplement. CandiTrol™ nutritionals include the following products:

- Serodex™ Scan, allergenic extracts of infectious yeast, supplied as homeopathic dilutions
- Serostatin™ SST, a broad spectrum, orally administered, fatty-acid mycostat (antifungal) containing a variety of nutrients effective in the control of *Candida albicans*
- Serodophilus™, a stable, high-potency lyophilized concentrate of symbiotic *Lactobacillus acidophilus/bifidus* culture
- Sero-Immuno Forte™, a multiple LyphoGland™ concentrate of proteins, hormones, and nucleic acids
- Mucovata™ EB-O, an all-natural bulking agent and hydrophilic mucilloid intestinal cleanser—herbs, fruit, and vegetable extracts, and digestive aids that tend to remove heavy metals, accumulated proteins, organic toxins, nonabsorbed food particles, and other waste products

- Hypo-Allervites™, nutritional supplements allergen- and excipient-free
- Sero-Garlic™ LG, odorless extract of garlic suspended in a base of soybean and dill oil
- Sero-Detox™ AMD, nutritional agents intended to aid "oral chelation" of heavy metals
- Sero-Aseptic™ SMW, an antiseptic/anesthetic blend of natural herbs and organic ingredients for oral or topical applications where antimicrobial action is desired.

NOTES

1. William G. Crook, "The Coming Revolution in Medicine," *Journal of the Tennessee Medical Association*, March 1983, 76:145–149.

2. E. Metchnikoff, *The Prolongation of Life*, New York: Arna Press, 1977.

3. Carl S. Hangee-Bauer, "Lactobacilli and Human Health," *Townsend Letter for Doctors*, December 1985, 33:335–340.

4. K. M. Shahani and A. D. Ayebo, "Role of Dietary Lactobacilli in Gastrointestinal Microecology," *American Journal of Clinical Nutrition*, 1980, 33:2448–57.

5. K. M. Shahani and B. A. Friend, "Nutritional and Therapeutic Aspects of Lactobacilli," *Journal of Applied Nutrition*, 1984, 36:125–152.

6. K. M. Shahani, J. R. Vakill, and A. Kilara, "Natural Antibiotic Activity of *Lactobacillus acidophilus* and *bulgaricus*," *Cultured Dairy Products Journal*, 1977, 12:8–11.

7. E. B. Collins and P. Hardt, "Inhibition of *Candida albicans* by *Lactobacillus acidophilus*," *Journal of Dairy Science*, 1980, 63:830–832.

8. B. J. Horowitz, S. W. Edelstein, and L. Lippman, "Sugar Chromatography Studies in Recurrent Candida Vulvovaginitis," *Journal of Reproductive Medicine*, 1984, 7:441–443.

9. R. E. Hargrove and J. A. Alford, "Growth Rate and Feed Efficiency of Rats Fed Yogurt and Other Fermented Milks," *Journal of Dairy Science*, 1978, 61:11–19.

10. Ibid.

11. V. D. Sharma et al., *Journal of Experimental Biology*, 1977, 15:466–468; M. G. M. Johnson and R. H. Vayaghna, *Applied Microbiology*, 1969, 17:903–905; M. Amer et al., *International Journal of Dermatology*, 1980, 19:285–287; R. A.

Fromtling and G. S. Bulmer, *Mycologia*, 1978, 70:397–405; Z. Tynecka and Z. Gos, *Annals of the University of Mariae Curie Sklodowska*, 1975, 30:5.

12. G. Prasad and V. D. Sharma, *British Veterinary Journal*, 1980, 136:448.

13. Amer et al., *op. cit.*

14. Y. Yamada and K. Azuma, *Antimicrobial Agents and Chemotherapy*, 1977, 11:743–749; F. E. Barone and M. R. Tansey, *Mycology*, 1977, 69:793–825.

15. Yamada and Azuma, *op. cit.*

16. Barone and Tansey, *op. cit.*

17. Eric Block, "The Chemistry of Garlic and Onions," *Scientific American*, March 1985, 252:114–119.

18. M. A. Adetumbi and B.H.S. Lau, *Medical Hypothesis*, 1983, 12:227–237; E. D. Wills, *Biochemical Journal*, 1956, 63:514–520; Fromtling and Bulmer, *op. cit.*

19. Adetumbi and Lau, *op. cit.*

20. Johnson and Vayaghna, *op. cit.*

21. Fromtling and Bulmer, *op. cit.*

22. I. F. Huddleston et al., *Journal of the American Medical Association*, 1944, 105:394.

23. P. C. Royal, "Herbally Yours," *Sound Nutrition*, 1982, p. 43; L. Tenney, *Today's Herbal Health*, Provo, Ut.: Hawthorne Books, 1982, p. 123.

12

The Antiyeast Wholistic Therapy Program—Part Two

Lucinda Damon is a thirty-eight-year-old waitress living in a tiny rural town in Washington State. Like most patients finally diagnosed with the Candida syndrome, Mrs. Damon was troubled with many health complaints that previous doctors could not help. She had recurrent pelvic infections punctuated by a dull aching in her lower abdomen. Soreness in the vagina gave her great discomfort; unusual dryness created difficulties with sexual intercourse.

Each morning the woman noticed a sticky secretion holding together her eyelids. Her calves felt tight and stiff just after arising, relaxing only after she had stood for several minutes. Mrs. Damon's bowel movements were a distressing combination of constipation followed by "the runs," followed again by another solid movement, all in one day. When her stomach began to grip, she frequently would have diarrhea so urgently that she was forced to find a toilet immediately. Her bladder was easily aggravated by tea and coffee, further necessitating frequent trips to the bathroom.

Her sinuses were always congested: a steady postnasal drip appeared whenever she encountered cedar dust, aerosols, or common household solvents. Strong cleaning agents caused an instant headache. At one time Mrs. Damon had been diagnosed as having hypoglycemia, yet a strict antihypoglycemic diet offered no control of the symptoms.

In September 1982, the patient took her complaints to wholistic physician Jonathan Collin, M.D. Dr. Collin practices preventive medicine, using nutritional approaches and chelation therapy, in Washington State, in both the city of Kirkland and the suburban area of Port Townsend. At the time Dr. Collin performed her physical examination, Mrs. Damon was taking on her own many food supplements in a desperate attempt to relieve her troubles—but not getting the results she was seeking. Her physical findings were essentially normal, with no notable signs of disease. Blood tests revealed normal white and red blood cell counts, normal liver and kidney function, and normal calcium, potassium, and other electrolyte levels. Blood sugar and cholesterol readings were also within acceptable values. Remember that it is common for a person suffering from the Candida syndrome to display "normal" findings on clinical and laboratory examination.

Based on yeast scoring (Y-score) of questionnaires, the diversity of her disorders, antibody-titer laboratory testing, and an educated clinical hunch, Dr. Collin offered a tentative diagnosis of yeast-related illness. He prescribed the antiyeast drug nystatin both as an oral tablet and as a vaginal suppository. Mrs. Damon found that her sinuses cleared after only two days. When she stopped using the vaginal suppositories, sinus symptoms and headache returned within twelve hours. Nystatin effects on the infection in her vagina were being reflected in other body areas, and nystatin tablets by mouth were insufficient by themselves.

Dr. Collin also recommended that she follow a yeast-controlling diet. Two such diets, one developed by Dr. William G. Crook and another, more stringent, perfected by Dr. John Parks Trowbridge, omit sugar and higher-content starches, caffeine, alcohol, yeasty foods, fruits, nuts, and pickled foods. Mrs. Damon conceded that the diet was "hell" to stay on. She maintained her adherence by dreaming of eating a sandwich with yeast-risen bread . . . instead of the rice cakes required.

Now, two and one-half years later, the woman reports continued success in treatment of her candidiasis. She still requires a stringent yeast-control diet including avoidance of yeast, sugar, and wheat. She no longer requires the nystatin prescription. Instead, she uses food supplements—including capsules of liquid aged garlic extract, *L. acidophilus* capsules, and herbs—to support her system. And she uses no other prescription medications.

The sinusitis and heavy-nose feeling that Lucinda Damon once experienced have disappeared. An early morning cough that she neglected to mention when first starting treatment—a symptom that had become a "normal condition" for her after twenty years—is now nonexistent. Itching is completely alleviated. Chronic indigestion, formerly soothed by daily doses of Rolaids®, is only a memory. She no longer has feelings of unreality and now shows confidence in coping with stress. Previously she was excessively prone to colds and the flu; today she can nursemaid friends and family who are ill with colds without herself succumbing to respiratory infection. She doesn't retain extra water now. But if she forsakes the Candida-control diet for any period of time, Mrs. Damon finds herself urinating incessantly when she resumes it. Her weight has decreased thirty pounds in one year—and the pounds have stayed off! She affirms that a change of diet is basic to the antiyeast wholistic therapy program. She insists that this habit change is absolutely necessary and must last until all signs and symptoms of the Candida syndrome have permanently disappeared.

THE ANTIYEAST NUTRITIONAL APPROACH OF JONATHAN COLLIN, M.D.

Representing the approach of the typical candidiasis-treating physician, Jonathan Collin, M.D., emphasizes the value of employing low doses of nystatin both as therapy and as a diagnostic marker. Dr. Collin told us:

> A patient's response to nystatin does provide a confirmation to the diagnosis of polysystemic chronic candidiasis. If I did not have that nystatin verification, I might be wary of labeling the patient's health problem a yeast-type of disturbance. So I usually prescribe 1,000,000–2,000,000 units of nystatin a day [four to eight oral

tablets], unless the patient turns out to be among those 7 percent of people who show a nystatin intolerance. [Such an intolerance is the patient's personal hypersensitivity and not a drug side effect.] Immediately with the nystatin therapy I initiate dietary improvements.

Assuming that I'm not dealing with an alcoholic who would be creating an entirely different set of circumstances, the first thing is my removal of white sugar and the reduction of dairy products and yeasted food products from the candidiasis patient's eating patterns. I want the person off caffeinated and decaffeinated coffee, but contrary to the standard anti-Candida diet I don't limit the ingestion of fruit. Each candidiasis-conscious physican varies antiyeast treatment in accordance with his or her personal belief system, and allowing fruit to remain on the menu is mine. Of course, I do encourage the eating of vegetables, fish, fowl, seeds and the drinking of pure spring water.

I find that prescribing *L. acidophilus* is the best and most efficient way of reestablishing the normal flora in a patient's gut. Based on stool analysis showing decreased pancreatic enzymes and undigested protein and fat plus an elevated indican score [a urine test confirming poor protein digestion in the upper gut], a dose of acidophilus is required at least twice a day. If there is increased indication of putrefaction in the bowel, I will have the patient use digestive enzymes and aged garlic extract. These detoxify the intestines. Variations on this treatment involve the addition of betaine hydrochloride, bromelain, aloe vera, and a combination of other nutrient items. Someone not adequately absorbing B vitamins from his diet must receive nonyeast-based multiple vitamins with special emphasis on vitamin B_6 (pyridoxine). I have been doing enzyme research which assesses the red blood cell pyridoxine level on these yeast syndrome patients, and frequently I find that their vitamin B_6 level is diminished. But I consider supplementation with most of the vitamins quite useful to the patient.

Trace minerals are recommended by me, particularly calcium, magnesium, potassium, and zinc. That way the patient will be covered for any potential deficiency without having to deal with a lot of sophisticated mineral manipulations and intense investigations. But I do screen my candidiasis patient with a hair mineral analysis. Looking for toxic metals is a must, since so many patients with yeast-related illness have heavy metal toxicity as well. It's a health problem that must be addressed by the prescribing doctor. It might involve chelation therapy or simply a nutrient program to dilute the individual metallic poisonings.

Caprylic acid is useful for yeast control. Taheebo tea is a secondary line of treatment that I do suggest patients should add to their anti-Candida armamentarium. But besides altering the diet to one which is nonadvantageous to yeast growth, nutrient support for the patient's immune system is absolutely vital. Certain supplemental nutrients plus extra protein are needed in the ongoing battle to human host balance with the ever present *Candida albicans*.

NUTRIENT ADJUNCTS TO ANTIYEAST THERAPY

The Candida syndrome causes an increased need for protein, but often the protein is poorly absorbed in the body. Jeffrey Bland, Ph.D., Professor of Nutritional Biochemistry at the University of Puget Sound, now on leave to be a Senior Research Fellow at the Linus Pauling Institute of Menlo Park, California, says,

Incompletely digested dietary proteins may be delivered to the blood through the portals of entry of the intestinal tract produced by the invasive mycelia of the fungal form of *C. albicans*. This may explain why many individuals who have chronic Candida overgrowth and a high percentage of the mycelial form of the organism commonly show a wide variety of food and environmental allergies. These incompletely digested dietary proteins can then travel into the bloodstream and exert a powerful antigenic assault on the immune system, which is seen as allergy, even producing a wide variety of effects such as cerebral allergy, with depression, mood swings, and irritability being a result.

Recent work from the National Institutes of Health in the United States and other work from W. A. Hemmings, M.D., in England, indicate that some of the incomplete protein-breakdown products, if absorbed, may have endorphinlike activity. Endorphins are a group of chemical compounds that occur naturally in the brain and have pain-relieving properties similar to those of the opiates (e.g. codeine and morphine). They change mood, mind, memory, and behavior. These incomplete protein-breakdown products have been given the name of exorphins, meaning that they are produced outside systemic circulation and become introduced into the blood by way of absorption across the gastrointestinal (GI) mucosa.

"The proliferation of the fungal form of *C. albicans* would provide the route of absorption of these exorphin materials. The breakdown of the GI mucosa can also lead to the introduction of the Candida organism into the bloodstream so that it then finds its way into other tissues, resulting in far-ranging systemic effects, including soreness of joints, chest pain, and skin problems," Dr. Bland added.

As a remedy for incomplete protein breakdown, the wholistic physician may suggest supplementing the patient's diet with particular free-form amino acids. Among them may be included L-taurine, L-ornithine, lysine, arginine, phospho-ethanolamine, aspartic, threonine, serine, asparagine, glutamic, D-amino adipic, glycine, glutamine, alanine, a-amino-n-butyric, valine, cystine, methionine, cystathionine, isoleucine, tyrosine, phenylalanine, ethanolamine, L-methylhistidine, histidine, 3-methylhistidine, leucine, tryptophane, and the remaining essential amino acids.

Efforts to correct a protein-calorie malnutrition (PCM) in the Candida syndrome are mandatory. Uncorrected PCM may cause atrophy of the thymus gland with associated decrease of T- and B-cell immunity. Lower levels of immunoglobulins and complement in blood can also occur.[1]

Modified immunity and lowered blood components allow for increased unpleasant symptoms of the Candida syndrome to occur. Nutritional intervention with micronutrients can improve the situation. In a 1981 nutritional workshop conducted by the American Medical Association, dysfunction of immunocompetence was shown to result from inadequacy of just a single nutrient, whether or not the condition is combined with PCM.[2]

Biotin, one of the B vitamins, can help to prevent the conversion of the yeast form of Candida to its fungal form. Under the proper conditions, biotin is manufactured by the friendly bacteria in the intestine. But over time, a deficiency may arise from the average person's exposure to antibiotics, particularly sulfa drugs.

It's generally known among orthomolecular psychiatrists, chelating physicians, naturopaths, and others who use nutritional approaches in the reversal of degenerative diseases that biological deficiencies of biotin reduce human production of antibodies, resulting in reduced resistance to disease. Biotin deficiency also lowers your resistance to stress, diminishes your reproductive ability, and increases your cholesterol synthesis. Therapeutic doses of biotin, which wholistic physicians treating candidiasis often prescribe, are advantageous in reversing all of these conditions. A usual dosage is 300 micrograms (mcg) of biotin taken orally, three times a day. Swallowing the biotin with two teaspoonsful of olive oil, a source of oleic acid, also seems to help prevent the conversion of proliferating yeast to the mycelial form of spreading and penetrating fungus.

Other supplements which are sometimes used to treat candidiasis include tea tree (te-tre) oil, linseed oil, vitamin E, beta-carotene, and catalyst-activated water. Chiropractic adjustments greatly assist some patients to restore a natural ability to fight off the results of a suppressed immune system.

Most people in the industrialized West, according to U.S. government studies, could use basic daily food supplements taken to boost the nutrition supplied by usual foods. Supplements are advisable in order to adequately meet the needs of coping with the everyday stresses of living in modern society. These vary somewhat from one person to another, depending on factors such as age, sex, medical condition, occupation, food selection, and so on. As a person becomes healthier, basic nutrients may decrease in dosage but probably should never be discontinued altogether. Usually prescribed at a much higher dosage than the inadequately low U.S. recommended daily allowances, such basic nutrients might consist of beta-carotene or vitamin A (25,000–30,000 IU per day), vitamin E (400–800 IU per day), calcium pantothenate (pantotheic acid; 200–1,000 mg per day), selenium (about 200 mcg per day), vitamin C (1,000–4,000 mg per day), and possibly a digestant with added hydrochloric acid. If you elect to supplement your nutrition without supervision of a wholistic physician, be sure to acquire "hypoallergenic" food supplements prepared from sources other than yeast.

Furthermore, if you are suffering with the Candida syndrome, certain nutrients will be part of your total program aimed specifically at solving your Candida-connected health problems. These particular nutrients, prescribed by your wholistic physician, will likely include those working more directly on the immune system, since that is always the basic underlying difficulty with regard to the Candida overpopulation. Prescribed nutritional supplements consist of adjunctive support for various systems, organs, tissues, cells, or body parts.

Glandular function, especially thymus, appears important to immune integrity. Thymus gland supplements, along with the amino acids L-ornithine and L-taurine, might be advised to enhance thymus function directly and indirectly through stimulating the production of growth hormone. A combination of thymus, adrenal, pancreas, and spleen extracts (raw glandulars) is a basic endocrine support. Thyroid glandular, iodine, or seaweed extract may be needed as well. Other glandular products such as pituitary or ovary or testis might also be recommended by your wholistic physician.

Many people victimized by candidiasis cannot process essential fatty acids efficiently. Candida toxin (canditoxin), the poison produced by *C. albicans*, gets absorbed into the bloodstream and carried throughout the body. It interferes with an enzymatic protein that is a vital processor of long-chain fatty acids, important in maintaining membranes, in conducting metabolism, and in producing local hormones called prostaglandins (PGs). Since interference with such a critical pathway can be associated with vague symptoms throughout the body, Candida-conscious physicians often advise supplementation with long-chain fatty acids of the omega-3 and omega-6 series. MaxEPA™ is the brand name of a widely accepted purified form of the omega-3 fatty acids, eicosapentanoic acid (EPA) and docosahexaenoic acid (DHA). MaxEPA™ capsules are available from R.P. Scherer, N.A., of St. Petersburg,

Florida. Each capsule contains 18 percent EPA, 12 percent DHA, 100 IU per gram of vitamin A, 1 IU per gram of vitamin E, and 0.1 percent free fatty acids. A usual dosage is one capsule daily, although several per day might be needed. The product may be purchased from health and nutrition outlets selling food supplements.

Evening primrose oil is known as the only source—other than mother's milk—of both linoleic acid and gamma-linolenic acid. These two acids help your body to manufacture the beneficial PGs. David Horrobin, Ph.D., of the Institute for Innovative Medicine in Montreal, Canada, an acknowledged expert on evening primrose oil, says that a fall in the level of prostaglandins will lead to increased blood clotting, elevated cholesterol level in the blood, diabeticlike changes in insulin release, weakening of the immune system, susceptibility to depression, greater risk of inflammation, disruption in the transmittal of nerve impulses, deregulation of calcium ions in the blood, and disruption of all types of cellular responses to stimuli. As a food supplement, evening primrose oil appears to stimulate the production of T-cells from the thymus as well as balance out prostaglandin production. A daily dose of 200 mg or more of evening primrose oil is recommended by Candida syndrome–treating doctors.

Vitamin A has been referred to as the anti-infective vitamin because of its prime function of maintaining the structural integrity of the skin and the functionality of the mucous membranes.[3] So-called pro-vitamin A, or beta-carotene, serves the same purpose when it is converted to vitamin A in response to body needs. In addition, beta-carotene seems to be virtually nontoxic and furnishes protection against certain damaging free radicals, the chemicals that are responsible for injury and illness at the molecular level. The wholistic physician is constantly seeking ways to direct his treatments at the most basic health problem—using the correct molecules for the right job at the best time. The practice of orthomolecular medicine ("orthomolecular" means "correct molecule") was designated by Nobel Laureate Linus Pauling to describe this sophisticated approach to medical therapy using nutrition.

Vitamin E intake, at a level increased ten times over the recommended dietary allowance of the National Research

Council of the National Academy of Sciences, can enhance immune antibody response. The alpha tocopherol form of vitamin E at high levels also helps to increase the removal of waste by the reticuloendothelial system, reduce the mortality associated with infections, and provide other immune and adjuvant-type support functions.[4]

The B vitamin folacin (folic acid) aids in normalizing the response to skin test antigens, thus aiding immune defense functions.[5]

Vitamin C (ascorbic acid) increases the percentage of B-lymphocyte cells and enhances humoral (antibody) immunity response.[6]

Vitamin B_6 (pyridoxine) improves cellular and humoral immunity.[7] The activated chemical form of vitamin B_6 is pyridoxal-5-phosphate (P-5-P). The body performs particular reactions to convert pyridoxine into the active form P-5-P. These reactions are magnesium-dependent, and a total body low-magnesium status—as is commonly found in Candida syndrome patients—may contribute to a lowering of active vitamin B_6. Canditoxin is also thought to interfere with vitamin B_6 activity. Candidiasis patients often respond well to relatively high doses of vitamin B_6 or P-5-P early in their treatment course; lower dosages are satisfactory after the first few weeks of care.

Vitamin B_5 (pantothenic acid), vitamin B_2 (riboflavin), and vitamin B_{12} (cobalamin) elevate the antibody response.[8] Pantothenic acid is also important in supporting the function of the adrenal glands, which help to "key" your body to an appropriate stress response posture.

Magnesium is a required mineral prescribed by physicians for candidiasis patients. As a result of diarrhea, vomiting, and other gastrointestinal symptoms, magnesium often is lost so that symptoms of weakness, confusion, personality changes, muscle tremor, anorexia, nausea, lack of coordination, skin lesions, and more gastrointestinal disorders may be added to the Candida syndrome. The usual adult food supplementing dose of magnesium is 500–1,000 mg a day. To much magnesium can be toxic. Toxicity is indicated by weakness, drowsiness, and lethargy. People with compromised kidney function should take magnesium supplements only under the direction of a physician.

Zinc deficiency can cause a depression of cell-mediated (lymphocyte) immune responses. Lack of this mineral may bring about lymphoid atrophy with a slight decrease in T-cell numbers in the peripheral blood. Not only is the number of T-helper cells decreased, but also noted is a decrease in the activity of *facteur thymic serique* (from the French, meaning thymus blood factor). Therefore, zinc supplementation with 20–30 mg per day or more is advised, preferably taken apart from other mineral supplements.

Be aware that nutritional dosages for food supplements which exceed the recommended dietary allowances of the National Research Council of the U.S. National Academy of Sciences represent a therapeutic intervention and should be taken only under the direction of a properly trained and experienced wholistic physician. Accordingly, the coauthors and the publisher offer this disclaimer: Information presented in this book is not to be construed as the practice of medicine or the giving of medical advice. We are not practicing nutritional therapy, which is illegal in certain states of the United States. We believe and so advise that therapeutic recommendations must be advanced only by your personal physician, who is directly responsible for your care and well-being. As for the education you have received on these pages, we suggest that you ask your doctor about the nutrients, nutritional supplements, other food supplements, and their various dosages, and how or whether any of these might be useful for you.

Additional nutrients known to stimulate the immune system and to counteract yeast include essential fatty acids, manganese, iron, chlorophyll, vitamin B_3 (niacin), and vitamin B_1 (thiamine). Of course, basic to the wholistic treatment program for candidiasis is a change of diet. Yeast thrives on carbohydrates, so a reduced carbohydrate diet is believed to be essential by most Candida-conscious physicians. Carbohydrate-rich foods are often the ones that Candida syndrome patients crave but must give up until better. These carbohydrates consist of sugars of all types, honey, grains, chocolate, fruit (especially orange juice, which can be high in yeast content), and nuts (an exception is sometimes made for those nuts that are low in carbohydrates, such as pine and macadamia nuts).

MINIDOSE CANDIDIASIS IMMUNOTHERAPY

The permanent wholistic correction for candidiasis first involves dietary control—eating the right foods to boost the patient's immune system and avoiding yeast-stimulating foods; second is nutritional supplementation with garlic extract, magnesium, vitamin B_6, fatty acids, and other nutrients; third is antifungal medication including nystatin, ketoconazole, and others; fourth are the "medication-type" nutritional supplements, such as caprylic acid. When the Candida syndrome patient is poorly responsive to these usual measures, the treating physician must reconsider his therapeutic approach. Since the patient's immune system is the primary problem in candidiasis, the doctor may choose to influence the immune system's reactivity directly with regard to *C. albicans*. An appropriate immune response to yeast may be stimulated by applying minidose candidiasis immunotherapy—with an added potential benefit of neutralizing inappropriate responses.

Minidose or neutralizing dose immunotherapy is a procedure frequently practiced by specialists in environmental medicine. This highly complicated process takes advanced training and experience for the doctor to succeed with it. Provocative neutralization, the technique applied by Dr. Pannathpur Jayalakshmi in the case of Cynthia Farris described in Chapter Eleven, is useful to offset discomforts caused by the toxins created by yeast. The effect is to reduce or eliminate allergic disorders distressing a patient. The specialist physician prepares serial dilutions from concentrated solutions of protein antigens from three organisms: trichophyton, Candida, and epidermophyton (T-C-E). Using the concentrate and dilutions, the physician can make up a treatment solution containing neutralizing doses for each of these fungal organisms.

The antigen concentrate is diluted so as to create a linear series of one-to-five (1:5) solutions—the first is a 1:5 dilution of the concentrated solution; the second is a 1:5 dilution of the first; the third, a 1:5 dilution of the second; the fourth, a 1:5 dilution of the third; and so on all the way to fifteen dilutions or more. C. Orian Truss, M.D., discoverer of the Candida syndrome, has perfected a specific minidose immunotherapy technique for neutralizing *C. albicans*. The dosage range that he administers to patients as immunotherapy often is between the seventh and the fifteenth dilutions. He usually starts at the highest number (weakest potency) and, as required, works toward the seventh (greater potency). The doctor has to search for the correct neutralizing dose for his patient, and this will change over time as the patient's condition changes, so retesting is advisable every few weeks. During the course of diagnostic testing with these solutions, the therapist may create an underdose or overdose reaction—stimulation of the patient's symptoms. When the neutralizing dose is applied, symptoms resolve. Knowing the correct neutralizing dilutions allows for preparation of a patient's treatment formula, which is then used as needed—either weekly, every few days, daily, or even several times a day at first, for the sickest patients.

The whole purpose of minidose immunotherapy is to utilize incredibly small amounts of Candida antigen to stimulate body defense reactions, stopping just below the level of what would cause reactions (symptoms) at the injection site or in distant organs. The attention of the immune defense system is thus directed toward the antigen-injected skin site and away from the place in one's body where dysfunction is occurring—in the gut, endocrine glands, brain, genitals, or elsewhere. These subclinical dilutions of antigen may be utilized for the patient as subdermal or intradermal injections (under or into the skin) or as sublingual (under the tongue) drops. Medical practitioners using Candida provocative neutralization techniques must receive one-to-one, hands-on instruction from experienced environmental medicine specialists. Many candidiasis-treating physicians use a variation on Dr. Truss's technique, employing neutralizing doses at much stronger potencies (dilutions closer to the concentrate). This is an illustration of the harmonics of the immune system. The minidose Candida immunotherapy method is not advisable for the acutely "overloaded" patient, and it is rarely used as a technique of first choice.

YOUR NEED FOR BODY DETOXIFICATION

Consumption of concentrated nutrients, described in this and the previous chapter as part of the antiyeast wholistic therapy program, makes a broad range of nutritional factors available. Your cells probably haven't been bathed by this much cellular nutrient since childhood years. At that early time in life, your cells were not blocked by accumulated wastes; nutrient assimilation was easy because there were few obstacles. Advancing years bring blockage. So now, pure and highly concentrated nutrition suddenly speeds up cellular metabolism, removing blockages for more normal function. An increased amount of metabolic waste is freed from the cells and dumped into the bloodstream. A larger pool of waste products now must be eliminated quickly.

Many people suffering with the yeast syndrome have poorly functioning organs of elimination, so they're challenged by this increased waste. Indeed, the average industrialized Western diet tends to disable the bowel, liver, and kidneys. Second only to painkillers (e.g., aspirin and acetaminophen) are bowel laxatives as the most frequently purchased over-the-counter pharmaceutical products in the United States. Liver disease is the seventh-ranked killer in the developed countries. Kidney disease is steadily increasing; in 1985, it killed 78,000 Americans, approximately 4 percent of deaths. When cellular waste products accumulate in the bloodstream, the individual feels ill and the cells cannot utilize as well the fresh nutrients being provided by the Candida control diet and nutritional supplementation.

Proper and thorough detoxification, in fact, is just as important as good nutrition—especially for those of us living in the mainstream of modern technological civilization. Detoxification measures are therefore advisable for almost everyone who has developed symptoms of chronic generalized candidiasis.

The liver is the major organ of detoxification and also the one most stressed by our modern lifestyle. You can live only briefly without the heart, brain, kidneys, or pancreas—yet proper liver function is the key that helps to prevent these organs from becoming diseased. In addition to usual metabolic wastes, the liver helps to remove from the body chemical pollutants, environmental contamination, food preservatives, and other toxins to which we are exposed daily. You should be as much concerned about the condition of your liver as you are about the condition of your heart. If you ever have been the victim of hepatitis (regardless of the cause), cirrhosis, severe infectious mononucleosis, or other liver damage (such as from medications), you must become respectful and protective of this vital organ.

Our society puts undue stress on the liver with various unnatural items such as chemicals, drugs, synthetic foods, artificial food additives (coloring, preservatives, emulsifiers, stabilizers, sweeteners, and more), alcoholic beverages, carbonated beverages, hair sprays, chemical deodorants, and reheated vegetable oils used in frying (especially at "fast food" restaurants). Functions of the liver include metabolizing different nutrients, synthesizing blood proteins, breaking down and eliminating toxins, and secreting bile. The obvious solution to toxic congestion of the liver, gall bladder, small intestine, colon, kidneys, lungs, or skin is detoxification.

One important procedure of detoxification utilized in the antiyeast wholistic program is the enema. The coffee cleansing enema and the nystatin retention enema may be quite useful. However, information that we are supplying here about enemas is unacceptable to many practitioners of so-called orthodox medicine.

Consequently, what we have written here must also be accompanied by our strong recommendation that you should check with your personal physician first before including enemas as part of your anti-Candida therapeutic regimen. Determine whether your doctor is wholistic in his knowledge. Regardless of your physician's agreeing or disagreeing with us, we advise that you follow his or her advice as related to anything you read in this book. We provide information here about body detoxification techniques strictly for your general education and not as medical advice for you to follow. Details about detoxification and coffee cleansing enemas that are presented derive from the research of William Donald Kelley, D.D.S., and his Dallas, Texas, organizations, the International Health Institute and the Computer Health Service.

THE COFFEE CLEANSING ENEMA

The coffee cleansing enema stimulates functioning of the liver and provides aid in eliminating the liver's toxic wastes. Moreover, the coffee enema seems to have beneficial effects in cleaning the colon, too. Coffee is an excellent solvent for encrusted wastes accumulated along the walls of the large bowel. The caffeine content probably directly activates peristaltic (gut wall muscle) contractions more powerfully, helping to loosen deposits that are likely to be hard "shingles" of mucus. As the body's protein metabolism improves, the muscle tone of the colon gradually increases. Elimination through the bowel becomes normal without the aid of the enemas.

Coffee enemas are said to help the liver perform tasks for which it was not originally intended. With careful nutritional coordination, you might eliminate, in one to two years, the wastes accumulated over many years of living in ignorance of the laws of nature. *We believe that the only way that coffee should be used internally is as an enema!* Coffee is more beneficial as a therapeutic agent that way and not as a beverage. Drinking coffee, in fact, is hazardous to your health.

Some people have an aversion to the idea of enemas. Reeducating them to the functions of an enema and teaching the proper procedure to follow will help them to reverse their prejudices. Taking a couple of enemas in the correct way can make you an avid supporter of the technique. An enema often relieves distress and gives you a sense of well-being and cleanliness never before experienced. Proper removal of toxins and debris from the colon and liver are thought to be absolutely essential as a disease prevention measure in many conditions of ill health.

For instructions on how to make and take a coffee enema, adults may consult Dr. William Donald Kelley at the International Health Institute, P.O. Box 802607, Dallas, TX 75380; (800) 527-0453.

THE NYSTATIN RETAINED ENEMA

Adults should review these instructions for taking nystatin retained enemas with their physicians prior to engaging in the procedure or using it with their children. Before taking a retention enema with nystatin, consider giving yourself a cleansing enema such as with a Fleet's enema bottle (available from almost any pharmacy). If constipation is a problem, you might be advised to use special digestive enzymes or pharmacy bulk agents and/or laxatives such as one called Per Diem™. To do the nystatin retained enema, consider following these guidelines:

1. Mix one-quarter to one-half teaspoonful of sea salt or ordinary table salt and one-quarter teaspoonful of nystatin in one cup (eight ounces) of warm (spring, distilled, or purified) water. Because of its small volume, the eight-ounce quantity of solution is easily retained while you do the necessary rotations described next.

2. Allow the enema solution to cool to body temperature.

3. Gently insert the plastic enema nozzle into the rectum. While lying on your back, gently squeeze the enema bag to allow the solution to flow into the rectum.

4. After the solution is in, remove the enema nozzle, roll onto your left side, lie there for about five minutes to allow the solution to travel to the left side of your colon.

5. Now lie again on your back but prop your bottom up on pillows, to allow the solution to travel up the left side of your colon.

6. Now roll onto your right side and lie there for about five minutes, to allow the solution to travel across your mid-colon.

7. You are now free to get up and walk around. Standing or sitting will allow the solution to travel down the right side of your colon.

8. Retain the solution as long as you are comfortable. Evacuate when you must.

The purpose of the nystatin retained enema is to bring the killing power of nystatin into direct contact with yeast presumed to be growing in your colon. This enema procedure is sometimes extremely effective in helping to rid your body of fungus infestation.

Helpful hint: If you get a sudden gas bubble causing an urge to expel the enema solution, breathe very fast through your nose using your abdominal muscles as bellows. This usually helps the colon wall break up the gas bubble and allows the spasm to pass.

OFFSETTING THE HERXHEIMER REACTION

T. Daniel Pletsch, M.D., Medical Director of the Riverview Medical Clinic in Vancouver, Washington, advises us that he recommends a colon cleanse to minimize Herxheimer reaction effects in his anti-Candida treatment program. "I do not use this colon cleanse on all patients," he writes,

> but I recommend it and use it in those patients in whom a die-off [Herxheimer] reaction might be detrimental to their health. Examples are patients with bronchial asthma, multiple sclerosis, or panic attacks, and some with severe depression. These patients we place on a modified colon cleanse for seven days. Then after three or four days of having been on this cleanse, they start taking the oral nystatin; initial dose is always one-quarter teaspoonful [of powder] four times a day.

For the exact anti-Herxheimer colon cleansing directions provided to patients at the Riverview Medical Clinic in Vancouver, Washington, please contact T. Daniel Pletsch, M.D., directly. His full address and phone number appear in Appendix 4.

Clinical ecologist Alfred V. Zamm, M.D., of Kingston, New York, coauthor of *Why Your House May Endanger Your Health* (Simon & Schuster, 1980), wrote to us endorsing the colon cleanse approach as an antidote to the Herxheimer reaction. Dr. Zamm said,

> Many physicians have been faced with patients who are unable to increase their dose of nystatin to a therapeutically efficacious level because of the Herxheimer reaction. Every time that they raise the dose beyond a modicum (in some patients almost a homeopathic dose

[exceedingly diluted]), the patients complain of an exacerbation of their symptoms and are reluctant or unable to proceed to higher dose levels.

Up to now we have been directing our attention to increasing the amount of nystatin. Another approach would be to lower the Candida concentration. The solution to the Herxheimer problem, as I see it, revolves not so much in subjecting the patient to months of prolonged discomfort in the hope of achieving a higher dose of nystatin by gradually increasing the dose, but to also direct one's attention to the physical removal of as much gastrointestinal yeast as possible. The method I have found successful is similar to that employed in the preparation of patients for fiberoptic colonoscopy. I have found this method to be useful for patients who are unable to achieve therapeutic doses [of nystatin] even after trying for a year. They have been able to achieve therapeutic doses within a week or two and have had less discomfort.

THE COLON CLEANSING TECHNIQUE
RECOMMENDED BY ALFRED V. ZAMM, M.D.

1. Consume clear, moderately salted meat and vegetable broth for the first day. Take no solid foods.

2. On the second day, add solid foods; they should be proteinaceous and fatty with a minimum of complex carbohydrates (starches) and no simple carbohydrates (sugar, honey, fruit, fruit juice, and so forth). Your food should be highly pureed in a blender to maximize absorption, thus minimizing the food residue in the gastrointestinal (GI) tract.

3. Starting the second day, solid foods are gradually added over a four- to five-day period, until the original diet is resumed.

4. Twice a day for two days take enemas of clear, room temperature warm water (purified water or tap water without chlorine, of course). These help to physically remove a substantial amount of the yeast present in the colon. The magnitude of the Herxheimer response can be expected to be proportional to the amount of yeast remaining. Many physicians will be surprised at the relatively smaller Herxheimer responses when compared to previous experiences.

5. Use the powdered form of nystatin. Increase the amount of nystatin used as quickly as possible: start with one-eighth teaspoonful three times a day and increase to one-quarter teaspoonful as quickly as you can, within three days to a week. You are, in essence, establishing a wave of nystatin that travels down a gut essentially emptied of solid material and lowered in the amount of yeast—hence the Herxheimer reaction will be less.

"Under the above-mentioned circumstances," wrote Dr. Zamm,

> I have found that the efficacy of nystatin powder is substantially greater than that of nystatin pills. Warning: This procedure is not to be done in patients who are metabolically fragile in regard to their electrolytes, who are on diuretics, or who have otherwise compromised systems incapable of dealing with a temporary stress as outlined (unless they can be adequately compensated for their instability [by the use of other forms of therapy]).

Again, we caution anyone considering the use of these aggressive food restriction and colon cleansing programs to be carefully monitored by a skilled Candida-conscious physician. These are medical treatment programs, and they should not be undertaken (or modified) without continuing counsel of your personal physician. Your physician might wish to contact Drs. Zamm or Pletsch for further discussion about these anti-Herxheimer reaction techniques (see their addresses and telephone numbers in Appendix Four).

SALT WATER SNIZZLES

Here is a technique for the relief of certain yeast-related common upper respiratory maladies such as coryza, congestion, allergic and various other forms of rhinitis, postnasal drying, and pharyngitis (sore throat).

First, obtain from your local pharmacy an infant nasal

syringe. The bulb narrows to a small plastic nozzle, just the size of a nostril.

Second, mix the warm salt water to be used in the following way: take one-half teaspoonful of sea salt or ordinary table salt and mix well into one cup of warm water. Allow the solution to cool to body temperature.

Third, suck up the salt water solution to fill the bulb syringe.

Fourth, while leaning forward over the sink, with your face pointing down, not up, and with a towel nearby, insert the bulb syringe into the right nostril (never the left first!). Gently squeeze the solution well back into the nose. Hold your breath: do *not* breathe in while squeezing. Gently blow out the congestion onto a tissue. The final step is to sniffle strongly to clear up the salt water remaining in the very back of the nose.

Fifth, repeat step four, now with the left nostril.

Sixth, use the remaining solution as an excellent throat gargle for relieving harsh discomfort and irritation.

Many advantages to the use of salt water snizzles can be clearly seen. For instance:

Dr. Trowbridge has applied his snizzles at any hour and as often as needed.

Snizzles don't have nasty drug side effects, so they can be used by people with otherwise limiting diseases such as hypertension.

Snizzles are cheap and cost less than "medicine."

Snizzles can be employed for young and old.

Snizzles can aid with many kinds of nasal congestion and often prevent small respiratory problems from becoming big ones that require a doctor's care.

NOTES

1. S. Sirishna, "Immunoglobulins and Complement in Protein-Calorie Malnutrition," in R. E. Olson, ed., *Protein-Calorie Malnutrition*, New York: Academic Press, 1975, pp. 369–375.

2. W. R. Beisel, R. Edelman, K. Nauss, and R. M. Suskind, "Single Nutrient Effect on Immunological Functions," *Journal of the American Medical Association*, 1981, 245:53–57.

3. R. K. Chandra, "Vitamin Deficiencies," in *Immunology of Nutritional Disorders*, Chicago: Yearbook, 1980, pp. 55–106; B. E. Cohen, and R. J. Elin, "Vitamin A–Induced Nonspecific Resistance to Infection," *Journal of Infectious Diseases*, 1974, 129:597–600.

4. R. H. Heinzerling, C. F. Nockels, C. L. Quarles, and R. P. Tengerdy, "Protection of Chicks Against *E. coli* Infection by Dietary Supplementation with Vitamin E," *Proceedings of the Society of Experimental Biological Medicine*, 1974, 146:279–283; K. N. Prasad and S. Romanujam, "Vitamin E and Vitamin C Alter the Effect of Methylmercuric Chloride on Neuroblastoma and Glioma Cells in Culture," *Environmental Review*, 1980, 21:343–349.

5. R. L. Gross, J.V.O. Reid, P. M. Newberne, B. Burgess, R. Marsten, and W. Hift, "Depressed Cell-Mediated Immunity in Megaloblastic Anaemia Due to Folic Acid Deficiency," *American Journal of Clinical Nutrition*, 1975, 28:225–232.

6. R. C. Fraser, S. Pavlovic, C. G. Kurahara, A. Murata, N. S. Peterson, K. B. Taylor, and G. A. Feigen, "The Effect of Variations in Vitamin C Intake on the Cellular Immune Response of Guinea Pigs," *American Journal of Clinical Nutrition*, 1978, 33:839–847.

7. R. E. Hodges, W. B. Bean, M. A. Ohlson, and R. E. Bleiler, "Factors Affecting Human Antibody Response *v.* Combined Deficiency of Pantothenic Acid and Pyridoxine," *American Journal of Clinical Nutrition*, 1962, 11:187–199.

8. Chandra, *op. cit.*

SECTION III

The Yeast Control Diet, Foods Lists, and Recipes

13

The Yeast Control Diet:
A Celebration of Healthy Eating

In this chapter, we will explain the yeast control diet that is incorporated into the four-phase Celebration of Healthy Eating program used extensively at The Center for Health Enhancement in Humble (Houston), Texas. In the next chapter we give you the long list of foods (by family and alphabetically) available in the four sequential phases. In Chapter Fifteen we supply you with a starter selection of yeast control diet recipes.

By itself, the phase one, or MEVY (Meat, Eggs, Vegetables, and Yogurt), diet counteracts candidiasis almost as well as nystatin. Even more dramatic in therapeutic effect is the realization that, when the four-phase Celebration of Healthy Eating program (4-phase CHE) is followed fully, it can eliminate or control most or all of the symptoms of the Candida syndrome. The 4-phase CHE furnishes excellent lifestyle maintenance guidelines, even in the face of yeast-connected illness, and assists in restoring the yeast–human interaction to an appropriate level of balance.

RATIONALE OF THE YEAST CONTROL DIET

In a lecture delivered in 1982 to the Price-Pottinger Foundation of La Mesa, California, Shirley Lorenzani, Ph.D., Director of the Life Care Center, Inc., of Pompano Beach, Florida, laid out the rationale for using the yeast control diet. Dr. Lorenzani said that the foremost condition with which most of us supply *C. albicans* with a wonderfully luxurious home is our diet. Those who have been advocates of eating health foods (natural foods) will be surprised to note that much of what they have been consuming may also have been feasts for their yeasts. For example, health food enthusiasts often are exponents of supplementing with brewer's yeast because it is loaded with B vitamins. While health food proponents are correct about the B vitamins, any yeast-containing food can feed or stimulate one's own internal yeast organisms. If you have the Candida syndrome, we strongly advise against taking brewer's yeast. Get your B vitamins from other sources.

Don't forget that yeast is put into bread to make it rise. Moreover, flour often worsens symptoms for candidiasis victims, too. Gluten grains can exacerbate fungal growth by providing a ready food source for yeast, by irritating the intestinal tract, and by provoking tissue, organ, and blood system disorders in those people known to have the Candida syndrome.

Next, *C. albicans* love sweets. If they don't get fed the sucrose of white sugar, honey will do—or molasses. With no access to simple sucrose, fructose (the "natural" sugar from fruits) will be acceptable. Dried fruits such as raisins, apricots, prunes, pears, dates, and figs are not only concentrated sweets but also are frequently moldy. Dr. Lorenzani cautioned, "The irony here is that often this yeast creates constipation, and then people eat prunes to relieve the constipation—and keep the vicious cycle going."

Most commercial soups, alcoholic beverages, nuts, vinegar, pickled products, and some condiments can nourish internal yeast.

Milk products encourage yeast overgrowth, too. The only dairy products not forbidden are yogurt, because live cultures in it restore *L. acidophilus* to a gut depleted of this friendly bacteria, and certain cheeses, as listed in the four-phase Celebration of Healthy Eating program of Chapter Fourteen.

Commercial breads, including those made from whole wheat, rye, and other "health food" types, should be set aside. Of course, even if you are not a victim of the Candida syndrome, white flour breads, pasta, and cakes must never be eaten. These so-called foods have almost no nutritional value, except the minimal vitamin supplementation added by the baker to the depleted flour. White flour pasta encourages yeast growth. An Italian with candidiasis might be attracted to spaghetti and cheese; the Candida-infested white Anglo-Saxon Protestant may go for German chocolate cake; a Jewish person with the Candida syndrome will possibly favor bagels, lox, and cream cheese. All of these are examples of foods that can feed their yeast. Each food attraction is often related to the individual's cultural heritage.

The Candida control diet temporarily (but sometimes permanently) holds back foods in our typical Western civilization diet that are high in yeast, sugars, and refined starches. These unsuitable edibles, even though attractive to people affected by the Candida syndrome, are hearty meals for their voracious yeasts. The four-phase Celebration of Healthy Eating program first eliminates yeast-stimulating foods and later allows their reintroduction, after a person progresses in his battle against yeast illness. In a series of steps or "phases" (the first phase being the most radical and the fourth phase the closest to "usual eating") the 4-phase CHE modifies Western civilization's standard approach to food consumption.

FIFTEEN GUIDELINES FOR FOLLOWING THE FOUR-PHASE CELEBRATION OF HEALTHY EATING PROGRAM

There are fifteen guidelines to most easily and effectively lead you into the four-phase Celebration of Healthy Eating program for counteracting the Candida syndrome. Extensive food lists are given in the next chapter as well, to help your efforts to stay within these guidelines.

1. Eat real food at every meal, never skip a meal, and snack on vegetables between meals. Take small bites and chew your food thoroughly.

2. Every day eat at least one selection (preferably two or more different choices) from each of the following vegetable groups: green leafy; red, orange, purple; green; yellow, white; and roots. A portion, or serving, is three or more tablespoonsful.

3. Eat vegetables raw, juiced at home, or steamed (about five to seven minutes). Vegetable juices should be considered a treat—you need the bulk that comes from the whole food. Consider using a juicer that can pulverize the whole vegetable, peeling and all.

4. About ten to fifteen times a week, eat one serving from any of the following protein food groups: poultry, eggs/egg products, fish/mollusks/crustaceans, and red meats. Choose white meat (fish or fowl) more often than red meat. If you have a problem handling sugar, you may be advised to consume protein foods three or more times a day.

5. Eat meats steamed, broiled, baked, or microwaved—not fried, grilled, or boiled. Meat cooked medium or medium rare is better for you than well done. Trim off as much fat as possible and avoid fatty skins and meats highly marbled with fat.

6. Drink at least one eight-ounce glass of water just before or with every meal, between meals, and before or at bedtime—a total of seven to eight or more glasses daily.

7. For beverages, drink bottled or mineral water (you may add fresh-squeezed lime for flavoring), herbal tea such as the noncaffeine selection available from Celestial Seasonings™, Lipton™, other herb teas, or regular tap water. (But we strongly advise you to use a water purifier when drinking tap water.) If you feel the compulsion to drink coffee or regular tea, ask your physician for recommendations relating to these beverages.

8. Use sea salt sparingly—or a salt substitute (such as Mrs. Dash™), if you are limiting your salt intake. Use unsalted, sweet butter sparingly (instead of margarine). Try various seasonings to add flavor to meats and vegetables: black pepper, caraway, chives, cloves, curry, garlic, ginger, olives, paprika, sage, and additional ones. Use the following oils with lemon juice as a salad dressing (definitely avoid vinegar): virgin olive oil, sesame oil, or cold-pressed vegetable oils such as safflower.

9. Away from home, "brown-bag-it" or order vegetable

platters or salads—*no* "fast foods," *no* "junk foods." Avoid fruits as snacks.

10. Eat natural foods—no sugar, soda pop, diet soft drinks, candy, cookies, or pastries. After you have eaten healthily for a few weeks, your cravings for sweets will decrease markedly.

11. Buy fresh meat and vegetables—no packaged, preserved, canned, bottled, or prepared foods. When you go grocery shopping, confine most of your selections to items available around the outer walls of the supermarket; avoid the temptations lurking in the middle aisles.

12. At every meal, leave the last little bite on your plate— try to avoid seconds (unless your first portions were small) and never eat desserts. If you get hungry later, take a proper snack so that you stay in control.

13. Eat only those foods you know are healthy for you—if you have questions or doubts, ask your physician.

14. Your age, the presence of the Candida syndrome, your health habits (such as smoking), your medical condition, and even your sex and occupation will influence your nutritional needs. Consult your wholistic physician for appropriate adjustments to account for these highly individualistic factors.

15. Make sure you take your personal nutritional supplements every day, employing the proper program for your own needs as prescribed by your physician.

THE FOUR-PHASE CELEBRATION OF HEALTHY EATING PROGRAM

For several reasons, the mainstay of therapy for any of the yeast-connected illnesses must be directed at dietary changes:

1. An incorrect diet has been one of the major reasons you have gotten into trouble with your commensal organism, yeast.

2. Until your immune system is strong enough to handle the insults of Western living, foods that stimulate yeast growth must be eliminated.

3. Nourishment must be provided to rebuild or replace your damaged "people parts"—rather than strengthening the pervasive Candida-parts—in order to restore or rejuvenate cells and metabolic systems that are dysfunctioning. This rebuilding sets the stage for resolution of many signs you may be showing of yeast-related illnesses, such as dry skin, dandruff, endless itching, nose congestion, and other troubles.

4. If you intend to work toward long-term wellness, feeling better faster depends on rebalancing your body's yeast–human interaction. You can't escape from yeast or eliminate it altogether from the mouth, the vagina, the area under the foreskin, the rectum, the intestines, or other body sites. But you can return to an acceptable level of commensalism. Of all the therapies, following an appropriate eating plan does this rebalancing best.

To achieve a higher level of wellness, we urge you to comply seriously with the four-phase Celebration of Healthy Eating program under your personal physician's direction. This 4-phase CHE provides you with a progression of foods, adding more as you steadily get better. After the toughest and more restrictive part of the 4-phase CHE is over—the MEVY diet that serves as phase one—you will notice much less disturbance to your usual food habits, physiology, or psyche. Phase-4 eventually brings you back almost to standard Western fare.

The MEVY diet, which, as indicated, is limited to meat/eggs/vegetables/yogurt, usually will not be continued for more than three or four weeks, inasmuch as it does not supply you with the broad range of nutritional factors in a proper balance. In brief, phase one fails as a complete nutritional eating program; therefore, *it is strictly a therapy employed against candidiasis*. Just as when you take a drug, you should consult with your physician if you are considering embarking on the 4-phase CHE. As your health responds positively, your Candida syndrome–trained physician will advise you on when to advance into phase-2 CHE and the subsequent phases three and four. Each succeeding phase adds foods to the prior phases. However, take special note: Your physician will advise you on including or omitting foods, regardless of which phase you are in.

The MEVY diet of phase-1 CHE is a highly limited eating program that disallows exposure to yeast and to foods that provide direct nourishment for the stimulation of yeast growth. As mentioned, phase one is truly a therapeutic eating program. Please understand that your physician and the authors know the limited selection of only meat/eggs/vegetables/yogurt is less appetizing. Bear with the brief discomfort of following this MEVY diet for three or four weeks, under the direction of your doctor, and you will find you have a lot more options in later phases. You will feel better, too.

Phase-2 CHE adds some food items that could encourage yeast growth if they were consumed in excess—so you will avoid eating a pound of cheese or a loaf of bread or other obvious indiscretions.

Phase-3 CHE lets you add (in moderate amounts) some foods associated with yeast or with a higher sugar/carbohydrate content, such as pears, apples, and bananas. Obviously, you must avoid excessive consumption of fruits and other foods listed, especially at one sitting.

Phase-4 CHE finally adds yeast-containing foods or foods with such an elevated sugar/carbohydrate content that they would dramatically encourage more *C. albicans* growth in a susceptible person who has a weakened immune system.

Your physician may choose to have you start with phase one and some selections from phase two. Depending on the doctor's personal preference, he might even include some parts of phase three at the beginning of your treatment program. As mentioned, this 4-phase CHE represents the full dietary plan for treating the yeast syndrome at The Center for Health Enhancement. Different anti-Candida diets may be recommended at other medical centers throughout North America or in other parts of the world. Your individual physician should be relied on for advice on which eating program you should follow.

The 4-phase Celebration of Healthy Eating program requires that you select items from many different "food families" in each particular phase, rather than narrowing your choices to just your few favored foods. In Chapter Fourteen, there are extensive lists of foods that fit into each phase. There is an alphabetical listing for ready referencing, too, to use for meal planning and to take along shopping. Here are some hints about using those lists:

- If an item you are planning to use as part of your menu is similar to one in another allowed group, select an alternative food from the second list. We recommend a wide variety in your eating as the best way to reduce any tendency toward developing food allergies.
- Don't be concerned with the fancy "food family" names that you may not recognize on the alphabetized foods list; these are merely biological classifications. Some members of a single food family may appear in phase one, while others show in phase two and phase three. Some food families actually have separate foods listed all the way across the four phases. The placement partly depends on whether the food items contain yeast (either in their native form or processed form) or whether their carbohydrate content will encourage yeast growth. The key to your success with this therapeutic menu plan is to follow the grouping of foods into four distinct phases.
- Most foods that have an increased tendency to create allergic responses in people have been pushed into phases three and four. In the alphabetized foods list, abbreviations inserted beside these reactive foods flag them for your attention. (See the key for an explanation of each abbreviation used.) People with the Candida syndrome often have food allergies, apparently resulting from damage to their gut lining and, subsequently, to their immune defenses. Why do we push these reactive foods to later phases? We'll answer the question with another question: If you already suffer from food allergies, why would you consume those same antagonizing foods in your therapeutic diet? You would not! You don't want to stimulate your allergic response pattern, which would continue your symptoms for a longer period of time.

What we have done early in the 4-phase CHE is to eliminate those items to which people are characteristically allergic. Reactant foods are pushed to a later stage, when your immune system will have had time to recover lost abilities. You should then be able to handle the reintroduction of more provocative foods. As a result, you should be less symptomatic, even if you eat items to which you formerly had been allergic. This principle is one foundation upon which the four-phase Celebration of Healthy Eating program is based.

If you know that you are allergic to one or more of the foods in a particular food family grouping listed in the next chapter, you have an increased likelihood of being allergic to other foods in the very same food family. Realize that you probably should avoid those additional foods, at least until your immune defense system (hence, your candidiasis) improves.

14

Four-Phase Yeast Foods Lists

PHASE ONE
CELEBRATION OF HEALTHY EATING PROGRAM

You may freely select from all of the Phase-1 CHE foods when you begin this dietary program, depending on the recommendations of your own physician.

Phase-1 Agricultural Products

Vegetables
Alfalfa sprouts
Artichoke, Chinese
Asparagus
Bamboo sprouts
Banana pepper
Bavarian endive (escarole, chicory escarole)
Bean sprouts
Beet greens
Bell pepper (sweet green)

Cabbages
Bok choy
Broccoli
Cabbage kraut
Cauliflower
Celery cabbage
Chinese cabbage (Pe Tsai)
Collard greens
Head (green, red)
Kale

Kohlrabi
Savoy
Cardoon
Carrot
Chayote
Celery
Celeriac (celery root, knob
    celery)
Cucumber
Curly cress
Curly endive (chicory)
Dandelion greens
Dulse
Eggplant
Fennel (finocchio)
Garden cress
Garlic
Gherkin
Jalapeno pepper
Jicama
Kelp (seaweed)
Lamb's quarters
Leek
Lettuces
    Butterhead
        Bibb
        Boston
        Butterscotch
    Celtuce (stem)
    Iceberg (crisphead)
    Loose-Leaf
        Lamb's
        Matchless
        Oakleaf (green, bronze)
        Prizehead
        Salad bowl
    Red-leaf chicory
        (Arugula)
    Romaine (cos)
    Roguette
Mung bean sprouts

Onion
Okra
Parsnip
Pumpkin
Rape
Radish
Red sweet pepper
Sea kale
Shallot
Spinach
Squashes
    Acorn
    Alligator
    Banana
    Boston marrow
    Bush
    Buttercup
    Butternut
    Caserta
    Cheese
    Cocozelle
    Connecticut field
    Crookneck
    Cushaw
    Delicious
    Golden nugget
    Hubbard varieties
    Mammoth
    Melopepo
    Mirliton
    Pattypam
    Pumpkin
    Quaker pie
    Queensland blue
    Small sugar
    Spaghetti
    Straightneck
    Table queen
    Turban
    Vegetable spaghetti
    Virginia mammoth

(*continued*)
   Whitebush scallop
   Zucchini
String bean
Swiss chard
Tomatillo
Tomato
Turnip greens
Upland cress
Water celery
Watercress
Whitloof chicory (Belgian
      or French endive)
Yucca

Herbs and Spices
Allspice
Althea root (tea)
Angelica
Anise
Apple mint
Balm
Basil
Bergamot
Boneset (tea)
Borage
Burdock root (tea)
Burnet (cucumber flavor)
Caraway
Cardamom
Cassia
Celery seed
Chamomile (tea)
Chervil
Chicory (in coffee, tea)
Chive
Clove
Comfrey (tea)
Coriander
Cumin
Dill
Dittany

East Indian arrowroot
Fenugreek
Ginger
Ginseng (tea)
Goldenrod (tea)
Hibiscus (roselle) (tea)
Horehound
Horseradish
Lavendar
Lemon balm (melissa)
Licorice
Lovage
Mace
Marjoram
Menthol
Mint
Nutmeg
Oregano
Paprika
Parsley
Peppercorns (black, white)
Peppermint
Pimiento
Rosemary
Saffron
Sage
Savory
Sorrel (dock)
Spearmint
Tarragon
Thyme
Tumeric
Vanilla (bean, extract)

Miscellaneous
Agar-agar
Aloe vera
Carrageen (Irish moss)
Green tea
Ground cherry
Guava
Herbal teas

Pepino (melon pear)
Rhubarb
Safflower oil

Salt (table salt, sea salt)
Sunflower (seed, oil, meal)
Tamarind

Phase-1 Animal Products

Amphibians
Frog (frog legs)

Birds
Chicken and eggs
Dove
Duck and eggs
Goose and eggs
Guinea hen
Peafowl
Pheasant
Pigeon (squab)
Prairie chicken
Quail
Ruffed Grouse (partridge)
Turkey and eggs

Crustaceans
Crayfish
Dungeness crab
Lobster
Shrimp (prawn)
Snow crab

Mammals
Antelope
Bear
Beaver
Beef
  Beef byproducts
    Gelatin from beef
    Rennin (rennet)
    Sausage casings
    Snet
  Milk products

Butter
Casein (protein)
Yogurt
Muscle meats (steak, roast, tongue, and others)
Organ meats (liver, kidney, tripe, and others)
Veal
Beefalo
Buffalo (bison)
Caribou
Deer (venison)
Elk
Goat (kid)
  Goat's milk
  Goat's milk cheese
Horse
Lamb
Moose
Opposum
Pork
  Gelatin from pork
  Ham
  Miscellaneous meats
  Sausage
Porpoise
Pronghorn antelope
Rabbit (hare)
Squirrel
Miscellaneous (frankfurters, sausage, salami, bologna)

Mollusks

Abalone
Clam
Cockle
Mussel
Octopus
Oyster
Quahog
Scallop
Snail
Squid

Reptiles

Alligator
Snake (rattlesnake)
Terrapin (diamondback
    terrapin)
Turtle (green, snapping)

Salt Water Fish

Albacore tuna
Amberjack
Anchovy
Barracuda
Bluefish
Bonito
Butterfish
Coal Fish
Cod (scrod)
Cusk
Dab
Dollarfish
Drumfish
Eel
Flounder
Grouper
Gurnard
Haddock
Hake
Halibut

Harvestfish
King Whiting
Lingcod
Mackeral
Mahi-mahi
Menhaden
Monkfish
Mullet
Northern scup (porgy)
Ocean catfish
Ocean perch
Petrale
Pilchard (sardine)
Plaice
Pollack
Pompano (jack)
Rosefish (scorpionfish)
Sailfish
Sandab
Sea bass
Sea herring
Sea robin
Sea trout
Shad
Shark
Sheephead
Silver perch
Silverside (whitebait,
    shiner)
Skipjack
Sole
Spot
Spotted bass
Striped bass (rockfish)
Swordfish
Tarpon
Tilefish
Tuna

Turbot
Weakfish (spotted sea
    trout)
White perch
Whiting
Yellow jack (yellowtail)

Fresh Water Fish
Beluga
Black bass species
Bluegill
Bullhead
Carp
Catfish species
Caviar (roe)
Crappie (crappy)
Croaker
Chub
Fresh water drumfish
King whiting
Minnow

Muskellunge
Northern pike
Paddlefish
Pickerel
Salmon species (all)
Sauger
Sea trout
Shad (roe)
Silver perch
Smelt
Sturgeon (caviar)
Sucker
Sunfish species
Trout species (all)
Walleye pike
Weakfish
Whitefish
White perch
Yellow bass
Yellow perch

PHASE TWO
CELEBRATION OF HEALTHY EATING PROGRAM

Add these foods to your Phase-1 CHE program when advised
by your physician.

Phase-2 Agricultural Products

Vegetables
Artichoke, globe
Artichoke, Jerusalem
    (sunchoke)
  Flour
Avocado
Brussel sprouts
Chinese water chestnuts
Chufa (groundnut)
Mustard greens

Peas
  Black-eyed (cowpea)
  Chickpea (garbanzo)
  Cream
  Field
  Green
  Purple-hull
  Split
Potato (waxy white, waxy
    red, mealy)

(*continued*)
Rutabaga
Salisfy (oyster plant)
Soy products
  Soybean
  Soy flour
  Soy milk
  Soy oil
  Tofu
Turnip

Fruits
Melons
  Canang
  Casaba
  Cassabanana
  Christmas
  Crenshaw
  Honeydew
  Muskmelon
  Persian
  Santa Claus
  Spanish
  Watermelon

Grains
Cornmeal

Corn oil
Corn starch
Popped corn
Rice
Triticale
Wheat germ
Wild rice

Miscellaneous
Bay leaf
Capers
Cayenne pepper
Cinnamon
Mustard seed
Nasturtium (leaves,
  flowers, seeds)
Olives (black, green, ripe)
Olive oil
Red pepper
Sassafras
Sesame (seed, oil)
Tabasco sauce
Tahini

Phase-2 Animal Products

Cheese
Soft
  American (white,
    yellow)
  Cream cheese
  Neufchatel
Hard
  Colby
  Edam
  Gouda

Monterey Jack
Whey Cheese
  Gyetost
  Mysost
  Primost
  Ricotta
  Sapsago

Honey bee pollen

PHASE THREE
CELEBRATION OF HEALTHY EATING PROGRAM

Add these foods to your Phase-1 and Phase-2 CHE program when advised by your physician.

Phase-3 Agricultural Products

Vegetables

Beans
  Aduki
  Black Turtle
  Fava
  Great Northern
  Green
  Jack
  Kidney
  Lima
  Mung
  Navy
  Pinto
  Beet Snap
Carob
Hearts of palm
Lentil (plain, pink)
Masur bean
Palm cabbage
Sago palm (starch)
Sugar beet
Swamp cabbage
Sweet corn (immature)

Grains

Barley
Barley malt
Buckwheat
Grits (hominy)
Kafir
Maltose
Millet
Oats
Rye
Sorghum syrup
Wheat
  Bran (farina)
  Bulgur
  Flour
    Gluten
    Graham
    Patent
    Whole wheat

Nuts

Almond
Beechnut
Chestnut
Chinquapin
Filbert
Hazelnut
Peanut
Peanut oil
Pine nut
Pinyon (pinon)

Fruits

Apple
Bearberry
Blackberry
Blueberry
Boysenberry
Cherry, West Indian
    (Barbados, acerola)
Citron
Crabapple

(continued)
Cranberry
Dewberry
Elderberry
Gooseberry
Huckleberry
Kumquat
Lemon
Lime
Longberry
Loquat
May apple
Murcot
Papaya
Pawpaw (custard apple)
Peach
Pineapple
Pomegranate
Rosehips

Sapota
Saskatoon
Satsuma
Sloe plum
Strawberry
Tangelo
Ugli fruit
Wineberry
Youngberry

Miscellaneous
Angostura (bitters)
Apple pectin
Arrowroot
Coffee
Juniper berry
Mate
Wintergreen

Phase-3 Animal Products

Cheese
Soft
  Cottage Cheese
Cheddar
  Cheddars
  Cheshire
Granular
  Grana
  Parmesan

Reggiana
Romana
Sardo
Stretched curd
  Caciocavallo
  Mozzarella
  Provolone
  String Cheese

PHASE FOUR
CELEBRATION OF HEALTHY EATING PROGRAM

Add these foods to your Phase-1, Phase-2, and Phase-3 CHE
Program when advised by your physician.

Phase-4 Agricultural Products

Fruits
Apricot
Banana

Breadfruit
Cantaloupe
Cherry (sour, sweet)

Coconut (oil, meal, milk, meat)
Currant (red, black, white)
Date
Date plum
Fig (all varieties)
Grape (all varieties)
Grapefruit (all varieties)
Kiwi fruit
Loganberry
Mango
Mulberry
Muscadine
Nectarine
Orange (all varieties)
Pear
Persimmon (American, Japanese)
Plum
Pomelo
Prune
Quince
Raisin (all varieties)
Raspberry (black, purple, red)

Vegetables
Agave
Castorbean and oil
Chinese yam (potato)
Dasheen
Malanga
Manioc
Morel
Mushroom
Name (yampi)
Plantain
Poi
Prickly pear
Tapioca
Taro (root)
Truffle

Yam (sweet potato)
Yautia
Yuca

Nuts
Brazil nut
Butternut
Cashew
Cola nut (cola, kola)
Heartnut
Hickory nut
Litchi nut
Macadamia nut
Pecan
Pistachio
Walnut (black, English)

Sugars
Beet sugar
Cane sugar (turbinado)
Corn sugar ("Cerelose," dextrose, "Dyno")
Corn syrup ("Cartose," glucose, "Sweetose")
Honey and related products
  Honey (commercial blended, raw, Tupelo)
  Honeycomb
  Beeswax
Maple Syrup, sugar
Molasses

Miscellaneous
Apple cider
Baker's yeast
Black tea
Brewer's yeast (nutritional yeast)
Buckthorn (tea)
Chocolate (cacao)
Cocoa
Cocoa butter

Cream of tartar
Hops (alcohol)

Pickles (cucumber,
   gherkin)
Vinegar (cider, wine)

Phase-4 Animal Products

Cheese (bacteria-, mold-,
   or yeast ripened)
Asiago
Bel Paese
Bleu/blue
Brick
Brie
Camembert
Emmental

Gorgonzola
Gruyere
Limburger
Muenster
Port de salut
Roquefort
Stilton
Swiss

THE FOUR-PHASE CELEBRATION OF HEALTHY EATING COMPREHENSIVE, ALPHABETICAL FOODS LIST

The Four-Phase Celebration of Healthy Eating comprehensive, alphabetical foods list is furnished for your convenience in determining into which of the four phases a particular food fits. We suggest that you use this list for food shopping, meal planning, recipe preparation, and question answering. It will aid you in knowing, first, in which phase the food is placed; second, in what food family it is classified, should you want to substitute other foods from the same family; third, the food's carbohydrate content, where applicable; fourth, the food's allergy-causing potential, where applicable.

Key to Abbreviations

The following four classifications of allergy-causing potential for foods are adapted from *Basics of Food Allergy* by James C. Breneman (Springfield, Ill.: Charles C. Thomas, 1978):

VHAP = very high allergy-causing potential
MHAP = moderately high allergy-causing potential
MAP   = moderate allergy-causing potential
LAP   = low allergy-causing potential

The following classifications of carbohydrate (sugar, starch) content in foods are adapted from *Hope for Hypoglycemia* by Broda A. Barnes, M.D., Ph.D., and Charlotte W. Barnes

(Fort Collins, Colo.: Robinson Press, 1978) and *Scientific Tables* (edited by K. Diem and C. Lentner, 7th ed., Basel: Ciba-Geigy, 1970). Note that many of the vegetables listed have less than 5 percent carbohydrates content, so no indication is made beside their names:

5-CHO	=	5 percent carbohydrate content
10-CHO	=	10 percent carbohydrate content
15-CHO	=	15 percent carbohydrate content
20-CHO	=	20 percent carbohydrate content

ALPHABETIZED FOOD	CHE PHASE	FOOD FAMILY	CARBOHYDRATE CONTENT [CHO]	ALLERGY POTENTIAL
Abalone	1	Mollusks		
Acorn squash	1	Gourd	10	
Aduki bean	3	Legume		
Agar (agar agar)	1	Algae		
Agave	4	Amaryllis		
Albacore tuna	1	Mackerel		
Alfalfa (sprouts)	1	Legume	5	
Alligator	1	Reptiles		
Alligator pear	1	Gourd		
Allspice	1	Myrtle		
Almond	3	Rose		
Aloes (aloe vera)	1	Lily		
Althea root (tea)	1	Mallow		
Amberjack	1	Jack		VHAP
American eel	1	Eel		VHAP
American cheese (white, yellow)	2	Cheese		VHAP
Anchovy	1	Anchovy		VHAP
Angelica	1	Parsley		
Angostura (bitters)	3	Citrus		
Anise	1	Parsley		
Apple	3	Rose	10	LAP
Apple cider	4	Rose		LAP
Apple mint	1	Mint		
Apple pectin	3	Rose		LAP
Apricot	4	Rose	15	LAP
Arrowroot	3	Arrowroot		
Artichoke, Chinese	1	Mint		
Artichoke, Common (globe)	2	Composite	10	

ALPHABETIZED FOOD	CHE PHASE	FOOD FAMILY	CARBOHYDRATE CONTENT [CHO]	ALLERGY POTENTIAL
Artichoke flour (Jerusalem)	2	Composite		
Artichoke, Jerusalem (Sunchoke)	2	Composite	10	
Asiago	4	Cheese		
Asparagus	1	Lily	5	
Avocado	2	Laurel	5	
Baker's yeast	4	Fungus		MHAP
Balm	1	Mint		
Bamboo (shoots)	1	Grains		
Banana	4	Banana	20	MAP
Banana pepper	1	Potato		
Banana squash	1	Gourd		LAP
Barracuda	1	Barracuda		VHAP
Barley	3	Grains	75	LAP
Basil	1	Mint		
Bavarian endive (escarole, chicory escarole)	1	Composite		
Bay leaf	2	Laurel		
Bear	1	Mammals		
Bearberry	3	Heath		MHAP
Beechnut	3	Beech		MHAP
Beef	1	Mammals		
Beefalo	1	Mammals		
Beeswax	4	Miscellaneous		
Beet	3	Beet	10	LAP
Beet greens	1	Beet	5	LAP
Bel Paese cheese				
Bell (sweet, green) pepper	1	Potato		
Beluga	1	Sturgeon		
Bergamot	1	Mint		
Berries	3,4	Rose		MHAP
Bibb lettuce	1	Composite	5	LAP
Black bass	1	Bass		
Black-eyed pea (cowpea)	2	Legume	15	MHAP
Black olive	2	Olive		
Black pepper	1	Pepper		
Black tea	4	Tea		

ALPHABETIZED FOOD	CHE PHASE	FOOD FAMILY	CARBOHYDRATE CONTENT [CHO]	ALLERGY POTENTIAL
Black turtle bean	3	Legume		
Blackberry	3	Rose	10	MHAP
Bleu/blue cheese	4	Fungus/ Mammal		
Blueberry	3	Heath	15	MHAP
Bluefish	1	Bluefish		VHAP
Bluegill	1	Bass		
Bok choy (bok choi)	1	Mustard	5	
Boneset (tea)	1	Composite		
Bonito	1	Mackerel		VHAP
Borage	1	Borage		
Boston lettuce	1	Composite	5	LAP
Boston marrow squash	1	Gourd		LAP
Boysenberry	3	Rose		MHAP
Bran (farina)	3	Grains	75	VHAP
Brazil nut	4	Lecythis		MHAP
Breadfruit	4	Mulberry		
Brewer's yeast (nutritional yeast)	4	Fungus		MHAP
Brick cheese	4	Fungus/ Mammal		
Brie cheese	4	Fungus/ Mammal		
Broccoli	1	Mustard	5	
Brussels sprouts	2	Mustard	10	
Buckthorn (tea)	4	Grape		
Buckwheat	3	Buckwheat	70	MHAP
Buffalo (bison)	1	Mammals		
Buffalofish	1	Sucker		
Bulgur (wheat)	3	Grains		VHAP
Bullhead	1	Catfish		
Burdock root (tea)	1	Composite		
Burnet (cucumber flavor)	1	Rose		
Bush squash	1	Gourd		LAP
Butter	1	Mammals		
Buttercrunch lettuce	1	Composite	5	LAP
Buttercup squash	1	Gourd	10	LAP

ALPHABETIZED FOOD	CHE PHASE	FOOD FAMILY	CARBOHYDRATE CONTENT [CHO]	ALLERGY POTENTIAL
Butterfish	1	Flounder		VHAP
Butterhead lettuce	1	Composite		LAP
Butternut	4	Walnut		MHAP
Butternut squash	1	Gourd	10	LAP
Cabbage (green, red)	1	Mustard	5	
Cabbage kraut	1	Mustard	5	
Caciocavallo cheese	3	Mammals		
[Caffeine— substance of abuse]	2	Cocoa		
Camembert cheese	4	Fungus/ Mammal		
Canang melon	2	Gourd	5	MAP
Cantaloupe	4	Gourd	10	
Capers	2	Caper		
Caraway (kummel liqueur)	1	Parsley		
Cardamon	1	Ginger		
Cardoon	1	Mustard		
Caribou	1	Mammals		
Carob (St. John's bread)	3	Legume		
Carp	1	Minnow		
Carrageen (Irish moss)	1	Algae		
Carrot	1	Parsley	10	LAP
Casaba melon	2	Gourd	5	MAP
Casein	1	Mammals		
Caserta squash	1	Gourd		LAP
Cashew	4	Cashew		MHAP
Cassabanana melon	2	Gourd	5	MAP
Cassava	4	Spurge		
Cassia (in curry)	1	Legume		
Castor bean and oil	4	Spurge		
Catfish	1	Catfish		
Catnip	1	Mint		
Cauliflower	1	Mustard		
Caviar (roe)	1	Sturgeon		

ALPHABETIZED FOOD	CHE PHASE	FOOD FAMILY	CARBOHYDRATE CONTENT [CHO]	ALLERGY POTENTIAL
Cayenne pepper	2	Potato		
Celeriac (celery root, knob celery)	1	Parsley		
Celery	1	Parsley	5	MAP
Celery cabbage	1	Mustard	5	
Celery seed	1	Parsley		MAP
Celtuce (stem) lettuce	1	Composite	5	LAP
Chamomile (tea)	1	Composite		
Chard	1	Beet	5	
Chayote	1	Gourd		
Cheddar cheese	3	Mammals		
Cheeses	2,3,4	Mammals		
Cheese squash	1	Gourd		LAP
Cherry, West Indian (Barbados, acerola)	3	Rose		MAP
Cherry, sour	4	Rose	15	MAP
Cherry, sweet	4	Rose	20	MAP
Chervil	1	Parsley		
Cheshire cheese	3	Mammals		
Chestnut	3	Beech		MHAP
Chicken	1	Birds	for females, for males,	MAP LAP
Chicken eggs	1	Birds		VHAP
Chickpea (garbanzo)	2	Legume	15	MHAP
Chicory (coffee, tea)	1	Composite		
Chili pepper	2	Potato		
Chinese cabbage	1	Mustard	5	
Chinese water chestnut	2	Chinese water chestnut		
Chinese yam (potato)	4	Yam		LAP
Chive	1	Lily	5	
Chocolate (cacao)	4	Cocoa		MHAP
Christmas melon	2	Gourd	5	MHAP
Chub	1	Minnow		
Chufa (groundnut)	2	Chinese water chestnut		
Cider, apple	4	Rose		LAP

ALPHABETIZED FOOD	CHE PHASE	FOOD FAMILY	CARBOHYDRATE CONTENT [CHO]	ALLERGY POTENTIAL
Cinnamon	2	Laurel		
Citric acid (used as a food preservative)	4	Citrus		
Citron	3	Citrus		
Clam	1	Mollusks		
Clove	1	Myrtle		
Coal fish	1	Codfish		VHAP
Cockle	1	Mollusks		
Cocoa	4	Cocoa		
Cocoa butter	4	Cocoa		
Coconut (oil, meal, milk, meat)	4	Palm		MHAP
Cocozelle squash	1	Gourd	5	LAP
Cod (scrod)	1	Codfish		VHAP
Coffee	3	Madder	in adults	MHAP
Cola nut (cola, kola)	4	Cocoa		
Colby cheese	2	Cheese		
Collard greens	1	Mustard	5	
Comfrey (tea)	1	Borage		
Connecticut field squash	1	Gourd		LAP
Coriander	1	Parsley		
Corn (sweet)	3	Grains	20	VHAP
Cornmeal	2	Grains	75	VHAP
Corn oil	2	Grains		VHAP
Cornstarch	2	Grains		VHAP
Cottage cheese	3	Mammals		
Cottonseed (meal and oil)	3	Mallow		MAP
Crabapple	3	Rose		
Cranberry	3	Heath	10	LAP
Crappie (crappy)	1	Bass		
Crayfish	1	Crustaceans		
Cream cheese	2	Cheese		
Cream of tartar	4	Grape		
Cream peas	2	Legume	15	MHAP
Crenshaw melon	2	Gourd	5	MAP
Croaker	1	Croaker		VHAP
Crookneck (summer crookneck)	1	Gourd	5	LAP

ALPHABETIZED FOOD	CHE PHASE	FOOD FAMILY	CARBOHYDRATE CONTENT [CHO]	ALLERGY POTENTIAL
Cucumber	1	Gourd	5	
Cucumber pickles	4	Gourd		
Cumin	1	Parsley		
Curly cress	1	Mustard		
Curly endive (chicory)	1	Composite	5	
Currant (red, black, white)	4	Beet	15	MAP
Cushaw squash	1	Gourd		LAP
Cusk	1	Codfish		VHAP
Dab	1	Flounder		VHAP
Dandelion (greens)	1	Composite	10	
Dasheen (upland taro)	4	Arum		
Date	4	Palm		
Date plum	4	Ebony		
Deer (venison)	1	Mammals		
Delicious squash	1	Gourd	10	LAP
Dewberry	3	Rose		MHAP
Dill	1	Parsley		
Dittany	1	Mint		
Dock	1			
Dollarfish	1	Flounder		VHAP
Dove	1	Birds		
Drumfish	1	Croaker		VHAP
Duck and eggs	1	Birds		
Dulse	1	Algae		
Dungeness crab	1	Crustaceans		
East Indian arrowroot	1	Ginger		
Edam cheese	2	Cheese		
Eggs	1	Birds		
Eggplant	1	Potato	5	
Elderberry	3	Honeysuckle	15	MHAP
Elk	1	Mammals		
Emmenthal cheese	4	Cheese		
Endive	1	Composite	5	

ALPHABETIZED FOOD	CHE PHASE	FOOD FAMILY	CARBOHYDRATE CONTENT [CHO]	ALLERGY POTENTIAL
Fava bean	3	Legume		
Fennel (finocchio)	1	Parsley	5	
Fenugreek (in curry)	1	Legume		
Field peas	2	Legume	15	MHAP
Fig	4	Mulberry	20	
Filbert	3	Birch		MHAP
Flounder	1	Flounder		VHAP
Flour artichoke	2	Composite		
Fluke	1	Flounder		
Fresh water drumfish	1	Croaker		
Frog (frog legs)	1	Frog		
Garbanzo (chickpea)	3	Legume	15	MHAP
Garden cress	1	Mustard	5	
Garlic	1	Lily		MAP
Gelatin from beef	1	Mammals		
Gelatin from pork	1	Mammals		MHAP
Germ from wheat	2	Grains	45	VHAP
Gherkin	1	Gourd		
Gherkin pickles	4	Gourd		
Ginger	1	Ginger		
Ginseng (tea)	1	Ginseng		
Gluten flour	3	Grains		VHAP
Goat's milk cheese	1	Cheese		
Goat (kid)	1	Mammals		
Goat milk	1	Mammals		
Golden nugget squash	1	Gourd		LAP
Goldenrod (tea)	1	Composite		
Goose and eggs	1	Birds		
Gooseberry	3	Beet	10	MHAP
Gorgonzola cheese	4	Fungus/ Mammal		
Gouda cheese	2	Cheese		
Graham flour	3	Grains		VHAP
Grana cheese	3	Mammals		

ALPHABETIZED FOOD	CHE PHASE	FOOD FAMILY	CARBOHYDRATE CONTENT [CHO]	ALLERGY POTENTIAL
Grape (all varieties)	4	Grape	15	LAP
Grapefruit (all varieties)	4	Citrus	15	
Great northern bean	3	Legume		
Green bean	3	Legume		MAP
Green olive	2	Olive	10	
Green peas	2	Legume	15	MHAP
Green tea	1	Tea		
Grits (hominy)	3	Grains	20	
Ground cherry	1	Potato		
Grouper	1	Sea bass		VHAP
Gruyere cheese	4	Cheese		
Guava	1	Myrtle		
Guinea hen	1	Birds		
Gurnard	1	Gurnard		VHAP
Gyetost cheese	2	Cheese		
Haddock	1	Codfish		VHAP
Hake	1	Codfish		VHAP
Halibut	1	Flounder		VHAP
Ham	1	Mammals		MHAP
Hard cheese	2	Cheese		
Harvestfish	1	Harvestfish		VHAP
Hazelnut	3	Birch		MHAP
Hearthnut	4	Walnut		MHAP
Hearts of palm	3	Palm		
Hibiscus (roselle) (tea)	1	Mallow		
Hickory nut	4	Walnut		MHAP
Honey (commercial, raw Tupelo)	4	Miscellaneous	80	
Honey bee pollen and related products	2	Miscellaneous		
Honeycomb	4	Miscellaneous		
Honeydew melon	2	Gourd	5	MAP
Hop, alcohol	4	Mulberry		
Horehound	1	Mint		

ALPHABETIZED FOOD	CHE PHASE	FOOD FAMILY	CARBOHYDRATE CONTENT [CHO]	ALLERGY POTENTIAL
Horse	1	Mammals		
Horseradish	1	Mustard		
Hubbard squash	1	Gourd	10	LAP
Huckleberry	3	Heath	15	MHAP
Iceberg (crisphead) lettuce	1	Composite	5	LAP
India gum	2	Cocoa		
Jack bean	3	Legume		
Jalapeno pepper	1	Potato		
Jerusalem artichoke (sunchoke)	2	Composite	10	
Jicama	1	Legume		
Juniper berry	3	Pine		
Kafir	3	Grains		
Kale	1	Mustard	5	
Karaya gum	2	Cocoa		
Kelp (seaweed)	1	Algae		
Kidney bean	3	Legume	60	
King whiting	1	Croaker		VHAP
Kiwi fruit (Chinese gooseberry)	4	Actinidia		LAP
Kohlrabi	1	Mustard	5	
Kumquat	3	Citrus		
Lamb	1	Mammals		LAP
Lamb's lettuce	1	Composite	5	LAP
Lamb's quarters	1	Beet		
Lecithin	2	Legume	in adults, MHAP in children, LAP	
Leek	1	Lily	10	
Lemon	3	Citrus	10	
Lemon balm	1	Mint		
Lentil (plain, pink)	3	Legume		
Lettuce	1	Composite	5	LAP
Licorice	1	Legume		
Lima bean	3	Legume	20	

ALPHABETIZED FOOD	CHE PHASE	FOOD FAMILY	CARBOHYDRATE CONTENT [CHO]	ALLERGY POTENTIAL
Limburger cheese	4	Fungus/ Mammal		
Lime	3	Citrus	10	
Lingcod	1	Codfish		VHAP
Litchi nut (lichi)	4	Soapberry		MHAP
Lobster species	1	Crustaceans		LAP
Loganberry	4	Rose	15	MHAP
Longberry	3	Rose		MHAP
Loose-leaf lettuce	1	Composite	5	LAP
Loquat	3	Rose		
Lovage	1	Parsley		
Macadamia nut	4	Macadamia		MHAP
Mace	1	Nutmeg		
Mackerel	1	Mackerel		
Mahi mahi	1	Dolphin		
Malanga	4	Arum		
Malt	3	Grains		LAP
Maltose	3	Grains		LAP
Mammoth squash	1	Gourd		
Mango	4	Cashew		LAP
Manioc	4	Spurge		
Marjoram	1	Mint		
Marlin	1	Marlin		VHAP
Masur bean	3	Legume		
Matchless lettuce	1	Composite	5	LAP
Mate	3	Holly		
May Apple	3	May Apple		
Mealy potato	2	Potato		MHAP
Melons	2,4	Gourd	5	MAP
Melopepo squash	1	Gourd		LAP
Menhaden	1	Herring		VHAP
Menthol	1	Mint		
Millet	3	Grains		
Mint	1	Mint		
Minnow	1	Minnow		
Mirliton squash	1	Gourd		LAP
Molasses	4	Grains	60	
Monkfish	1	Shark		VHAP

ALPHABETIZED FOOD	CHE PHASE	FOOD FAMILY	CARBOHYDRATE CONTENT [CHO]	ALLERGY POTENTIAL
Monterrey Jack cheese	2	Cheese		
Morel	4	Fungus		
Moose	1	Mammals		
Mozzarella cheese	3	Mammals		
Muenster cheese	4	Fungus/ Mammal		
Mulberry	4	Mulberry	15	
Mullet (fish)	1	Mullet		VHAP
Mung bean sprouts	1	Legume		
Mung beans	3	Legume		
Murcot	3	Citrus		
Muscadine	4	Grape		
Muscle meats (steak, roast, tongue, and others)	1	Mammals		MAP
Mushroom	4	Fungus	5	MAP
Muskellunge	1	Pike		
Muskmelon	2	Gourd	5	MAP
Muskrat	1	Mammals		
Mussel	1	Mollusks		
Mustard greens	2	Mustard	5	MHAP
Mustard seed	2	Mustard		MHAP
Mutton	2	Mammals		
Mysost cheese	2	Cheese		
Name (yampi)	4	Yam		LAP
Nasturtium	2	Nasturtium		
Navy bean	3	Legume		
Nectarine	4	Rose	20	
Neufchatel cheese	2	Cheese		
Northern scup (porgy)	1	Porgy		VHAP
Nutmeg	1	Nutmeg		
Oakleaf (green, bronze) lettuce	1	Composite	5	LAP
Oats (flakes)	3	Grains	70	LAP
Ocean catfish	1	Sea catfish		VHAP
Ocean perch	1	Rosefish		VHAP

ALPHABETIZED FOOD	CHE PHASE	FOOD FAMILY	CARBOHYDRATE CONTENT [CHO]	ALLERGY POTENTIAL
Octopus	1	Mollusks		
Okra	1	Mallow	5	
Olive	2	Olive		
Olive oil	2	Olive		
Onion	1	Lily	10	MAP
Opposum	1	Mammals		
Orange (all varieties)	4	Citrus	15	MHAP
Oregano	1	Mint		
Organ meats (liver, kidney, tripe, and others)	1	Mammals		
Oyster	1	Mollusks		
Paddlefish	1	Paddlefish		
Palm cabbage	3	Palm		
Palmetto cabbage	3	Palm		
Papaya	3	Papaya		
Paprika	1	Potato		
Parmesan cheese	3	Cheese		
Parsley	1	Parsley		
Parsnip	1	Parsley	15	
Patent flour	3	Grains		VHAP
Pattypan squash	1	Gourd		LAP
Pawpaw (custard apple)	3	Papaya		
Peach	3	Rose	10	LAP
Peafowl	1	Birds		
Pear	4	Rose	15	
Peas	2	Legume	15	MHAP
Peanut	3	Legume		MHAP
Peanut oil	3	Legume		MHAP
Pecan	4	Walnut		MHAP
Pepino (melon pear)	1	Potato		
Peppercorn	1	Pepper		
Peppermint	1	Mint		
Persian melon	2	Gourd	5	MAP
Persimmon (American)	4	Ebony		
Persimmon (Japanese)	4	Ebony	20	

ALPHABETIZED FOOD	CHE PHASE	FOOD FAMILY	CARBOHYDRATE CONTENT [CHO]	ALLERGY POTENTIAL
Petrale	1	Flounder		VHAP
Pheasant	1	Birds		
Pickerel	1	Pike		
Pigeon (squab)	1	Birds		
Pike, northern	1	Pike		
Pilchard (sardine)	1	Herring		VHAP
Pimiento	1	Potato		
Pineapple	3	Pineapple	15	LAP
Pine nut	3	Pine		
Pinto bean	3	Legume		
Pinyon (pinon)	3	Pine		
Pistachio	4	Cashew		MHAP
Plaice	1	Flounder		VHAP
Plantain	4	Banana		
Plum	4	Rose	15	MAP
Poi	4	Arum		
Pollack	1	Codfish		VHAP
Pomegranate	3	Pomegranate		
Pomelo	4	Citrus	15	
Pompano	1	Jack		VHAP
Popped corn	2	Grains	75	VHAP
Pork	1	Mammals		MHAP
Porpoise	1	Mammals		
Port du Salut cheese	4	Fungus/ Mammal		
Potato	2	Potato	20	MHAP
Prairie chicken	1	Birds		
Prickly pear	4	Amaryllis		
Primost cheese	2	Cheese		
Prizehead lettuce	1	Composite	5	LAP
Provolone cheese	3	Cheese		
Prune	4	Rose	70	MAP
Pulque	4	Amaryllis		
Pumpkin	1	Gourd	5	
Pumpkinseed	1	Bass		
Pumpkin squash	1	Gourd		LAP
Purple hull peas	2	Legume	15	MHAP
Quahog	1	Mollusks		
Quail	1	Birds		

ALPHABETIZED FOOD	CHE PHASE	FOOD FAMILY	CARBOHYDRATE CONTENT [CHO]	ALLERGY POTENTIAL
Quaker pie squash	1	Gourd		LAP
Queensland blue squash	1	Gourd		LAP
Quince	4	Rose	15	
Rabbit (hare)	1	Mammals		
Raccoon	1	Mammals		
Radish	1	Mustard	5	
Ragweed and related inhalants	4	Composite		
Raisin (all varieties)	4	Grape	75	
Rape	1	Mustard		
Raspberry (black, purple, red)	4	Rose	15	MHAP
Red-leaf chicory (arugula)	1	Composite	5	LAP
Red pepper	2	Potato		
Red-sweet pepper	1	Potato		
Reggiana cheese	3	Cheese		
Rennin (rennet)	1	Mammals		
Rhubarb	1	Buckwheat		
Rice	2	Grains	75	LAP
Ricotta cheese	2	Cheese		
Ripe olive	2	Olive	5	
Romaine (cos) lettuce	1	Composite	5	LAP
Romano cheese	3	Cheese		
Roguette lettuce	1	Composite	5	LAP
Rosefish	1	Rosefish		VHAP
Rosehips	3	Rose		
Rosemary	1	Mint		
Ruffed grouse (partridge)	1	Birds		
Rutabaga	2	Mustard	10	
Rye	3	Grains	75	LAP
Safflower (oil)	1	Composite		
Saffron	1	Iris		

ALPHABETIZED FOOD	CHE PHASE	FOOD FAMILY	CARBOHYDRATE CONTENT [CHO]	ALLERGY POTENTIAL
Sage	1	Mint		
Sago palm (starch)	3	Palm		
Sailfish	1	Marlin		VHAP
Salad bowl lettuce	1	Composite	5	LAP
Salmon	1	Salmon		LAP
Salsify (oyster plant)	2	Composite	15	
Salt (table, sea)	1	Miscellancous		
Sandab	1	Flounder		VHAP
Santa Claus melon	2	Gourd	5	MAP
Sapodilla	1	Sapodilla		
Sapota (edible fruit)	3	Sapodilla		
Sapsago cheese	2	Cheese		
Sardine (pilchard)	1	Herring		VHAP
Sardo cheese	3	Cheese		
Sarsparilla	1	Lily		
Saskatoon	3	Rose		
Sassafras	2	Laurel		
Satsuma	3	Citrus		
Sauger	1	Perch		
Sausage	1	Mammals		MHAP
Sausage casings	1	Mammals		
Savory	1	Mint		
Savoy cabbage	1	Mustard	5	
Scallop	1	Mollusks		
Sea Bass	1	Sea Bass (grouper)		VHAP
Sea herring	1	Herring		VHAP
Sea kale	1	Mustard		
Sea lion	1	Mammals		
Sea robin	1	Gurnard		VHAP
Sea trout	1	Croaker		VHAP
Sesame (seed, oil)	2	Pedalium		
Shad	1	Herring		
Shad roe	1	Herring		VHAP
Shallot	1	Lily		
Shark	1	Shark		VHAP
Sheephead	1	Croaker		VHAP

ALPHABETIZED FOOD	CHE PHASE	FOOD FAMILY	CARBOHYDRATE CONTENT [CHO]	ALLERGY POTENTIAL
Shrimp (prawn)	1	Crustaceans		
Silver perch	1	Croaker		VHAP
Silverside (whitebait, shiner)	1	Silverside		VHAP
Skipjack	1	Mackerel		VHAP
Sloe plum	3	Rose		LAP
Small sugar squash	1	Gourd		
Smelt	1	Smelt		
Snail	1	Mollusks		
Snake (rattlesnake)	1	Reptiles		
Snap bean	3	Legume		
Snow crab	1	Crustaceans		
Soft cheese	2	Cheese		
Sole	1	Flounder		VHAP
Sorghum grain	3	Grains		
Sorghum syrup	3	Grains		
Sorrel	1	Buckwheat		
Soybean	2	Legume		in adults, MHAP in children, LAP
Soy flour	2	Legume	30	in adults, MHAP, in children LAP
Soy grits	2	Legume		in adults, MHAP in children, LAP
Soy milk	2	Legume		in adults, MHAP in children, LAP
Soy oil	2	Legume		in adults, MHAP, in children, LAP
Soy sauce	4	Legume		in adults, MHAP, in children, LAP
Spaghetti squash	1	Gourd		LAP
Spanish melon	2	Gourd	5	MAP
Spearmint	1	Mint		
Spinach	1	Beet	5	MAP
Split peas	2	Legume	15	MHAP
Spot fish	1	Croaker		VHAP
Spotted bass	1	Sea Bass		VHAP
Sprouts, beans	1	Legume	5	
Squash	1	Gourd		LAP
Squid	1	Mollusks		

ALPHABETIZED FOOD	CHE PHASE	FOOD FAMILY	CARBOHYDRATE CONTENT [CHO]	ALLERGY POTENTIAL
Squirrel	1	Mammals		
Stilton cheese	4	Fungus/ Mammal		
Strawberry	3	Rose	5	MHAP
String cheese	3	Mammals		
Straightneck (summer straightneck) squash	1	Gourd	5	LAP
String beans	1	Legume	5	
Striped bass (rockfish)	1	Sea bass		VHAP
Sturgeon (caviar)	1	Sturgeon		
Sucker	1	Sucker		
Sugar beet	3	Beet		LAP
Sugar from beet	4	Beet		
Sugar from cane (turbinado)	4	Grains	99.5	MHAP
Sugar from corn ("Cerelose," dextrose, "Dyno")	4	Grains	99.5	
Sugar from maple	4	Maple	99.5	
Sunfish	1	Bass		
Sunflower (seed, oil, meal)	1	Composite		
Swamp cabbage	3	Palm		
Sweet corn	3	Grains		
Sweet potato (yam)	4	Yam	25	LAP
Swiss chard	1	Mustard	5	
Swiss cheese	4	Cheese		
Swordfish	1	Swordfish		VHAP
Syrup (corn) ("Cartose," glucose, "Sweetose")	4	Grains		VHAP
Syrup (maple)	4	Maple	65	
Syrup (sorghum)	3	Grains		
Tabasco	2	Potato		
Table queen squash	1	Gourd		LAP

ALPHABETIZED FOOD	CHE PHASE	FOOD FAMILY	CARBOHYDRATE CONTENT [CHO]	ALLERGY POTENTIAL
Tahini	2	Pedalium		
Tamarind	1	Legume		
Tangelo	3	Citrus		
Tapioca	4	Spurge		LAP
Taro (root)	4	Arum		
Tarpon	1	Tarpon		VHAP
Tarragon	1	Composite		
Tea, black	4	Tea		
Tea, green	1	Tea		
Terrapin (diamondback terrapin)	1	Reptiles		
Thyme	1	Mint		
Tilefish	1	Tilefish		VHAP
Tofu	2	Legume	in adults, in children,	MHAP LAP
Tomatillo	1	Potato		
Tomato	1	Potato	5	MHAP
Triticale	2	Grains		
Trout species	1	Salmon		
Truffle	4	Fungus		
Tuna	1	Mackerel		VHAP
Turban squash	1	Gourd	10	LAP
Turbot	1	Flounder		VHAP
Turkey and eggs	1	Birds		
Tumeric	1	Ginger		
Turnip	2	Mustard		
Turnip (greens)	1	Mustard	5	
Turtle (green, snapping)	1	Reptiles		
Ugli fruit	3	Citrus		
Upland cress	1	Mustard		
Vanilla (bean, extract)	1	Orchid		LAP
Veal	1	Mammals		
Vegetable spaghetti squash	1	Gourd		LAP
Vinegars (cider, wine, rice, etc.)	4	Fungus		LAP

ALPHABETIZED FOOD	CHE PHASE	FOOD FAMILY	CARBOHYDRATE CONTENT [CHO]	ALLERGY POTENTIAL
Virginia mammoth squash	1	Gourd		
Walleyed pike	1	Perch		LAP
Walnut (black, English)	4	Walnut		MHAP
Walrus	1	Mammals		
Water celery	1	Parsley		
Watercress	1	Mustard	5	
Watermelon	2	Gourd	5	MAP
Waxy red potato	2	Potato		MHAP
Waxy white potato	2	Potato		MHAP
Weakfish (spotted sea trout)	1	Croaker		VHAP
Wheat	3	Grains		VHAP
Wheat flour	3			VHAP
Wheat germ	2		45	VHAP
Whey cheese	2	Cheese		
White mustard	2	Mustard		MHAP
White perch	1	Bass		
White perch	1	Sea Bass		VHAP
Whitebush scallop squash	1	Gourd		LAP
Whitefish	1	Whitefish		
White pepper	1	Pepper		
Whiting	1	Codfish		VHAP
Whitloof chicory (Belgian or French endive)	1	Composite		
Whole wheat flour	3	Grains	70	VHAP
Wild rice	2	Grains		LAP
Wineberry	3	Rose		MHAP
Wintergreen	3	Heath		
Yam	4	Yam	25	LAP
Yautia	4	Arum		
Yellow bass	1	Bass		
Yellow jack (yellowtail)	1	Jack		VHAP

ALPHABETIZED FOOD	CHE PHASE	FOOD FAMILY	CARBOHYDRATE CONTENT [CHO]	ALLERGY POTENTIAL
Yellow perch	1	Perch		
Yogurt	1	Mammals		
Youngberry	3	Rose		MHAP
Yuca	4	Spurge		
Yucca (soap plant)	1	Lily		
Zucchini squash	1	Gourd	5	LAP

If you have suggestions for additions to, deletions from, or modifications of this listing, please contact Dr. Trowbridge through the publisher.

Four-Phase
Yeast Control Recipes

Candidiasis victims who are faithful to the yeast control diet described in this section often find relief from the pressures and unhappiness of their disorders while those merely taking antiyeast medication may not. The yeast control diet combined with the extensive 4-phase CHE food lists furnish you with ingredients for menu plans and recipes. We suggest that you apply the information for daily food shopping, preparation, and consumption—enjoyable living.

Among food preparation methods our foremost choice is to prepare and eat freshly picked and washed raw vegetables. Next best is consuming freshly washed store-bought raw vegetables from a health foods or organic gardening store (or from a grocery store or supermarket). We urge you to employ steamed or minimum-moisture (waterless) cooking. You might consider (as less preferred methods) using microwave, broiling, roasting, wokking, boiling, and dry frying, but never deep frying.

We recommend the minimum-moisture, or "waterless," cooking method to maintain the natural nutritional value of your food. In minimum-moisture cooking the food is tenderized by heating but kept below its boiling point, without adding water. Thus, many nutrients that might otherwise be boiled away or thrown away in the cooking water are retained instead for the better nourishment of your body. By utilizing the most advanced engineering and technology in minimum-moisture cookware, maximum nutrition is maintained. A study performed at the Yale Nutrition Laboratory, Yale University School of Medicine in New Haven, Connecticut, and published in the *Journal of the American Dietetic Association* (December 1983) measured the average retention of eight vitamins and minerals in twelve vegetables after they were cooked by the minimum-moisture method, as compared to the water-to-cover method. Their results are shown in the table below:

| NUTRIENT MEASURED AFTER COOKING | PERCENTAGE OF NUTRIENT RETAINED IN THE COOKED FOODS: | |
	Minimum-Moisture Method	Water-to-Cover Method
Calcium	94.4	77.8
Iron	90.4	76.7
Phosphorus	92.3	72.1
Thiamine (vitamin B_1)	91.0	62.6
Riboflavin (vitamin B_2)	87.9	63.1
Niacin (vitamin B_3)	91.3	59.2
Ascorbic acid (vitamin C)	73.3	52.7
Carotene (vitamin A)	94.7	79.1

You can obtain up to 54 percent more nutritional value from properly cooked foods, almost as much real food value as is found in uncooked vegetables.

Cookware used in the minimum-moisture method of cooking has been available for a long time. Some manufacturers of the cookware are VolRath™, Temp-Tone™, Colonial™, and Carico™. Nutri-Tech™, manufactured by Carico Distributors, Inc., of Fort Lauderdale, Florida (not available in stores; sold only by direct marketing) is the cookware we personally use for taking advantage of minimum-moisture cookery. For information on the Nutri-Tech™ system of cooking, please consider contacting our foods preparation consultant, J. J. Wetz, Superior Home Products, 1101 Forest Cove Drive, Kingwood TX 77339; (713) 358-3253.

Our focus in this chapter is mostly on the more difficult

phase-one aspect of Candida control eating to help introduce you to the whole dietary program. Phase one consists nearly exclusively of meat, eggs, vegetables, and yogurt—the MEVY diet—to starve your invading yeast for four weeks or so. The MEVY diet provides very little nourishment for fungi, along with yogurt, the natural antiyeast antidote. It is true that the phase-1 CHE *is* quite stringent, less appetizing, not too varied, and rather different from the diet you have followed until now. But your former diet most likely has contributed to your infestation with *Candida albicans*. Remember, the MEVY diet is actually therapeutic, so we encourage you to decide to "take your medicine" in the form of the phase-one menu plan and progress on the path to getting well. Before getting started, don't forget to seek your physician's advice.

Our seven days' menus that follow provide a simple guideline for easy-to-fix, fun foods. When most people first see the phase-1 CHE, they become discouraged that "there is nothing to eat." Such thinking may be considered as an illustration of how distorted our eating patterns have become in modern Western society. As with other diet plans, wholesome meats and vegetables are part of the MEVY diet, but you must omit the gravies, sauces, breads, biscuits, and fruits.

Most people know what vegetables they prefer in salads and with main courses at meals. We suggest that you start with these preferences. Add any others that are in season or available in your area. (Try to eat only fresh vegetables.) We advise that your experimentation with the MEVY diet is valid—and fun. Try new and different flavors. You will surprise yourself with how much enjoyment you get from eating healthfully. Eat as many vegetables in a day as you wish—with meals, for snacks, as "desserts."

Prepare new types of beverages as special treats, too. We recommend that you try the many excellent flavors of herbal teas to add variety to your eating. Bottled sparkling waters add a refreshing pause to a tiring day. Add lime or lemon juice to the sparkling water to create a little zest. Coffee substitutes are useful for those people weaning themselves from drinking caffeinated and decaffeinated coffee; health food stores often have a fine selection of coffee substitutes.

Spices add zest to vegetables, meats, eggs, soups, salads,

dips, and other items. We suggest you use them in combinations to create new taste sensations all your own. Be mindful, however, of many spice mixtures that have a yeast base or otherwise depend on yeast flavoring for their uniqueness. Stay away from anything having to do with yeast until you are into the phase-4 CHE program.

SEVEN DAYS' MENUS FOR PHASE-1 CHE: THE MEVY DIET

An asterisk indicates the recipe for this food is provided below.

DAY ONE

Breakfast	Lunch	Dinner
Ranch Omelet*	Steamed broccoli,	Spinach Salad*
1 cup yogurt	carrots,	Gumbo*
Coffee substitutes	cucumbers	Cauliflower
sold in health food	Baked chicken	Quick Dip*
stores such as		
Cafix™, Inka™,		
Pionier™, Pero™,		
Postum™, Bambu™,		
and the		
noncaffeinated		
herbal teas.		

DAY TWO

Breakfast	Lunch	Dinner
2 scrambled eggs	Vegetable soup	Lettuce Salad
1 cup yogurt	Salad of choice	Lo-Cal Mexican
Coffee substitute	Shrimp Dip*	Fish
		Asparagus
		Turnips

DAY THREE

Breakfast	Lunch	Dinner
Hogan's Breakfast* Coffee substitute	Raw vegetables with Herb Dressing* Tuna salad made with Mayonnaise Our Way* Nine Vegetable Cocktail*	Lemon-Fried Chicken* Raw or steamed cabbage, squash, and carrots Salad Dressing and Vegetable Marinade* Yogurt Shake*

DAY FOUR

Breakfast	Lunch	Dinner
Broiled breakfast steak Carrots Squash Coffee substitute	Broiled veal Collard greens Italian-style Zucchini Squash or Eggplant*	Scampi* Curried Cauliflower* Cole Slaw*

DAY FIVE

Breakfast	Lunch	Dinner
2 hard- or soft-boiled eggs Celery and carrots with Quick Dip* Coffee substitute	Chuck Wagon Stew* Spro-gurt* Total Juice with Tomatoes*	Meatless Vegetable Soup* "Stir-Fry" Vegetables* Herbal tea

DAY SIX

Breakfast	Lunch	Dinner
2 fried eggs 1 cup yogurt Mineral water	Zucchini and Tomatoes* Deviled Eggs* Yogurt "Popsicles"™ ("Yo-sicles")	Vegetables of choice with Homemade Chicken Stock* Roller-Dippies* Salad of choice Basic Vege-Yogurt Dip*

DAY SEVEN

Breakfast	Lunch	Dinner
2 hard- or soft-boiled eggs	Chicken Egg Drop Soup*	Veal steak
Broiled fish	Zucchini Supreme*	Tomato Sauce*
"Almost Tartar" Sauce*		Salad of choice
Coffee substitute		Mayonnaise Our Way*

PHASE-1 CHE RECIPES: THE MEVY DIET

Ranch Omelet

½ bell pepper, chopped
½ onion, chopped
parsley sprigs, minced
1 tomato (or any other vegetable you like)
Ham or baked fish, minced (optional)

1 tbs butter
3 eggs
½ tsp sea salt
1 tsp white pepper

Sauté pepper, onion, parsley, tomato, and ham in ½ tbs butter until onions are clear.

Put eggs, salt, and pepper in a small mixing bowl and mix together. Melt ½ tbs butter in pan, heat, and pour in egg mixture. When bubbles appear, place sautéed vegetables down center of omelet. Fold omelet in thirds over filling, remove, and serve.

Spinach Salad

1 head spinach, torn or sliced to desired size
1 cucumber, sliced
1 tomato, diced
2 eggs, hard-boiled

½–1 cup cauliflower, cut up (optional)
1–2 stalks celery, chopped (optional)
6 radishes sliced (optional)

Toss all ingredients together. Flavor as desired with herbs and spices. Serve with lemon and oil dressing. Fresh sprouts may be added to give extra "crunch."

Gumbo

2–3 tbs butter or safflower oil
1 medium onion, chopped
2–3 stalks celery, chopped
2 lb fresh okra, chopped
4 fresh tomatoes
8 oz tomato sauce
salt and pepper to taste

1–2 tbs chili powder
¼ bell pepper, chopped
1½ lb shrimp, cleaned
½ lb crab meat (may be canned if fresh is not available)
10 oz oysters (optional)

Melt butter in saucepan. Sauté onion until clear. Add celery. Then add cut okra and brown slightly. Add whole tomatoes and tomato sauce, salt and pepper, chili powder, and bell pepper. Simmer 20 minutes. Add cleaned shrimp, crab meat, and oysters; simmer another 10–20 minutes.

Note: Chicken may be substituted for the seafood for a chicken gumbo. When you have advanced to phase-3 CHE eating, use ¼ cup of whole wheat flour to cover the cut okra before adding; also, serve over brown rice in phase 2.

Quick Dip

1 pt yogurt
1 envelope French onion soup mix or "ranch-style" dressing or fresh/dehydrated ingredients, if available

1 tbs lemon juice
few drops tabasco sauce

Mix all ingredients together. Chill or serve immediately at room temperature, with slices, chunks, or cubes of any vegetable.

Shrimp Dip

1 cup tomato sauce
1 envelope unflavored gelatin
¼ cup water
8 oz shrimp, cleaned and coarsely chopped

½ cup cooked green onion, chopped
½ cup celery, chopped
1 cup yogurt
salt and pepper to taste
herbs and spices to taste

Heat tomato sauce. Add gelatin which has been dissolved in ¼ cup water. Let cool, then add remaining ingredients and spoon into oiled mold. Let set overnight, or until firm.

Note: After you have passed through Phase-1 CHE, an 8 oz package of cream cheese may be added to the shrimp dip to give it a richer, creamier consistency. Add the cream cheese to the heated tomato sauce and blend well; then add the gelatin.

Lo-Cal Mexican Fish

1–2 lb fish (such as snapper, trout, flounder, or farm-raised catfish), whole or fillets
1 clove garlic, freshly chopped
1 lime, freshly juiced
1 small onion, chopped
pepper to taste (black or white)

2 cups (1 lb) peeled tomatillos (green Mexican tomatoes)
2 pinches comino seed
1 clove garlic
½ onion, minced
2 serrano chilis

Pierce fish on each side with fork. Rub garlic into fish. Put fresh lime juice on inside and outside of fish. Sprinkle on black pepper (white is hotter). Marinate for 2 hours. Place in cold skillet with chopped onions. Leave on medium heat for 8 minutes. Turn fish over and cook until done, approximately 10 minutes more.

Blend tomatillos, comino seed, whole garlic clove, minced onion, and chilis and heat in a separate skillet until onions and tomatillos are clear. Pour on platter. Serve fish on top. Or place in bowl and eat like relish. Keep in refrigerator and serve with other meals as well.

Note: When you have advanced to phase-4 CHE, use ½ cup white wine when cooking fish.

No-salt variation: Mix garlic, lime, and pepper together, rub into fish, and marinate for 2 hours. Put in with 1 tsp butter (just enough to coat bottom of pan) and cook for 10 minutes. Turn fish over. Place cover on skillet and cook about 10–12 minutes more on low heat, or until fish is white and tender.

Note: This recipe contains no salt; the garlic and lime make salt unnecessary. We recommend you use a skillet that maintains an even temperature to keep the fish from burning.

Hogan's Breakfast

1 tbs safflower oil	pepper (black or white) to taste
1 tbs butter	parsley (a few sprigs, or dehydrated) to taste
2 small onions, sliced or chopped	basil (fresh or dehydrated) to taste
½ bell pepper, sliced or chopped	lean ham, chopped (optional)
3–4 medium tomatoes, sliced	4 eggs
6 oz tomato sauce	

Melt safflower oil and butter in skillet; add onions, bell pepper, tomatoes, tomato sauce, and ham. Season to taste with pepper, parsley, and basil. Cook 10–12 minutes uncovered, until the juice is thickened. Break eggs on top, whole. Cover; cook until eggs are poached just as you like them, soft, medium, or hard.

Note: This recipe can be adjusted to fit the number of people you are serving. Add any fresh vegetables you prefer—cauliflower, carrots, broccoli, whatever. When you have advanced to phase-3 CHE, serve over whole wheat toast.

Herb Dressing
(for salads and vegetables)

1 tsp dry mustard	1 tbs fresh parsely
1 tsp dillweed	½ tsp sea salt
¼ tsp tarragon	¼ tsp freshly ground black pepper
pinch thyme	⅓ cup virgin olive oil
pinch oregano	

Stir together all ingredients except olive oil until mustard is dissolved. Allow to sit for 10 minutes, then blend in olive oil, starting with ⅓ cup and adding additional oil to taste.

Note: When you have advanced to phase-3 CHE, you may also add 1 tsp soy sauce and 2 tbs vinegar.

Tuna Salad

½ cup "Mayonnaise" recipe
(see below) or plain
yogurt
1 tbs lemon juice
¼ tsp sea salt or Mrs. Dash™

7 oz tuna, crumbled
few drops tabasco sauce
1 slice small onion
1 stalk celery, coarsely cut
jalapeno peppers (optional)

Lightly blend all ingredients. Makes about 1½ cups.
Note: Chill and serve with slices, chunks, or cubes of any
vegetable.

Mayonnaise Our Way

2 eggs at room temperature
2 tbs freshly squeezed
lemon juice

¼ tsp sea salt
1¼ cup safflower or virgin
olive oil

Combine all ingredients except oil in blender at high speed
for 1 minute. Slowly add oil. Store in glass jar. Refrigerate.

Nine Vegetable Cocktail

1 pt fresh tomatoes
1 cucumber, sliced
sprigs fresh parsley
1 radish

¼ onion, sliced
1 green pepper, sliced
1 lettuce leaf
1 pt ice cubes

In an electric blender, blend together all ingredients, adding
ice cubes a few at a time. If juice tends to freeze, allow to run
a little longer before adding rest of ice. Add, if desired, salt
and pepper and other herbs and spices, 1 slender carrot, 1
stalk celery.
Note: If you wish to have the juice colder or thinner, add
more ice with the carrot and celery. Makes 1½ quarts. Recipe courtesy of the VitaMix™ Corporation.

Lemon-Fried Chicken

1 fryer chicken, skin
   removed
¼ cup fresh lemon juice
¼ tsp garlic salt
¾ tsp sea salt

¼ tsp ground thyme
¼ tsp ground marjoram
⅛ tsp pepper
½ tsp grated lemon rind
2 tbs butter

Cut chicken into serving pieces and place in a large, shallow pan. Mix the lemon juice, garlic salt, salt, thyme, marjoram, pepper, and lemon rind and pour over chicken. Marinate in refrigerator for at least 3 hours, turning occasionally, then drain chicken on absorbent paper.

Preheat skillet, add butter, cook for 15 minutes with lid partially on. Turn chicken, cook for 10 minutes with lid partially on. Place cover on tightly and cook for 5 minutes more. Total cooking time is 30 minutes.

Note: If you use a skillet capable of "greaseless frying," do not add butter.

Salad Dressing and Vegetable Marinade

½ cup safflower oil
juice of 2 lemons

2 tsp oregano
1 tsp garlic powder

Mix all ingredients in a pint jar. Finish filling the jar with water. Shake well to mix, then pour over vegetables and marinate in refrigerator 2 hours or longer. Other herbs and spices may be added to flavor as desired.

Some vegetables from which to choose (sliced or chopped): squash, radishes, cucumbers, broccoli, carrots, bell pepper, cauliflower, onions.

Note: If spinach or lettuce is used, add just before serving.

Yogurt Shake ("Yo-Shakes")

1 cup plain yogurt
1 cup ice cubes
1 raw egg (optional)

dash of vanilla extract or
other natural flavor
extracts (optional)

Blend all ingredients well in electric blender; serve immediately. If extracts are not available, artificially sweetened
packages of Kool-Aid™ or Wyler's™ drinks may be used sparingly. When advanced to phase-3 and phase-4 CHE, fresh
fruits may be added.

Italian-Style Zucchini Squash or Eggplant

Italian seasoning, to taste
pepper, to taste
1 green tomato, sliced or
chopped
2 ripe tomatoes, sliced or
chopped
1 small onion, sliced or
chopped

1 tbs butter
3 zucchini squash or 1
eggplant, sliced
other spices and herbs to
flavor, as desired

Combine all ingredients in pan; cook for a few minutes (try
not to overcook).

Scampi
(Shrimp in Garlic Butter)

4 tbs butter
1 clove garlic, finely minced
1½–2 lbs large shrimp,
cleaned and deveined

salt and pepper to taste

Using an electric skillet, melt butter and add garlic; simmer 3 minutes. Turn up heat to 375 degrees and cook shrimp
5–7 minutes, stirring frequently. Shrimp is done when it
turns pink and white. Serve with attractive tossed salad.

Curried Cauliflower

1–2 cups cauliflower, cut up
2 thin slices onion
½ cup fat-skimmed chicken
  stock
½ tsp butter

1 tsp curry powder (or
  more, to taste)
½ tsp cumin seeds
  (optional)

Combine cauliflower, onion, chicken stock, butter, curry powder, and cumin seeds in a small pan. Cover and simmer over low heat for 5 minutes. Uncover and simmer until most of the liquid has evaporated.

Note: Other vegetables may be "curried" in this way too.

Cole Slaw

¼ head cabbage, grated
2 carrots, grated
6 radishes, sliced
½ turnip, sliced or chopped
  (optional)

1 stalk celery, chopped
Spices and herbs to flavor,
  as desired

Toss all ingredients together.

Note: For an interesting dressing, combine with any of the several yogurt-based dips described in this recipe section.

Chuck Wagon Stew

2 lb beef chuck, cut in
  1½-inch cubes
2 tsp sea salt
¼ tsp pepper (black or
  white)
1 tsp chili powder
¼ tsp thyme
1 bay leaf
6 small whole onions, or 1
  large onion, cut into
  small pieces

1 green pepper, coarsely cut
3–4 fresh tomatoes, sliced
8 oz tomato sauce
6 carrots, cut in 2-inch
  chunks
4 stalks celery, chopped

Preheat 6-quart roaster over medium heat until a paper towel scorches. Add cubes of beef chuck and brown. Add salt, pepper, chili powder, thyme, bay leaf, onion, and green pepper to meat after browning. Cook 45 minutes to 1 hour. Then add all other ingredients at one time. Gradually reduce heat to low. Cook another 1–1½ hours. Total cooking time is 2–2½ hours. No additional liquid should be needed. Serves 6 to 8 people.

Note: After you have advanced to phase-2 CHE, add 6 medium potatoes (quartered) when you combine the final ingredients.

Spro-Gurt

Mix fresh sprouts into your plain yogurt to provide a crunchy, tasty, change-of-pace breakfast, side dish, or anytime snack. Use spices or herbs to flavor, as desired.

Total Juice with Tomatoes

1 pt fresh tomatoes	2 radishes
1 pt ice cubes	½ cup fresh endive leaves
1 small carrot	½ cup fresh lettuce
½ cup fresh beets	½ cup turnip leaves
⅓ raw cucumber	⅓ cup fresh spinach
⅓ cup cabbage leaves	¼ cup parsley

In an electric blender, blend tomatoes; add ice cubes a few at a time.

If juice freezes, allow to run until thawed.

As blender runs, add any one or a combination of the remaining ingredients.

If juice becomes too thick, add more ice. If drink freezes, allow to run longer to thaw. Taste. Add salt and pepper and other herbs and spices to flavor, as desired. Recipe courtesy of the VitaMix™ Corporation.

Meatless Vegetable Soup

5 tbs or less butter
¼ cup diced carrots
¼ cup diced celery
¼ cup sliced onion
3 cups water
½ cup tomatoes, chopped
1 cup fresh spinach, chopped (optional)

1 bouillon cube (if available, use fresh beef stock in place of water and bouillon cube)
¾ tsp salt
¼ tsp paprika
3 tbs parsley, freshly chopped

Melt 3 tbs butter in medium-size saucepan. Add carrots, celery, and onion. Slowly cook for 10 minutes. Add water, cover, and simmer 1 hour. Melt remaining butter. Stir in tomatoes and cook, stirring until smooth. Simmer 15 minutes. Add spinach the last 5 minutes, if desired. Add beef stock or bouillon cube and water.

Beat the soup with a wire whisk or a fork to break up the vegetables (or blend before cooking and simmer only 5 minutes in all). Add salt, paprika, and parsley. Makes 3 cups.

Note: When advanced to phase-2 CHE, add ½ cup diced potatoes after cooking carrots, celery, and onions for 10 minutes; cook with potatoes for 2 more minutes, then simmer as instructed. When advanced to phase-3 CHE, stir in ½ tbs whole wheat flour with the tomatoes.

Stir-Fry Vegetables

1 cup cabbage, shredded
¼ cup onion, sliced
½ cup celery, sliced diagonally
1 tsp butter
1 tbs freshly squeezed lemon juice

garlic powder
sea salt
pepper
spices (Mrs. Dash™)

Place vegetables in skillet with the butter and lemon juice. Cover and simmer over medium heat for 3–5 minutes. Uncover and add garlic powder, sea salt, pepper, and Mrs. Dash™. Stir well and continue to cook 2 minutes, or until vegetables are tender crisp. Use other spices and herbs to flavor, as desired.

Note: This recipe is good served hot or cold. If you serve it cold, you may wish to add more lemon juice just before serving.

Zucchini and Tomatoes

2 zucchini, sliced
1 onion, sliced or chopped
2 tomatoes, sliced or
  chopped

sprigs of fresh parsley
pat butter or 1 tbs safflower
  oil (optional)

Sauté zucchini and onion until tender; waterless cookware will permit you to sauté without butter or oil. Add tomato; continue to stir until cooked. Add parsley (add sea salt and other spices and herbs as desired) and serve.

Deviled Eggs

6 hard-boiled eggs, halved
  lengthwise, yolks re-
  moved and reserved
salt and pepper

paprika
2 tsp ground mustard
  (optional)
2 tbs yogurt

In a small bowl mash the cooked egg yolks. Add salt, pepper, paprika, mustard, and yogurt. Mix well and spoon back into the cooked egg whites. Arrange on a platter and sprinkle more paprika over the tops.

Yogurt "Popsicles™" ("Yo-Sicles")

plain yogurt

dash of vanilla extract or
  other natural flavor
  extracts

Mix extract into yogurt until evenly distributed, then pour yogurt into popsicle molds. Insert wooden handle sticks. Place in freezer until frozen. Keep "Yo-sicles" handy for quick snacks, desserts. Especially enjoyed by children.

Homemade Chicken Stock

6 chicken breasts, skinned
and all visible fat
removed
6 stalks celery, including any
leaves
1 small onion, peeled and
studded with 3 whole
cloves

several sprigs fresh parsley
plus any available stems
1 tsp white pepper
3 bay leaves

Place all ingredients in a large pot. Cover with water. Bring to rapid boil. Cover, lower heat, and gently simmer for 30–40 minutes, until chicken is tender. Add more water if needed during the cooking. Remove chicken from the pot. When cool enough to handle, cut chicken meat from the bones and return bones to the stock pot. (After it cools to room temperature, refrigerate the chicken meat to use in salads, soups, etc.) Continue to simmer the stock for 1 hour. Remove from heat and let cool enough to strain the stock into covered containers and refrigerate. When all fat has congealed, carefully remove and discard. Stock may be frozen for future use.

Note: This is a basic chicken stock. Any fresh or dried herbs or spices may be added during cooking. A cup of stock heated then garnished with sliced scallions, chopped bell pepper, or chopped celery makes a good first course. Try it with a sprinkle of fresh mint and a few drops of fresh lemon juice. Use the stock freely in cooking.

Roller-Dippies

Roll thinly sliced meats (roast beef, tongue, luncheon meats, ham) around stalks or slices of vegetables (cucumber, squash, celery, carrots) and dip in plain yogurt or other dips as "finger food" snacks.

Note: When advanced to phase-2 CHE, add thin long slices of cheese with the rolled meat for an extra treat. The entire Roller-Dippy can be wrapped in a corn tortilla, making a quick and easy breakfast or lunch "sandwich" or any-time snack. When advanced to phase-3, use wheat tortillas, too.

Basic Vege-Yogurt Dip

½ cup plain yogurt
juice of ½ lemon

spices and herbs as desired
(garlic, chives, marjo-
ram, thyme)
sea salt to taste

Mix together all ingredients.

Note: In favorite recipes, try Basic Vege-Yogurt Dip in place of sour cream, cream cheese, or cottage cheese.

"Almost Tartar" Sauce

½ cup green onions, tops
and all, coarsely chopped
¼ cup parsley, no heavy
stems, coarsely chopped
¼ cup cucumber, finely
chopped
1 tsp capers

1 tsp sea salt
⅛ tsp pepper
¼–½ tsp Mrs. Dash™
juice of ½–1 freshly
squeezed lemon
few drops tabasco sauce
1 pint yogurt

Combine all ingredients except yogurt in a bowl and toss to blend. Put mixture through a meat grinder using the coarse blade, or use a blender on "chop." Stir into yogurt. Chill and serve with fish dish or with slices, chunks, or cubes of any vegetable.

Chicken Egg Drop Soup

1½ cups homemade chicken
stock

3 eggs, beaten

Bring chicken stock to boil, adding herbs and spices to flavor as desired. Remove from heat. Drop eggs into stock, stirring constantly. The heat of the soup stock will cook the eggs.

Zucchini Supreme

6 small zucchini, cut into
¼-inch slices
2 tbs butter

3 eggs, slightly beaten
1 tsp sea salt

Put zucchini into 8-inch skillet. Dot with butter. Cook covered for 10 minutes. Combine and pour remaining ingredients over zucchini and cook additional 10 minutes. Use spices and herbs to flavor, as desired.

Tomato Sauce

(for flavoring meats, vegetables; use as soup stock, use in dips, dressings)

½ cup onions, chopped
½ cup fat-free chicken or vegetable stock
3 cups tomatoes, coarsely chopped

½ tsp each oregano, thyme, and basil
1 tsp garlic powder
freshly ground pepper

Cook onions in stock until soft. Add remaining ingredients. Bring to boil, cover, and simmer 30–45 minutes. Add other herbs and spices to flavor, as desired. Makes about 3½ cups.

Note: Store in glass jar. Refrigerate until ready to use.

SECTION IV

Specific Local Disorders as Manifestations of the Yeast Syndrome

16

Curing Yeast
Vaginitis and Thrush

A sixty-year-old married housewife named Sylvia Holden, who resides in Princeton, New Jersey, had a long history of vaginal discomfort from repeated yeast infections. Since 1967, Mrs. Holden had attempted to cure her trouble by following her physician's advice: Swallow a nystatin tablet each day for one week, then take no medicine for the next week, then start another treatment cycle again. During the weeks without her daily nystatin, she noted a worsening of vaginal discharge and an increase in generalized body complaints. Seemingly chained to taking nystatin the rest of her life, she was distraught that nothing else was offered.

Mrs. Holden had been to many medical specialists— gynecologist, urologist, internist, family practice specialist, and others—but no cure for her vaginitis was found. Numerous trials with various treatments simply failed to correct her recurrent condition permanently. Hers was not an uncommon situation, according to Jack D. Sobel, M.D., Associate Professor of Medicine, Department of Infectious Diseases at the Medical College of Pennsylvania in Philadelphia. In a lecture delivered to the March 1985 Yeast–Human Interaction Conference in San Francisco, Dr. Sobel frankly stated,

"Throughout the world, Candida vulvovaginitis attacks about three-quarters of all adult females at some time in their lives and half of them have multiple episodes. . . . I estimate that 15 to 20 percent of all women [worldwide] have chronic, recurrent vulvovaginal candidiasis."

The affliction has no respect for income, education, social class, fastidious hygiene, chastity, or any other aspect of a woman's life or lifestyle. Given the right circumstances and a susceptible immunological status, any woman can get it. Some women experience yeast vulvovaginitis over and over again, even as frequently as every month. Unrelenting itching and discharge are the telltale symptoms and sign that they have joined the burgeoning ranks of those with the Candida syndrome.

The medical history of Mrs. Holden reveals that she never took oral contraceptives, she sustained two full-term, uneventful pregnancies, and she experienced much difficulty with abdominal gas, bowel constipation, and frequent sniffling colds. She was often confined to bed as a child with upper respiratory tract infections and sore throats. She had required a great deal of dental work for the correction of cavities, and eventually some teeth had to be removed.

Although Mrs. Holden's greatest discomfort came from chronic vulvovaginitis, she was also currently suffering from marked fatigue, insomnia, the tendency to wake at night without apparent cause and a subsequent inability to return to sleep, impaired memory, shortened attention span, and a wandering mind with difficulty concentrating. Her head seemed to "pound" incessantly; her ears had been aching for years; and frequent canker sores of the mouth persistently plagued her. Prunes and prune juice were taken daily for their laxative effect.

On June 1, 1985, Sylvia Holden consulted another internal medicine specialist, Milan J. Packovich, M.D., Medical Director of the Medical Nutrition Center in Paramus, New Jersey, who also has a second office in Wierton, West Virginia. She was fortunate that Dr. Packovich devotes his efforts to the wholistic methods of metabolic medicine, orthomolecular nutrition (vitamins and minerals), chelation therapy, and bariatrics (weight control). Combatting the Candida syndrome is one of his major medical interests, and he had studied with Dr. C. Orian Truss, discoverer of this emerging epidemic.

Dr. Packovich began a thorough search for the roots of Mrs. Holden's many problems with an electrocardiogram, echocardiogram, Pap smear, blood counts, blood chemistries, and other clinical and laboratory tests. They turned up normal results. But Dr. Packovich knew that normal physical examination findings and laboratory tests are usual for candidiasis patients. His careful clinical evaluation ruled out other likely illnesses for her. The vulvovaginitis was a main clue; indeed, diagnostic procedures for the presence of yeast showed that treatment for the Candida syndrome was required.

Dr. Packovich began Mrs. Holden on a precisely planned, low yeast, reduced processed food, no-sugar Candida control diet, similar to phase one of the four-phase Celebration of Healthy Eating program discussed in Section Three. Instead of nystatin tablets, he prescribed oral nystatin powder on a graduated dose regimen. Colonic-lavage enemas like those described in Chapter Twelve were advised. The doctor also employed immune stimulation methods similar to those explained in Chapter Eleven. Finally, the patient was given oral adrenal glandular extracts (Mil-Adregen™, produced by Miller Pharmaceutical Group, Inc., West Chicago, Illinois) to support her exhausted adrenals (stress glands).

Revisiting the physician six weeks later, Mrs. Holden reported that she felt much improved. Loss of memory was not a problem anymore; her energy was greater; the vague head pounding sensation had disappeared; her ears were no longer painful. Dr. Packovich continued his patient on the same anti-Candida treatment program.

At the next consultation on August 11, 1985, Mrs. Holden told Dr. Packovich that her ability to remember details of prior occurrences or things that she had read in the past seemed to have returned, and her energy had increased to a higher level than ever before. Abdominal gas was reduced as well. The doctor allowed his patient to add greater numbers of complex vegetable carbohydrates—the dietary additions listed as phase three of the Celebration of Healthy Eating. Only one glaring flaw in the woman's progress toward health remained: although improved, her vulvovaginal symptoms were still present.

Dr. Packovich sat down with Mrs. Holden and discussed the remote potential of liver problems developing from the use of ketoconazole. From Chapter Ten you may recall that Nizoral™, commercial brand of ketoconazole, has a variety of adverse reactions sometimes associated with it: nausea, vomiting, abdominal pain, itching, headache, dizziness, sleepiness, fever and chills, avoidance of light, and diarrhea. Only slightly worrisome, however, are infrequent transient increases in serum liver enzymes. Since Mrs. Holden still suffered with insomnia and constipation, she joked that she might welcome the side effects of sleepiness and diarrhea.

Arranging with his patient for follow-up blood chemistry tests for liver function to be done after a trial of thirty ketoconazole tablets, Dr. Packovich prescribed a nightly dose of 200 mg of the medication. On her own, Mrs. Holden also decided to drink the antifungal la pacho/taheebo tea (see Chapter Eleven) at the same time that she took her daily ketoconazole tablet. (Incidentally, douching with the taheebo tea—or dropping a little taheebo solution into one empty, no. 2, plain gelatin capsule for insertion into the vagina—is a sometimes useful remedy for vaginitis suggested by some wholistic physicians.)

After Mrs. Holden took the ketoconazole tablets for eighteen days, the accumulated side effects had become too distressing for her. Feeling quite unwell, she stopped using both the ketoconazole and the taheebo tea. Two weeks later, she kept her appointment for the blood tests, and, indeed, minor changes showed the medication probably had caused brief irritation to her liver. By electing to discontinue ketoconazole treatment, Mrs. Holden had correctly "listened to" her body. The liver irritation alarmed her, and she discontinued all medications for twenty-one days.

But vulvovaginitis and discharge returned intensely. She resumed the oral nystatin powder, using a gradually increasing amount. By November 24, 1985, Mrs. Holden had increased her dosage to one-half teaspoonful of nystatin three times a day, and her vaginal complaints had completely resolved themselves. (At this writing, March 23, 1986, they have not returned.) At a follow-up office visit for blood chemistry tests, she advised Dr. Packovich that all of her prior symptoms along with the troubling yeast vaginitis had finally disappeared. Mrs. Holden declared that she felt like a new woman!

FACTS ABOUT VULVOVAGINITIS

Symptoms of discomfort for a woman may occur in the vagina alone (vaginitis), the female external sexual organs of the vulva alone (vulvitis), or both the fleshy folds of the vulva (known as the *labia majora* and *labia minora*) and the vagina (vulvovaginitis).

This inflammation of the vulva and/or vagina has a number of causes, the most common of which are: (1) infection by *Candida albicans*, which produces the condition called vulvovaginal candidiasis (also known as moniliasis, vulvovaginal thrush, yeast vulvovaginitis, a "yeast infection," or a "monilia" infection); (2) infection by Gardnerella, a bacterium, which produces the condition known as bacterial vulvovaginitis (also called *Haemophilus vaginitis*); (3) infection by *Trichomonas*, a protozoa or single-cell animal parasite, also idiomatically referred to as "trich" (pronounced "trick"); (4) atrophic vaginitis (thinning of the lining of the vagina due to a decreased presence of hormones), psychosomatic vaginitis (physical discomfort because of psychological distress), and other incidental causes, including herpes (a virus), chlamydia (a viruslike parasite), gonorrhea (a bacterium), and physical trauma to the vulva or vagina (from intercourse, tight-fitting clothes, or foreign objects), frequent or strong douches, or allergy to vaginal deodorants, soaps, sprays, or pads, or to scented or colored toilet tissue. Any of these can bring on a vaginal discharge.

We will explain the lesser forms of vulvovaginitis first and then discuss the most prevalent reason for this worldwide scourge of women.

Herpes simplex virus (type II and occasionally type I) is increasingly the source of vulvovaginal infection, due to changes in sexual mores since the 1960s. This often shows a thin, watery discharge. Painful external ulcers are sometimes apparent on the vulva. Cultures can provide an accurate diagnosis, but these must be sent to a specialized laboratory. There is no known cure for herpes, but acyclovir (Zovirax™ capsules, ointment, and powder made by Burroughs Wellcome Company of Research Triangle Park, North Carolina) provides some symptomatic relief, shortens the course of the infection, and often appears to reduce the frequency of recurrent episodes.

Chlamydia is recognized as a rising source of sexually transmitted disease. Recently it has been isolated at venereal disease clinics in up to 31 percent of women. In men, the viruslike organism causes a slight discharge from the urethra. In women, usually no symptoms or signs are noted. Chlamydial infections can be treated effectively with the tetracycline antibiotics.

In gonococcal vulvovaginitis, itching, burning, and painful urination or a thick, yellow discharge may be present. Gonococcal testiculitis and prostatitis in men almost always is accompanied by a yellow-green discharge from the penis, with intense pain on urination. Because the disease organism is becoming more resistant to treatment, tetracycline or penicillin antibiotics are used in increasing dosages as recommended in updates issued by the U.S. Public Health Service Centers for Disease Control.

Psychosomatic vulvovaginitis is noninfectious but physically identical to any other type of vulvitis and vaginitis, characterized by itching of the vulva or vagina and a variable discharge. The condition commonly comes from "nervous tension," because stress weakens the body's natural defense systems. Relaxation techniques such as yoga, transcendental meditation, hypnosis, biofeedback, psychoanalysis, and other stress-reducing methods are employed in its treatment.

Atrophic vulvovaginitis is not an infectious condition. Rather, it is due to thinning and shrinkage of the tissues lining the vagina and vulva. Women past menopause or those who have had surgical removal of their ovaries can experience these changes due to decreased estrogen production. Symptoms include an inflamed, dry, and roughened vulva and vagina, with itching, burning, and a sticky, brownish discharge that discolors undergarments. This condition is often responsible for pain on urination, itching, and painful sexual intercourse. It is occasionally misdiagnosed as a urinary infection.

Vaginal atrophy leaves the vagina at risk for other kinds of vulvovaginitis. Treatment is aimed at improving the condition of the vulva and vagina to make the area less susceptible to infection. Vulvovaginal estrogen creams or oral estrogen pills can be administered for a short period of time. Estrogen replacement must be prescribed and monitored by a physician.

Trichomoniasis is found in both men and women and, like candidiasis, has worldwide distribution. Humans are the only known host for the causative protozoan parasite. An estimated 2.5 million Americans are afflicted with it each year. Up to 10 percent of females and virtually all males display no symptoms of the condition. The 90 percent of women having symptoms show a yellow-green or gray, frothy, foul-smelling discharge. Trichomoniasis patients are often sexually active. The causative organism can be transmitted during sexual intercourse or from any moist object. Symptoms come on suddenly. Besides the profuse discharge with an offensive fishlike odor, there may be itching around the vulva, vagina, and inner thighs, painful intercourse, and burning during urination. A pelvic and microscopic examination are necessary for a physician to diagnose a trichomonal infection.

Oral medication affecting the entire system is required to eradicate *Trichomonas* and discourage recurrence of the infection. Topical agents such as vaginal creams, vaginal tablets or suppositories, or medicinal douches are used, but frequently they provide only temporary symptomatic relief. If men developed such symptoms, the same medications would be applied for them. Metronidazole oral tablets (Protostat™ made by Ortho Pharmaceutical Corporation of Raritan, New Jersey, or Flagyl™ made by Searle & Company of San Juan, Puerto Rico) have been shown to be effective in treating this disorder, but are not recommended for use during pregnancy. The responsible physician should consider metronidazole treatment for the patient's sexual partner to prevent prompt reinfection.

Gardnerella vaginitis and infection, produced by the bacterium *Haemophilus vaginitis* (more recently named *Gardnerella vaginitis*), is the most frequent cause of vaginal discharge in sexually active women. Regarded as a disease of the reproductive years, it affects approximately 20 percent of women in this period of life, although many exhibit no symptoms. A physician must confirm the presence of bacteria with a culture taken from the vagina. An associate infection with *Trichomonas* in 25 percent of vaginitis patients, it is characterized by discharge with a bad odor, mild pain on urination, and occasional itching. The discharge often necessitates douching or changing of clothing. Treatment consists of vaginal creams or tablets and oral antibiotic medications. To prevent recurrences, the sexual partner may also be advised to receive treatment with ampicillin, an oral penicillin agent.

Although bacteria, more frequently than yeast, bring on repeated attacks of vulvovaginitis in women of developed countries, in developing areas candidiasis most often is the culprit in recurrent, chronic vulvovaginal disease. Up to 45 percent of women in Third World nations suffer repeated episodes as compared to 20 percent of women in Westernized societies. But in all cultural settings, vaginitis associated with *C. albicans* is the most persistent and most frustrating to treat.

Symptoms of Common Vulvovaginal Infections

TYPE OF INFECTION	DISCHARGE	ODOR	ITCHING	BURNING SORENESS	LESION BLISTER
Gardnerella (Haemophilus) vaginitis infection	Scant to profuse, gray or white	Unpleasant	Rarely	Mild, if any	None
Yeast infection (candidiasis)	Sometimes; white, thick, curdlike	None or rarely unpleasant	Intense	Sometimes	Rash, red spots
Trichomoniasis	Always; profuse, gray or yellow-green	Very foul	Often	Often	None
Herpes simplex II, rarely I	Not usually	None	None	Almost always	Painful, shallow, open sores

VULVOVAGINAL CANDIDIASIS

Vulvovaginal candidiasis can occur at almost any time of life—during childhood, the childbearing years, or after menopause. The increasing use of antibiotics has made it a serious problem among young and middle-aged women. Candidal infection is most commonly troublesome, however, during the childbearing years, probably because of occasional hormonal imbalances affecting the vagina. In fact, the disease is ten times more frequent in pregnant women than nonpregnant women. It is also markedly increased in those who are diabetic (a hormonal and chemical imbalance). If a woman has a vulvovaginal yeast infection when she gives birth, the infant may acquire the Candida infection, often first showing in the mouth as "thrush." Thrush is usually not serious and is easily treated. When promptly and completely treated, the chances are reduced that the child will develop further problems with the yeast syndrome from this first exposure.

Symptoms and signs of vulvovaginal candidiasis include external itching, redness and swelling of the vulva, burning, and pain sometimes so severe that the patient can neither sit nor walk. A distressing, often whitish, nonbloody discharge from the vagina is characteristic. It may range from scanty to profuse, watery to cottage-cheesy, with an odor that is not unpleasant but rather yeast- or vinegarlike. Discomfort during sexual intercourse may be experienced or might be the only symptom noticed. After fruitless attempts to rid themselves of vaginal problems, many women accept these symptoms as the price to be paid for being a woman. On the other hand, there are women whose vulvovaginal cultures show Candida colonies who may never experience any symptoms of local candidiasis. In his 1985 lecture, Dr. Jack Sobel offered these statistics:

Those women having four or more confirmed episodes of recurrent or chronic vulvovaginal candidiasis every year comprise about 20 percent of the current population. The morbidity [illness and distress] of chronic vulvovaginal candidiasis is enormous. Not only are these patients exposed to repeated attacks of disabling vaginal and perineal [vulva] symptoms, but the effect that the symptoms have on normal marital relations is often devastating. In no small way they contribute to major marital stress.

Moreover, take any 100 normal, healthy women off the street of an average American city, get a single vaginal swab of each for a "point-prevalent" study, and doctors will find that from 10 to 55 test subjects will have positive Candida cultures. The same species of vaginal Candida can be identified month after month in asymptomatic healthy women. But in those with recurrent conditions, the symptoms typically exacerbate in the week or ten days immediately prior to menses. This is a hormone-dependent infection.

Recurrent yeast vulvovaginitis frequently flares up in the second half of the menstrual cycle, between ovulation and menses. With the onset of menstruation, symptoms commonly subside on their own, but all too often return the next month, again following ovulation.

WHY YEAST VAGINITIS STRIKES
SOME WOMEN AND NOT OTHERS

Vulvovaginal candidiasis may be more readily excited into producing symptoms if the victim furnishes the organism with only a few of the following advantageous circumstances:

1. pregnancy
2. diabetes
3. malnutrition from a deficient diet (such as the common practices in average American dietary habits)
4. a high carbohydrate diet
5. physical or chemical stress
6. chronic fatigue
7. the presence of one or more other diseases or infections
8. the continued use of some medications such as hormones or certain broad spectrum antibiotics
9. the use of vaginal deodorants or cosmetic sprays, colored or scented toilet tissue, or noncotton crotch in underwear
10. too frequent douching or irritation from douche chemicals

11. the shifting of hormones during the last two weeks of the menstrual cycle in ways that encourage yeast growth

12. psychological factors such as mental stress

13. childbirth

14. vaginal cuts or abrasions

15. excessive frequency or duration of sexual intercourse in a short period of time

16. sexual intercourse without enough lubrication

17. the wearing of tight-fitting clothing such as jeans, slacks, pantyhose, and underpants.

Some women have allowed many of these adverse circumstances to be present simultaneously, even for a prolonged time, while still suffering no signs or symptoms of yeast vulvovaginitis. Why? Bacteriologist and microbiologist Stephen Witkin, Ph.D., M.S., Associate Research Professor in the Department of Obstetrics and Gynecology at Cornell University Medical College, has found an answer. In his excellent paper delivered before the same 1985 San Francisco Candida conference addressed by Dr. Sobel, Dr. Witkin described his own discoveries about T-lymphocyte (T-cell) function in women with severe intractable yeast vulvovaginitis. He and his associates at Cornell have concluded that a specific defect in the cellular immunity of affected women is the cause of chronic, recurrent vulvovaginal candidiasis.

Dr. Witkin designed an investigation using sixty-five vulvovaginitis patients with three or more vaginal yeast attacks in a year and thirty-six controls with no attacks. His studies demonstrated that some women with recurrent vulvovaginitis have a macrophage regulation defect in response to *C. albicans* but not to other antigens. Affected macrophages produce excessive PGE_2 that blocks the production of IL-2, thereby keeping their lymphocytes (T-cells) from responding to *C. albicans*. The women remain highly susceptible to repeated vaginal yeast infections. This is a particular immune system flaw in the patient who endures persistent vulvovaginitis. Her treatment must be directed toward a buildup of the immune system utilizing the various techniques that we describe throughout this book.

YEAST VULVOVAGINITIS AND FREQUENT INTERCOURSE

The implication from Dr. Sobel's 1985 report is that yeast vulvovaginitis is connected to frequency of intercourse. He said,

> Women having frequent intercourse with husbands whose occupations are in the military result in vulvovaginitis. For example, a military husband might go away for three to four weeks and come back to the base with a weekend pass. The wife, in turn, has no sexual intercourse during his absence but then over his two-day weekend at home engages in sex two or three times daily. She can then predictably guarantee an attack of symptomatic vulvovaginitis by Wednesday. This short-term frequency of intercourse resulting in symptoms is analogous to "honeymoon cystitis." The repeated microtrauma under these circumstances may create local weakness in the vaginal defense mechanism mucosa [surface layer] that allows the organisms previously there as commensals to become pathogenic.

IS YEAST VULVOVAGINITIS A SEXUALLY TRANSMITTED DISEASE?

Dr. Sobel also asked the audience of Candida-conscious physicians to consider sexual transmission as a source of recurrent infection. "If you do cultures of the penis of male partners of women having recurrent vaginal infections, the likelihood of colonization [of the penis by yeast organisms] is four times higher than in control males. But one is not sure if the strain of Candida isolated on the penis is the cause of the vaginal infection or the result of her candidiasis."

Candida-affected males who have balanitis (inflammation under the foreskin at the tip of the penis) appear to be spreading the yeast-connected condition. Dr. Sobel explained that if men are positive for penile-cultured *C. albicans*, 80 percent of their female sexual contacts will be positive as well. If males have no penile colonization with yeast, only 32 percent of their female sexual contacts will be positive for Candida vaginitis.

Studies of oral-genital sexual contacts also produce remarkable realizations about the spread of vulvovaginal candidiasis. Dr. Sobel's investigation of the oral cavities of male controls turned up only 10 percent with positive *C. albicans* cultures. In male partners of chronic, recurrent vulvovaginitis patients, 45 percent had positive oral *C. albicans* cultures. In *C. albicans* strain typing for candidiasis-affected women, 75 percent of their male sex partners had the very same Candida strain in their mouths as the women had in their vaginas.

A male who notes burning, itching, redness, and irritation around the glans penis (head of the penis) about an hour after sexual intercourse usually finds the condition is self-limiting. After a shower and the passing of a day, penile discomforts often resolve. This chain of events likely represents a hypersensitivity reaction to a toxic product of the woman's Candida organisms or to some specific Candida antigen.

CURING ORAL THRUSH

Most people know about vaginal thrush—vaginitis—arising from yeast infection, but there is also oral thrush. The yeastlike parasite we've been discussing can be responsible for fungus infection in the mouth. Common in infants and sometimes in the elderly, white patches on the tongue may spread all over the interior of the mouth and the throat. The disease causes a crop of white, slightly raised, adherent splotches resembling milk curds, beginning on the tongue and inside the mouth and spreading throughout to the palate, gums, tonsils, throat, larynx, and elsewhere.

Repeated use of antifungal antibiotic mouthwash may offer some relief for oral thrush. Better control for many people, however, comes from sloshing around the mouth and over the tongue a product from Wakunaga of America: concentrated aged, liquid garlic extract brand-named Kyolic™ (or the professional dispensing package brand-named SGP™). The dosage consists of one good squirt (about one teaspoonful, or one-quarter ounce, to one-half tablespoonful [one half ounce]) from the two-ounce bottle into the mouth. Hold the concentrate in your mouth and keep sloshing it as long as you can. The taste might be difficult for some to accept, but this remedy is quite effective in ridding nearly all the structures within the oral cavity of the yeast infection. No characteristic odor of garlic is left on the breath, since this product is deodorized. Sloshing must be repeated three or four times a day until the tongue feels less stiff from fungus patches. Don't waste the liquid by spitting it out. Swallowing it and drinking some cool purified water (distilled, bottled, filtered, or other types with lessened toxic agents than tap water) afterward will send the therapeutic ingredients of garlic coursing through your gastrointestinal tract, to do even more internal good.

As an alternative, slosh and gargle using a solution made with one-half teaspoonful of table salt plus one teaspoonful of Kyolic™ liquid garlic extract in an 8-ounce glass of warm purified water. This solution also can be swallowed to help provide internal benefits. Sipping la pacho/taheebo tea has also been employed by some as an effective treatment for oral thrush.

THE YEAST SYNDROME—A GREAT IMITATOR

Yeast is the great invader of mucous membranes. The sheathlike vaginal passage is covered over almost all of its length by mucous membrane. The invasion capability of *C. albicans* takes advantage of this inviting surface, since the vagina is exceedingly vulnerable to fungal infection. Vaginal candidiasis is so common that the patient often must make a point of complaining about the white cheesy discharge, itching, or other genital symptoms in order to have her physician offer treatment. Otherwise, the condition might be ignored as "normal." Although doctors most assuredly recognize localized candidiasis, it's not given much attention on women who don't complain of signs or symptoms.

Not to diagnose and treat every vulvovaginal *C. albicans* infection is a serious error in judgment, because this subtle indication of the yeast syndrome produces more misery among women than all other diseases combined (except perhaps for premenstrual syndrome, which also may relate to yeast infestation). Systemic candidiasis can mimic almost any recognized disease—from eye infection or allergy to colitis, cystitis, gastritis, neurological changes, multiple sclerosis, and even insanity. This is an extraordinary list of symptoms for an infection that is present in an overwhelming number of people to some degree and is considered unimportant by most establishment physicians. Such an unfortunate oversight is the reason so many women have come to accept the presence of a vulvovaginal yeast infection as their personal way of life.

Syphilis used to be called "the great imitator" because it affected nearly all major organs, and its signs or symptoms simulated virtually every other major disease state. Today, the Candida syndrome is the new great imitator. Our physicians must become more aware of the enormous range of disorders that represent yeast-connected illnesses. Awareness is vital because the yeast infection, which wreaks so much havoc, is a treatable and frequently curable disease.

TREATMENT OF VULVOVAGINAL CANDIDIASIS

The patient with yeast vulvovaginitis may be given nystatin by mouth, as cream for vaginal use, and liquid or powder for oral use, since thrush infestation of the mouth and throat occasionally accompanies the infection lower down.

Pure, yellow nystatin powder is taken orally and vaginally in females, orally in males. Some patients also apply it topically, either powdered directly on the body part or mixed with lanolin or a similar carrier. To give yourself vaginal therapy, consider following these rules recommended by Dr. Packovich:

1. Commit yourself to a duration of vaginal therapy for at least thirty to sixty days.

2. Acquire some plain, empty, no. 4 gelatin capsules from your local pharmacist. Fill the smaller-diameter end of the capsule with the yellow nystatin powder.

3. Insert the capsule nightly into the vagina. If needed, moisten the capsule to make insertion easier.

4. If you still have monthly menstrual periods, it is vital to use this vaginal nystatin capsule *during* the flow days as well. *C. albicans* grows heavily during your flow days and in the immediate premenstrual days.

5. Regular prescription nystatin vaginal suppositories probably should not be used, since the chemical ingredients of the suppository have caused painful vaginal irritation in some women.

Orally administered nystatin therapy is useful for both oral and vulvovaginal thrush. Dr. Packovich often advises his patients to proceed with oral application of nystatin powder in the following manner:

a. Although it does not taste delicious, most people can tolerate the medication "straight" or mixed in a small amount of purified water. Only rarely do patients request to mix it with a small amount of diet soft drink (or diluted fruit juice if absolutely necessary) to make it more palatable. (Check with your physician before mixing the powder with food items not on your present phase of the Celebration of Healthy Eating program.)

b. About one-quarter to one-half teaspoonful of powdered nystatin dissolved in water is ready for use as a mouthwash for oral thrush. Hold it in your mouth for a minimum of one minute or longer, sloshing extensively before swallowing. You can also gargle with the nystatin solution.

c. An ideal schedule is to take nystatin one hour after each meal, three times a day, and also at bedtime. Avoid eating or drinking for approximately one hour after taking the nystatin. If your work schedule, school attendance, or lifestyle does not make this dosage schedule possible, then take it whenever you have a chance. Although a haphazard schedule might be somewhat less effective, you still will get some benefit.

Remember, you are trying to kill the yeast infestation not only in the vulvovaginal areas but also throughout the digestive tract—the mouth, esophagus, stomach, and small and large bowels. Nystatin in tablet form has no effect on the mouth and esophagus, so this dosage form is less beneficial than the powder and is more expensive, too.

Nystatin douches and enemas are also recommended by Dr. Milan Packovich. Both the douche and the enema are made at the same strength: one teaspoonful of nystatin powder in a quart of plain purified water. Dr. Packovich recommends them to be self-administered once a week. Dr. Trowbridge considers these remedies in lower dosage to be sufficiently beneficial and nontoxic that they might be employed up to once a day when needed. The nystatin douche and enema will definitely, although temporarily, reduce the yeast population in the vulvovaginal region and the large bowel.

Fifty-four-year-old Vera Weido, a health food store owner in San Antonio, Texas, successfully makes use of another form of vaginal douche, one comprised of aged garlic extract. "For over four years, I have suggested Kyolic™ to a lot of my customers for the elimination of vaginal yeast infections," said Mrs. Weido in an interview.

> I have used it myself, as well, and my twenty-nine-year-old daughter has, too. We have inserted a tampon or sterile cotton moistened with garlic extract into the vagina and left it overnight. We advise changing the saturated material each morning and night for the fastest effect. Women report that they get good results. The yeast infection goes away within a week's time. It's really good to douche with purified liquid garlic as a preventive measure. That keeps yeast vaginitis away permanently. I haven't had such vaginal trouble since I was thirty-four.[1]

If therapy for the mucous membranes is not effective quickly, or if it is only partially effective, Candida extract injections (described in Chapter Twelve) may be advised to build the body's natural defense system. The combination antigen known as TCE (Trichophyton-Candida-Epidermophyton), or the Candida antigen alone, can work well to stimulate defense reactions against existing mucous membrane disease. The strengths of the extracts and their frequency of use are determined for each individual by the Candida-conscious physician and will vary widely among patients. Injections might be needed for weeks or several months to several years in rare cases.

Nizoral™ taken for two weeks (see Chapter Ten), along with simultaneous treatment of infected sexual partners, followed by low-dose maintenance therapy for three to six more months, can eliminate three-fourths of recurrent infections.

A newer and more convenient three-day dosage form of Monistat®, called Monistat 3® (200 mg miconazole nitrate), is a refinement of Monistat 7® vaginal suppositories. Responding to patient needs, the modified product has recently been introduced by the Ortho Pharmaceutical Corporation of Raritan, New Jersey. This three-day vaginal treatment gives rapid symptomatic relief of itching, burning, and irritation. Unfortunately, this miconazole nitrate product fails to do anything for the Candida syndrome as a whole.

Newly approved by the U.S. Food and Drug Administration for the topical treatment of yeast vulvovaginitis, Femstat™ is a 2.0 percent vaginal cream manufactured by Syntex Laboratories, Inc. of Palo Alto, California. Femstat™ is a broad spectrum antifungal agent generically known as butoconazole, derived from imidazol, a chemical similar to ketoconizole. Although introduced to the medical community as recently as April 28, 1986, butoconazole is thought to be more effective than ketoconizole with fewer side effects. It has a long shelf-life and is simple to use.

Femstat™ is packaged in a 28-gram tube with three disposable applicators. For three days at bedtime, fill the applicator until it stops taking cream. Apply the cream within the vagina and apply extra cream from the applicator to the vaginal lips. Simply throw away the used applicator. Some physicians have their patients use the cream intermittently if chronic systemic candidiasis continues to be present.

Orithrush® mouthwash and Orithrush® vaginal douche concentrate, produced by Ecological Formulas of Concord, California, consist of a stabilized and buffered derivative of sorbic acid. Salts of sorbic acid have shown excellent results in combating vulvovaginal candididasis. Their use is more appealing since sorbic acid appears on the U.S. Food and Drug Administration's GRAS (generally recognized as safe) list.

One or two tablespoons of Orithrush® mouthwash for treatment of oral thrush are used for gargling three times a day. Rinse the mouth, gargle, and swallow. Mint-flavored and nonmint mouthwash are available.

For douching, dilute one part of Orithrush® douche concentrate with twenty parts of distilled water, as directed on the bottle. Douche with approximately eight ounces once or twice daily. Severe vaginal candidiasis may respond to inserting a tampon saturated with diluted solution for two hours twice a day.

Another product, Orifresh™, is made by Advanced Medical Nutrition, Inc., of Hayward, California. This water-soluble powder premix contains aloe vera concentrate stabilized with buffered sorbic acid. Prepared as directed, it can be used as a mouthwash-gargle, body rinse, or vaginal douche.

THE YOGURT DOUCHE

Women of Third World countries have used a solution made with plain yogurt as a douche for centuries. In the last few decades it has become popular with women in Western societies, too. Yogurt used "straight" or mixed half and half with purified water has been found effective as a remedy and a preventative for vaginal yeast infections.

A 60 ml irrigating syringe can be purchased from your local pharmacy to aid in douching with yogurt. The tip is a narrow smooth cone, ideal for easy insertion into the vagina. You merely pull out the plunger and fill the syringe as desired with room temperature yogurt, yogurt and water, or the whey of yogurt. Place the plunger on the back end of the syringe barrel and carefully turn the syringe so that the tip end points skyward. When the yogurt drops away from the tip end, the plunger can be gently and carefully inserted into the syringe barrel, minimizing any squirting or spilling. To place the yogurt into the vagina, simply lie in the same position as you would for a douche, insert the tip end of the syringe into the vagina, and gently depress the plunger. Do not rinse inside afterward, just rinse outside and pat dry. Wear a mini- or maxi-pad and panties to minimize leakage. Most women prefer to insert the yogurt at bedtime. (Wait until after sexual intercourse if you wish.) Wash the vulva (outer vaginal area) with water (in a shower or bath) in the morning before dressing. Sometimes continued use of a mini-pad is needed during the day.

Instead of yogurt, *Lactobacillus acidophilus* powder may be mixed with water (one-half teaspoonful of the powder mixed into eight to sixteen ounces of water) to create a douche solution. As another alternative, consider filling a pure gelatin capsule with *L. acidophilus* or half and half nystatin powder and *L. acidophilus* and inserting the capsule into the vagina daily or as otherwise directed by your physician. Yogurt or acidophilus douching or the use of acidophilus capsules (with or without nystatin) have been determined by many physicians to be ideal for daily or twice-daily application. You apply it vaginally for up to several weeks, then usage is carried forward as needed or as advised by your personal doctor.

NOTES

1. Morton Walker, *Garlic, Nature's Healer*, Greenwich, Conn.: Devin-Adair, 1984, pp. 21, 22.

17

Reversal of Yeast-Related
Mental Illness

"A living death," is the way Donna Carson Harris of Tahlequah, Oklahoma, describes the schizophrenia label pinned to her for twenty years, when the true cause of her mental derangement was Candida infestation.

In 1960, Mrs. Harris slipped from her role as University of Oklahoma beauty queen, homemaker, wife of handsome Dallas Cowboys football star Jimmy Harris, and mother of two children into the darkness of overwhelming depression, anxiety, fear, mental collapse, and schizophrenia. It happened suddenly. "I was a prisoner of my bedroom. I was depressed all the time. I couldn't sleep, yet I was sleepy. I couldn't think, and when I tried, I couldn't stand the confusion. No matter how hard I tried, I wasn't me," she acknowledged in a 1982 *Oklahoma City Times* newspaper story.[1] During brief moments of sanity she attempted treatment, mostly with psychiatrists. They had diagnosed her as having schizophrenia and no therapy seemed to be effective, even after she wasted $100,000 on their psychoanalyses, drugs, and other nostrums. She also failed at suicide.

Then in 1980 the real source of her mental illness was uncovered. The cause was not buried in her mind at all; it was physical—a breakdown of her immune system by *Candida albicans*. Her nervous system was being assaulted by Canditoxin, and interruption of her normal metabolism took place.

Reading articles in health magazines that described the work of C. Orian Truss, M.D., Mrs. Harris recognized her own symptoms in the patients whom Dr. Truss was treating. "His approach intrigued me, but when I checked to see about getting in to see him I learned that I'd have to wait a year or longer for the opportunity. I was disappointed but knew his approach was the answer that I had been seeking," she said. Not able to wait a year, she brought information about the Candida syndrome to an open-minded osteopathic wholistic physician practicing in a suburb of Tulsa, Leon Anderson, D.O., of Jenks, Oklahoma. Dr. Anderson employs nutrition, preventive medicine, and chelation therapy as therapeutic tools for restoring health to his patients. Fortunately for Mrs. Harris, he was amenable to being educated about the Candida syndrome.

From interviewing Dr. Anderson, we learned that he first met Mrs. Harris in the latter part of 1981 and began her on antiyeast treatment early in 1982. A dramatic reversal of her schizophrenic symptoms began almost immediately. "She has had a lot of mental problems," admitted Dr. Anderson. "But she is so much better now that she isn't infested with yeast that it's really amazing. She was very chemically sensitive because of suppression of her immune system and the adrenal glands by toxin that the *C. albicans* produces."

Today, at forty-nine, Mrs. Harris is quite normal, and her mental wellness is completely restored. No longer mislabeled schizophrenic, the woman does not suffer from either depression or anxiety. Dr. Anderson's remedial procedure did not require psychiatric techniques—merely proper diagnosis and needed application of those methods we have described earlier: a low carbohydrate, no-sugar, no-yeast diet; no coffee or tea; much eating of yogurt; taking supplemental vitamins and minerals; using air purifiers and humidifers to control mold in the home; and other noncomplicated wholistic approaches.

Dr. Anderson additionally prescribed orally administered nystatin powder instead of tablets. "She started with one-

eighth of a teaspoonful of nystatin powder four times a day.
Now she maintains herself on one-half teaspoonful of nystatin
four times a day. She also took the Candida serial dilution
titration vaccines [immunotherapy] three times a week," Dr.
Anderson explained.

"Our world is so much better now," said twenty-two-year-
old David, Mrs. Harris's son, who also once took nystatin
because of potential immunological breakdown from *C. albicans*
infestation. He doesn't need the medicine anymore.

David's mother has come back to her family—restored to
mental health—as the result of remedying physical problems
in her gastrointestinal tract rather than presupposed psychological aberrations in her brain. How is that possible? How is
a physician able to reverse mental illness by prescribing for
the yeast syndrome?

BRAIN DYSFUNCTION
CAUSED BY THE YEAST SYNDROME

Donna Carson Harris had been misdiagnosed as schizophrenic. Schizophrenia, the most common mental illness, afflicts
about 25 percent of all patients admitted to mental hospitals
and about 60 percent of their permanent residents. Although
its major cause is unknown, heredity seems to be a main
contributing factor. Yet, with brain dysfunction shown to be
sometimes created by the Candida syndrome, imagine how
many thousands of expensive mental hospital beds could be
emptied merely from treatment of this condition.

Twenty-six years ago, when Mrs. Harris was in her early
twenties, she was in the most common age group for
schizophreniclike symptoms to strike. The course of schizophrenia is regressive, with worsening mind deterioration. Its
principal symptoms are a "split" personality, escape from
reality into a dream world, and emotional indifference. The
victim's behavior is determined by his or her imagined
thoughts, not by real surroundings. His answers to questions
often sound silly and meaningless. Speech can be garbled and
unintelligible, and a certain lack of concern with any serious
situation prevails. For instance, the schizophrenic cares little
that his words, deeds, and general behavior repeatedly bring

deep emotional hurt to those who care for him. He seems concerned only about himself.

For over two decades, Mrs. Harris suffered from chronic, severe distortion of brain function, until she was finally given treatment for chronic candidiasis and not for the resulting psychiatric problems. She has recovered now because of the correct therapeutic approach, designed to suppress her yeast overgrowth. Her old schizophrenia-like symptoms have been left to the past, a situation that confirms Dr. Truss's statements in *The Missing Diagnosis:*

> *Candida albicans* is capable of interfering with brain physiology in a way that results in an illness recognizable as schizophrenia by competent psychiatrists. . . . There might well be more than one cause of identical symptoms in different patients with brain disease. . . . There seems no logical reason why functional abnormalities of the brain, manifested by symptoms included in such labels as "schizophrenia" and "manic-depression," cannot be due to any one of many factors capable of interfering with the same set of brain functions. . . . At this time we can say only that *Candida albicans* can cause great difficulty with brain function, and that this type illness, when caused by this fungus, will respond to yeast suppression.[2]

When mental depression, schizophrenia, fear, anxiety, paranoia, manic-depression, and other erratic behaviors are present, these patients may be affected by generalized, chronic candidiasis. We believe that they should be given antiyeast treatment along with the required psychological, pharmaceutical, social management, and rehabilitation methods usually employed as mental health therapy. Our recommendation is predicated on allergy-hormone-acetaldehyde interactions produced in these mentally involved—not necessarily mentally ill—patients by fungal infestations.

Yeast toxins have been shown to stimulate allergic responses (see Chapter Eighteen). Neurologists have demonstrated that the central nervous system, as with most body organs, is a reactor to toxic allergens. Thus, the infested patient's brain might well be having a hypersensitivity reaction to products from the Candida organism.

Dr. Truss was the first to focus on the excitation effects on the human brain caused by *C. albicans* and its Canditoxin. He writes:

> Chronic yeast infection with systematic allergic and toxic effects is a widespread problem, especially in women, but one that is both correctable and preventable. . . . Because the allergic (or toxic) response in the brain leads to anxiety, crying, depression, and diminished intellectual function, almost all such women eventually are referred to the psychiatrist for diagnosis and treatment, after extensive diagnostic efforts have failed to establish a physical basis for the illness. . . . The psychiatrist, no matter how conscientiously he may try to solve the mystery of illness, will not succeed because the condition is physical rather than psychiatric in its cause. . . . Well-intentioned psychological explanations of the illness frequently serve only to create feelings of inadequacy and guilt, and to erode further the impairment of self-confidence and self-esteem already present as a result of the illness. . . . Endless years of mental and physical suffering ensue because, once the psychiatric path has been chosen, virtually all efforts cease in the search for physical correctable causes of the patient's problems. . . . Symptoms are so varied and changeable and so rarely associated with laboratory, X-ray, or other objective abnormalities, that each new symptom tends to be dismissed as just one more "psychosomatic" or "neurotic" complaint. . . . The patient eventually becomes reluctant to describe complaints, often preferring to answer simply, "I feel fine," rather than again be subjected to the response she has come to expect.[3]

C. albicans infestation causes hormonal alterations such as premenstrual difficulties (see Chapter Twenty). Referring to psychiatric drugs given to women with a Candida-related brain syndrome because of the mistaken belief that they are schizophrenic, Dr. Truss affirms, "Certain components in many of the 'anti-anxiety' drugs, despite any help conferred, may aggravate the hormonal imbalance."[4]

There is another dysfunction of the brain resulting from chronic, generalized candidiasis: the acetaldehyde effect. All yeasts convert sugar and digestible carbohydrates to acetaldehyde under anaerobic (absence of oxygen) conditions. The intestinal environment is sufficiently anaerobic for this process to occur. The potentially harmful acetaldehyde is transported to the liver just as though it were an absorbed foodstuff, via the portal circulation. There it is oxidized to harmless acetate by aldehyde dehydrogenase (a zinc-containing enzyme). The oxidation is very efficient. Under normal circumstances acetaldehyde cannot be detected in peripheral blood. When it is detectable the oxidizing capacity of the liver has been exceeded either by excessive and prolonged acetaldehyde production or lack of enzyme. A critical fact is that about 60 percent of Orientals and 5 percent of Europeans and Americans are unable to synthesize this protective aldehyde dehydrogenase enzyme.

Acetaldehyde binds strongly to human tissues, and, like the related substance formaldehyde, it has a significant potential to injure body organs by "pickling" them. During moderate acetaldehyde production, the compound can bind to the cells of the intestine, liver, brain, and portal blood vessels; to their contents such as nutrients, enzymes, vitamins, polypeptides; and to the blood constituents of platelets, leukocytes, erythrocytes, and circulating proteins. During excessive acetaldehyde production, these harmful bonds can be formed throughout the body. The bonding is cumulative and quickly becomes irreversible when exposure to acetaldehyde is prolonged. Thus, tissue injury as a result of polysystemic chronic candidiasis is a very real possibility. This explanation helps to make more understandable how Candida infestation can show such a broad range of symptoms, affecting virtually all body functions and symptoms.

At least part of the potency of acetaldehyde is within the brain, as a synaptic blocking agent. Acetaldehyde can lead to inhibition of the synthesis of acetylcholine, a key neurotransmitter. A disturbance in the availability of acetylcholine transmitter can unsettle the normal automatic functions of the autonomic nervous system. This will be a contributing factor to erratic thinking and deranged behavior. Defective short-term memory occurs as well. These mental disturbances are frequently encountered in people with the Candida syndrome. Many neurotransmitters are amines (derived from amino acids) and can be bound to acetaldehyde, forming "false neurotransmitters." Such false neurotransmitters may be the initiators of depression, anxiety, the vague uneasiness associated with stress, schizophreniclike symptoms, difficulties with concentration, and possibly lapses in memory.

Dr. Truss, in his "Acetaldehyde Hypothesis" article, has introduced his new concept of acetaldehyde produced by *C. albicans* as the basic cause for mental and physical disorders accompanying the Candida syndrome.[5] The combination of these false neurotransmitters, allergic responses, and hormonal imbalances serves to aggravate the potential for an underlying mental derangement in any nonsymptomatic individual. Although the cause of brain dysfunction may be the Candida syndrome, more often an ill person's misthinking and aberrant behavior are tagged with a wastebasket diagnosis—the all-encompassing label "schizophrenia."

RECOVERY FOR AUTISM

Duffy Mayo, the eight-year-old son of Gianna and Gus Mayo of Walnut Creek, California, had been diagnosed at the age of two as autistic. Today he is completely recovered from this serious disability. Duffy was finally discovered to be suffering with the yeast syndrome, but a true diagnosis and correct treatment weren't determined until he received a great deal of unnecessary psychiatric care for his "mental illness."

Autism is a severe disturbance of mental and emotional development in young children. It is characterized chiefly by withdrawal from reality and lack of responsiveness or interest in other people or in the normal activities of childhood. In spite of considerable research over the last few decades, the fields of genetics, neurology, neurochemistry, and biochemistry have offered little to our understanding about childhood autism. Some specialists are convinced that it is simply an abnormal way of behaving and reacting and has its roots in a vague combination of causes which vary from child to child.

Since authorities do not agree about the source of the illness, parents looking for help may be told that their youngster "lives in a world of his own" because of mental retardation, brain damage, emotional disturbance, schizophrenia, or psychosis—none of which may be true.

The most obvious and the earliest indication of autism— first seen in infancy—is extreme self-isolation. Even as a baby, the autistic child does not respond to either parent or to gestures of affection. Eye contact is avoided and there is a strong tendency to look through or past people. Toys and objects are used inappropriately and repetitiously. The child indulges in ritualistic and peculiar word repetitions or body movements (called perseveration), such as incessant rocking and head banging.

As the autistic infant approaches early childhood, speech may fail to develop, or if it does develop, it may soon disappear. Forms of speech are conspicuously bizarre and have little to do with communication. Imitation of the speech of others is usually limited to meaningless repetition rather than responsiveness. Other early indications of autism include a seeming insensitivity to pain, resulting in self-mutilation; laughing, crying, or tantrums for no apparent reason; and abnormal responses—either overly sensitive or extremely limited—to external stimuli.

Duffy Mayo exhibited some of these symptoms. He also bounced off walls as if he were drunk. "It was embarrassing," recalls his mother. "I would take him to the doctor's office and he'd stagger around, slump against the wall, giggle and then break into that silly laugh that drunks have, you know? And he'd have this strong alcoholic breath." We were attracted to this child's health history by a feature story in the *Los Angeles Times*.[6]

With a diagnosis of autism securely pinned on him, the child only got worse. "He would go into comas, and then get rigid. He'd swell up and discolor and, at the age of three and a half, he'd have so much adrenaline flowing through him that he could practically pick up his father," said Gianna Mayo.

"He would obviously turn violently allergic to any number of things, as if his immune system had entirely broken down," Gus Mayo said. "We had this lovely house then, in Kensington, overlooking San Francisco Bay, and we completely stripped it—disconnected the gas because Duffy seemed too sensitive to it. We began heating with wood, and threw out the carpeting because of the formaldehyde in the backing. We spent about $10,000 redoing the house." Still, there was hardly any improvement in the child's condition.

"And this was when Duffy's drunkenness got so bad," Mrs. Mayo said. The parents sought help from San Francisco immunologist and allergy expert, Alan S. Levin, M.D. (see Chapter Six). "Because Duffy, and I, too, had always been prone to thrush . . . and because diabetics seem to have this, too [Gus Mayo has diabetes], Dr. Levin decided that autism had nothing to do with the symptoms," the mother said. "Duffy had Candida!"

At first nystatin brought great improvement in the boy's condition. "His eyes were brighter and he was more alert and inquisitive, so we were encouraged," she added. And then, after an enjoyable trip to Italy, Mrs. Mayo's country of birth, her son had a relapse.

"Two weeks later," Gus Mayo said, "we rented out the house in Kensington and took a place in Walnut Creek [California], which was the driest area we could find in the San Francisco–Oakland area, but the drunkenness had come back, his energy was gone, and he would slip into these comas. It was obvious that the nystatin had lost its impact."

Then the Mayos read about the Japanese drunkenness disease experienced by Charlie Swaart of Phoenix. "The similarities to Duffy's drunkenness were uncanny, but what really excited us was that nystatin had lost its effect on Mr. Swaart, too, but then he'd recovered, anyway," Gianna Mayo said excitedly. Dr. Levin contacted Charles Swaart's doctors and adapted a proper dosage of similar medication for the child. Ketoconazole (Nizoral™) is what saved little Duffy from carrying his childhood autism into a lifetime of adult schizophrenia.

Duffy Mayo is no longer labeled autistic. His mental illness has disappeared as a result of the treatment for his Candida syndrome. "He's still got a lot of catching up to do," a happy mother agreed, "because he lost so much ground when he was sick. But with special speech therapy and reading lessons, he's closing the gap fast."

Autism, twice as common as childhood blindness and many times more devastating, may be conquerable—reversible—by directly treating its potential physical cause—the yeast syndrome.

NOTES

1. John Hopkins, "Living Without Immunity" (a five-part series), *Oklahoma City Times*, April 12, 1982.

2. C. Orian Truss, *The Missing Diagnosis*, Birmingham, Ala.: The Author, 1982, p. 86.

3. Ibid., p. 89.

4. Ibid.

5. C. Orian Truss, "Metabolic Abnormalities in Patients with Chronic Candidiasis—the Acetaldehyde Hypothesis," *Journal of Orthomolecular Medicine*, 1984, 13:66–93.

6. Don G. Campbell, "The Cruel Trick That Nature Played on Young Duffy Mayo," *Los Angeles Times*, September 25, 1983, pt. 8, p. 10.

18

Allergies, Chemical Hypersensitivities, and Yeast Infestation

While working in a hospital dental clinic early in 1984, forty-two-year-old Eric O'Meara, D.D.S., of Irondequoit, New York, developed classical chemical hypersensitivity symptoms. He found himself periodically unable to think, depressed, dizzy, exhausted, suffering with chest pains and headaches, and generally reacting adversely to an environment that has been altered by man's technology. Dr. O'Meara reacted to manmade surroundings such as nylon draperies, carpeting giving off formaldehyde vapors (designated as "outgassing"), soft plastic substances like packing materials, petroleum products, and numerous other items. To find some semblance of wellness, he consulted clinical ecologist (an environmental medicine specialist) Sherry A. Rogers, M.D., of Syracuse, New York. Dr. Rogers is a Diplomate of the American Board of Family Practice, Fellow of the American College of Allergists, Fellow of the American Association for Clinical Immunology and Allergy, and member of the Board of Directors of the American Academy of Environmental Medicine. She undertook to find the source of this dentist's hypersensitivity difficulties and swiftly uncovered that his main allergic factor was the Candida syndrome.

Dr. Rogers reported in written and recorded interviews:

Dr. O'Meara's allergy trouble was part of the man's total body load, a chemical burden resulting from his serious immune system breakdown. Candidiasis brought about part of that breakdown. In turn, his immunity impairment gave rise to the "spreading phenomenon," a term indicating the patient's general reaction to many allergens. *Candida albicans* became another one of these excitants which brought on more hypersensitivity responses. As soon as he moved from out of state to work in the dental clinic, two years ago, and also moved into a new home, his allergies flared. There's something present in that new house and new job that's causing Eric's trouble.

He was so highly chemically sensitive, in fact, that in order to reduce his total body load of chemicals, the only way I could return him to any kind of normal state for the first time in two years was to have him live outdoors in his garage with the garage door wide open for a year. Eric moved a cot with bedclothes made of cotton out there and slept in the garage summer and winter.

"I keep warm in these freezing New York State winters by using an electric blanket," Dr. O'Meara told us on February 22, 1986. "Besides, I've always had a feeling for camping out."

Dr. Rogers continued:

As soon as he walked into the house and remained for any length of time, all of his symptoms would recur. Obviously, he's preparing to buy a home that is more chemically suitable.

As well, Dr. O'Meara had to operate on his dental patients wearing a ceramic mask with metal tubing attached to the hospital clinic's wall oxygen system. Before treatment for the Candida syndrome he could not go upstairs in the hospital to make rounds on patients. The hospital corridors' ambient chemicals made him too sick and disoriented. His first sign of hypersensitivity was a reaction to the formaldehyde cold-sterilization solution used in the hospital dental office. He knew that the formaldehyde bothered him. Open formaldehyde trays may have triggered his chemical hypersensitivity.

Dr. Rogers treated the dentist's yeast infestation with nystatin. She added:

After nystatin, he could go upstairs in the hospital corridors and rooms to make rounds on patients with no difficulty and no symptoms whatsoever. It did lower his chemical hypersensitivity, and I see this happen in numerous people over and over again. People who have terrifically debilitating chemical and food hypersensitivities—once they go on nystatin—it knocks their level of sensitivity down by a third or more—up to 50 percent. But nystatin was just sort of the icing on the cake. It reduced Eric's level of sensitivity, what I designate as his "total load," even further than I had been able to already accomplish by addressing his other chemical, mold, and food hypersensitivities.

The most severely affected people with candidiasis do not merely have the Candida problem. Instead, as I've mentioned, they have Candida as one of many aspects of the total body burden that has made them victims of the twentieth-century disease—known to be environmental illness. It's naive to think that Candida is the only fungus or mold that can cause these symptoms in people who have received many antibiotics. There are many others that we are finding. Sometimes nystatin and even Nizoral™ do not work, but injections do. Just administering injections to a person for house dust, mites, Candida, and many molds that are found in the environment using mold plates (that are available to people throughout the country by sending fifteen dollars per mold plate to my office [and are available through other sources around the U.S.]), clear up the individual's chemical hypersensitivities. My mold cultures frequently pick up Candida in a person's ambient environment at home and at work.

Dr. Rogers suggests that people assess their environment to learn: (1) how mold is contributing to their total hypersensitivity load; (2) which molds are unusual and are not included in their anti-allergy injections—or which should now be addressed to bring about tighter environmental controls to get rid of that particular mold; (3) whether or not *C. albicans* is present.

Dr. Rogers is herself a victim of the yeast syndrome. She admitted:

> Many of us who are more understanding of the patient's candidiasis difficulties probably reach a higher level of empathy because we are burdened with the disease. Then we become highly motivated to know everything possible about it.
>
> The Candida syndrome is spreading among the populace. It's going to get worse, too, but conventionally practicing allergists don't believe so. They think we environmental medicine specialists are "nuttier than fruitcakes" or are "quacks" and that our patients are hypochondriacs.
>
> I just feel sorry for the individual candidiasis patient. It's bad enough to suffer from a disease in which very few people understand what you've got—it's not taught in medical school and not published in standard peer-reviewed medical literature—but then when relatives, friends, neighbors or doctors don't believe you, the condition is even more difficult with which to cope. Patients find that having the Candida syndrome is very lonely.

YOUR BODY'S TOTAL LOAD

William Rea, M.D., of Dallas, Texas, first advanced the "barrel concept" of resistance to environmental toxins and stressors, in which chemicals and infections, allergens and other stressors to which you are exposed, fill up "your resistance barrel" until it overflows with symptoms. Dr. Rogers introduces the similar concept of your body's total load, the amount of potential environmentally induced illness, or EI, to which you are exposed every day. Dr. Rogers says that knowing about EI is crucial to the healing of the immune system. Not only is EI a cause of illness, but it is basic to our wellness.

Dr. Rogers says,

> I like to think of the total load as being analogous to a boat filled with twelve marked boxes. All of us are set adrift in the sea in the same type of boat with the same twelve marked boxes. The only difference is the location of our boat's leak. Some of us have a leak up near the gunwhale so that we only have to throw one or two heavy boxes overboard in order for the boat to stop taking on water. Others have their leak further down toward the keel and must throw many boxes overboard before they stop the seepage. Only the very worst off have their leak located along the keel. Even if they toss all twelve boxes into the ocean and get rid of their entire total load, they still will continue to take in water and proceed to sink. Instead, they must go into dry dock for the full repair job. This dry dock is my metaphor for the environmental hospital unit, where everything that contributes to environmentally induced illness is left outside.

What is in Dr. Rogers's twelve mysterious boxes? The total environmental overload.

In the first box are the inhalants, pollens, dust, dust mites, molds, animal danders, and similar pollutants. Once this box is thrown overboard, it no longer contributes to the overload. That's usually as far as conventional-type allergists go. For the patient, once he utilizes the environmental controls and receives immunotherapy for his inhalant hypersensitivities, this no longer contributes to his symptom overload.

The second box contains food allergies. Let's look at the case of thirty-nine-year-old David Jurgenson of Danbury, Connecticut, who has consulted innumerable psychiatrists for his twenty years of depression. David has taken many different antidepressant medications, prescribed for years by those psychiatrists. Within two weeks of being treated for food allergies with specific food antigen injections and upon starting the rotation diet, he was able to discard his Elavil® prescription (an antidepressant with sedative effects). Not only did his depression lift, but David became a happier man because once again he experienced clear thinking—for the first time in two decades. Food was one of David Jurgenson's major heavy boxes. He carried it around in a boat that was in danger of sinking.

The third box is chemical sensitivity. For a year, Theresa Ballone of Utica, New York, had been suffering with severe rheumatoid arthritis, shown by test results of elevated rheumatoid factors and sedimentation rates. When Dr. Rogers tested her to phenol, the patient was completely neutralized free of pain and stiffness. "This event was filmed double-blind to teach other physicians," Dr. Rogers wrote to us. "It also served to prove to Theresa that chemical hypersensitivity was at the root of her symptoms and led us to know what chemicals she then had to remove from her home in order to attain a symptom-free state."

The fourth box contains the newer molds that have been the topic of Dr. Rogers's research published in the *Annals of Allergy* (July 1982, January 1983, and May 1984). Bill Wallensky was the chairman of a college theology department near Hanover, New Hampshire, and suffering from extreme depression, tiredness, and weakness. During a visit that Reverend Wallensky made to Syracuse, New York, he undertook an evaluation at the Syracuse Medical Center—complete with lumbar puncture and CAT scans. But the diagnostic tests could not establish any cause for his problems. Yet, two weeks after taking antigen injections of the newer molds, Bill's symptoms had totally disappeared. Now, whenever he is late with receiving the appropriate injections, his symptoms recur—upon injection, they disappear within ten minutes.

The fifth box is labeled "phenol-free." Some people never stop sinking until they are on phenol-free injections. They are just too chemically overloaded and sensitized to be able to improve without phenol-free injections. In Chapter Nine, Conrad G. Maulfair, Jr., D.O., of Mertztown, Pennsylvania, could not complete an allergy testing panel for his patient since she reacted to the phenol preservative used in all of the test antigens. Now meet Lenny Siegal, a twenty-seven-year-old television engineer from New York City. He prefaced his visit to Dr. Rogers with the information that all allergists' injections made his condition worse. "I assured Lenny that I would not worsen him because of the individualized serial dilution testing method that I use. When I did create a severe asthma reaction, I knew instantly why we all made him worse. Sure enough," wrote Dr. Rogers, "testing to phenol dropped his pulmonary function. Giving Lenny phenol-free inhalants left him symptom-free and medication-free for the first time ever."

The sixth box contains *C. albicans*. David Raleigh is a forty-two-year-old attorney from Buffalo, New York. He suffered with extreme lethargy, depression, weakness, and headaches for two years after a surgical procedure was performed and several antibiotics prescribed. Treatment for candidiasis got rid of his troubles in short order. Now David has a full sense of well-being.

The seventh box consists of nutrition. For thirteen years, Mary Sally O'Leary of Springfield, Massachusetts, was afflicted with eczema on her face, throat, arms, and upper torso. She saw several dermatologists and allergists but had never been cleared of the condition. Using the total load concept, Dr. Rogers drew her serum for a vitamin A level, rationalizing that Mary Sally's accelerated turnover of skin must be depleting her vitamin A faster than that of a normal person. Sure enough, her level was very low. Within one month of starting dust and mold injections and oral vitamin A supplementation, the patient's eczema went away entirely. She is now completely clear of the condition.

Vitamins, minerals, essential fatty acids, digestive enzymes, and other food supplements are often crucial factors in attaining complete health. Currently, many doctors sadly fail to employ nutrition as a therapeutic aid the way it should be used. But wholistic physicians are on the cutting edge of clinical research and patient care—they know that such nutritional treatment is mandatory.

The eighth total environmental overload box is hormone hypersensitivity. Paula Loedenheim of Manchester, New Hampshire, had severe premenstrual syndrome, becoming psychotic and extremely depressed for four days before her period. Progesterone neutralization injections brought Paula out of this trouble within three minutes. She used this hormone treatment every four hours for those four days to remain asymptomatic. Clinical ecologists and candidiasis-conscious physicians have also utilized estrogen, luteinizing hormone, and testosterone for such hormone hypersensitivities.

The ninth box is labeled "toxic." Such toxicity signifies people who are overloaded with heavy metal poisoning, such as cadmium from cigarette smoking, lead and other chemicals from auto exhaust, or pesticides. Levels of pesticides and other chemical compounds can now be determined from the blood, and heavy metal toxicity is often established by hair mineral analysis. Some people are never better until all of their dental silver-mercury amalgams are entirely replaced (see the conclusion of this chapter).

The tenth box contains emotional and mental stress and distress. Many people never experience EI until after sustaining serious emotional trauma such as the death of a spouse, a divorce, or some other significant distressing event. Medical scientists know that the immune system is extremely vulnerable to stress. For instance, men whose wives were dying of breast cancer showed lower numbers of T-suppressor cells in their bloodstream during the last month of their wives' illness. These T-cells are crucial in restricting the amount of potentially harmful antibodies that are produced.

The eleventh box that Dr. Rogers describes is a miscellaneous group of mediators such as histamine (a depressor protein breakdown product), serotonin (a blood chemical that constricts the vessels and serves as a neurotransmitter), heparin (a blood anticoagulant), and viral vaccine extracts that neutralize some people's symptoms.

The twelfth box of environmentally induced "total load" illness is a mystery. Dr. Rogers told us,

The twelfth box was a mystery to me for a long time, because I thought there was something extremely important in there and, indeed, there is. But it is not nearly as elusive as one would like to think. We've been looking for a long time for some magic final ingredient that will turn around our diseases, make us totally well, and not dependent upon such strict environmental and dietary controls as indicated by the Candida control diet in your Section Three. Well, I have finally figured out what the mystery box contains. It is patient compliance. Whenever I find someone who is not improving as I expect, it usually is that he or she still has a gas-heated house or some other tremendously potent overload that continues to sink the boat of wellness. Such people frequently have to go outside the home, as did Dr. Eric O'Meara, simply because they do not have a safe oasis to which they can escape. They frequently must fast to reduce their total load since often they cheat in their eating and don't rotate foods. They need the salts, ascorbate [vitamin C], frequent oxygen, and neutralizing doses to keep their illnesses under control.

By periodically reminding ourselves of the total load and the contents of each box, we will be able to attain a constant upward progress toward total wellness.

WHAT'S EATING YOU?—OR CANDIDA ALBICANS AS PART OF THE TOTAL LOAD

Is it hard to pinpoint the last time you felt really well? That's a question environmental medicine specialists frequently ask their patients. Here are a few others you might try answering as well:

Are you depressed soon after breakfast that includes toast, coffee, and sugar?

Does your temper flare unexpectedly when you come up from a damp and moldy basement or just finish working in the garden?

Have you wondered what's eating you?

It might be that *C. albicans* is your primary allergenic factor. That the yeast is, indeed, "eating you."

Allergy and hypersensitivity to chemicals, foods, molds, and additional aspects of our environment have become easier to diagnose and treat. Environmental medicine (clinical ecology) has arisen as a new discipline in the health sciences of allergy and immunology. An allergic person was once considered to be reactant to something with which no one else had a problem. This outdated concept is not accepted anymore. Most people respond to their surroundings adversely in some way, simply because these surroundings have undergone major changes in ecology as our technology has advanced. Medical scientists have established that 50 percent of all of us (including "healthy" and "unhealthy" individuals) have definite and well-demarcated allergies. To find yours merely requires looking by means of the new methods developed by clinical ecologists.

"Allergy" comes from the Greek word *állos* meaning "altered" or "other," and *érgon* meaning "work" or "action." About a century ago the Austrian pediatrician Clement Von Perquet, M.D., came up with this combined descriptive term. During the last twenty-five years medical science has learned that *C. albicans* alone can bring on allergic symptoms which might occur as a result of the toxins it produces.

In October 1961 A. Liebeskind, M.D., of Haifa, Israel, told the Fourth International Congress of Allergology, "*C. albicans* can evoke allergic reactions in a human organism [a person], which otherwise is in a normal condition." Using hyposensitization injections of an extract of *C. albicans* under the skin of subjects. Dr. Liebeskind first tested and then treated twenty-five patients suffering with various allergic illnesses: migraine headaches, vulvitis, chronic blepharoconjunctivitis (inflammation of the eye's covering membrane), bronchial asthma or rhinitis, gastrointestinal manifestations, and other conditions. The one thing that all of these patients had in common was the Candida syndrome. Treatment of their candidiasis meant remission of allergy symptoms for all of them.[1]

Studies on the mechanism of fungal infections have been carried out by Kazuo Iwata, Ph.D., Chief Microbiologist in the Department of Microbiology, Faculty of Medicine, University of Tokyo. In 1967, Dr. Iwata was the first scientist to isolate several high- and low-molecular-weight toxins from virulent strains of *C. albicans*.[2] He named this yeast's poison "Canditoxin," described its physical and chemical properties, and tested its toxicity on mice.[3] Over the ensuing years of research, Dr. Iwata, who summarized his findings as the featured speaker at the 1983 Yeast–Human Interaction Symposium in Birmingham, Alabama, showed that Canditoxin produces histopathological changes in the host's tissues and various internal organs.[4] It brings on toxicity that resembles an anaphylactic shock, related to its principal action as a histamine-releasing agent and its ability to cause extreme vascular permeability.[5] Canditoxin fractions also contain glycoprotein toxin and shock toxins.[6]

The same hypersensitivity response to Canditoxin that occurs in mice takes place in people in the form of allergies. Allergies are no respectors of age, sex, or economic situation and can manifest themselves in a number of ways. The following listing of sites and symptoms assumed by allergies has been collected by Yehuda Barsel, M.D., an allergist practicing in Colonia, New Jersey.

Head (Cerebral)

- Headache
- Inappropriate thought processes
- Depression—acute or chronic
- Learning disability—minimal brain dsyfunction; attention-deficit disease
- Neuritis; paresthesia (numbness, tingling)
- Tension fatigue syndrome
- Convulsion
- Hyperactive; irritable
- Hungry; thirsty
- Lethargy; disorientation
- Schizoid personality syndrome (mood swings)
- Schizophrenia

Eyes (Ophthalmologic)

- Allergic shiners (darkened "circles" under the eyes)
- Lid edema—varying (swelling eyelid)
- Blurring of vision—episodic (comes and goes)
- Transitory refractive changes (blurring)
- Itching; burning
- Photophobia (light bothering eyes)
- Redness; edema of the conjunctiva (white portion of eye)
- Allergic conjunctivitis

Ears (Otologic)

- Serous otitis (fluid in the middle ear)
- Ear popping
- Tinnitus (ringing, roaring, buzzing)

- Meniere's syndrome; vertigo (dizziness)
- Loss of hearing

Nose and Throat (Upper Respiratory Tract)

- Nasal salute (allergic salute: rubbing nose from mouth upward, often with palm of hand or with wrist, causing the mark of a crease across the nose)
- Frequent nosebleeds
- Rhinitis (runny nose)
- Postnasal drainage; cough
- Nasal itching
- Nasal speech
- Laryngeal edema; hoarseness
- Polyps
- Sinusitis

Bronchi and Lungs (Lower Respiratory Tract)

- Asthma
- Repeated bronchiolitis
- Asthmatic bronchitis
- Coughing

Digestion (Gastrointestinal Tract)

- Edema (swelling)
- Colic; cramps
- Foul odor to the breath
- Frequent canker sores
- Trouble swallowing
- Lump in throat
- Gas; belching; stomachache
- Nausea; vomiting
- Retasting (food taste reappearing in mouth, due to belching)
- Constipation; diarrhea
- Ulcer syndrome; gallbladder syndrome; appendiceal syndrome and ulcerative colitis syndrome
- Bloating
- Rectal itching; pain; fissure
- Proctalgia fugax (rectal pain)

Heart and Blood Vessels (Cardiovascular)

- Tachycardia
- Palpitation
- Edema—localized and generalized
- Chilling; flushing
- EKG (electrocardiogram) changes
- Ecchymosis—spontaneous bruising
- Vasoconstriction; vasodilation
- Vasculitis (inflammation of vessels)
- Anginal (heart) pain
- Arrhythmia

Skin (Dermatologic)

- Hives; urticaria
- Atopic dermatitis; eczema
- Erythema multiforma (large red welts)
- Pallor
- Contact dermatitis
- Dermatophytid—known idiomatically as an "Id" reaction
- Allergic eczema
- Contact eczema
- Atopic dermatitis (rashes)
- Seborrheic dermatitis (dandruff)
- Irritative changes
- Infectious eczematoid dermatitis (skin infection)
- Nummular dermatitis (rash)
- Neurodermatitis
- Psoriasis

Sex Organs and Urinary Tract (Genitourinary)

- Urination frequency—urgency
- Dysuria—abnormality with urination (painful or difficult)
- Enuresis (bedwetting)
- Albuminuria; hematuria (albumin and/or blood in urine)
- Prostatic edema (swelling of prostate gland)
- Vulvovaginitis (itching or infection of the vulva and/or vagina)
- Dysmenorrhea (painful menstruation)

Musculo-Skeletal

- Arthralgia (pain in joint)
- Myalgia; leg muscle ache; restless legs
- Edema of joints
- Rheumatoid syndrome

Blood (Hematological)

- Anemia (low red blood cell count)
- Neutropenia (low white blood cell count of neutrophils, the defenders against bacteria)
- Thrombocytopenia purpura (black and blue swelling due to decrease of blood platelets)
- Leukopenia (low white blood cell count)
- Eosinophilia (high white blood cell count of eosinophils, the defenders against allergens)

ALLERGIC SYMPTOMS FROM IMMUNE SYSTEM DYSREGULATION

In December 1985, a position paper explaining allergic symptomatology was drafted by a committee representing the American Academy of Environmental Medicine. The paper clarified the ways in which chemical and food sensitivities result in acute and chronic illnesses. Its central thesis is that such hypersensitivity becomes mediated (expressed) by the same body system that causes traditional allergic reactions to pollens, dust, animal dander, and molds. These allergens may bring about responses caused by a different malfunction of the immune system, named by the academy's clinical ecologists "immune system dysregulation" (ISD).

ISD may develop over a long period or very rapidly. Canditoxin or other aspects of infesting yeast are some of the several allergens known to trigger the condition. A susceptible individual's accumulated exposure to circumstances that favor the growth of *C. albicans* help to excite allergic disorders related to candidiasis: damp, moldy, and mildewed cellars; freshly plowed soil in the garden or the fields; yeast-risen bread; fermented beverages; dried fruits; most condiments; many cheeses; and other factors described in this book. ISD often remains undiagnosed because many physicians faced with its incredible array of seemingly unrelated symptoms are ignorant of newly available diagnostic methods. As you have seen from various case histories supplied by the numerous medical contributors to this book, a misdiagnosis of psychosomatic disease, mental illness, or just plain "psychic stress" is not uncommon for many patients afflicted with the Candida syndrome. While medications commonly prescribed for these false diagnoses to some extent may suppress symptoms, at times the drugs can further aggravate the patient's disorder without improving at all the underlying disease process. When the immune system is malfunctioning, a broad range of improper reactions occur, even in response to beneficial substances entering the body.

The body's malfunction commonly originates with the immune defensive lymphocyte T-cells. If their normal numbers are reduced or their ability to function is impaired, they can no longer properly regulate lymphocyte B-cell antibody production. Without adequate T-cell control, B-cells cannot readily distinguish harmless dust, pollen, animal dander, or nutritious foods from toxic chemicals or life-threatening microorganisms. The patient's restoration of normal immune function then becomes a long, slow process punctuated by exasperating short-term setbacks. These setbacks are part of the healing scheme. Fortunately, the frequency, duration, and severity of setbacks gradually diminish until symptoms are mild and occur only on occasion.

Poisoning by Canditoxin takes place in no small measure by the production of free radical pathology in a person suffering with the Candida syndrome. Free radicals damage the microsomal membranes (linings throughout your cells, responsible for synthesizing proteins), eventually resulting in a depletion of adenosinetriphosphate (ATP), the cofactor (described in Chapter Seventeen) that is the result of energy production in metabolism. Without ATP, our cells can't carry out their functions. This may explain the weakness seen in environmentally sensitive people. Their fat, sugar, and protein metabolism pathways are altered. Enzyme systems that detoxify chemicals entering their bodies and the sulfhydryl systems both become damaged. After repeated induction and constant stimulation, these two systems eventually become depleted with resultant end-organ failure. For example, the kidneys slow down their filtering or the liver reduces its detoxifying activities. When the systems no longer gather up and extrude pollutants coming into the body from surroundings, a person with the yeast syndrome will then experience a worsening of his immune system dysregulation.[7]

SILVER-MERCURY AMALGAM DENTAL FILLINGS AND THE YEAST SYNDROME

Since having her "silver"-mercury amalgam dental fillings removed, Diane Toombs, a thirty-six-year-old homemaker living in Indianapolis, Indiana, is much relieved of various disorders arising from the Candida syndrome. Her medical progress was supervised by David A. Darbro, M.D., and Sandra C. Denton, M.D., practicing together in Indianapolis. These two family practice physicians specialize in allergy, arthritis and other degenerative diseases, chelation therapy, and preventive medicine.

Drs. Darbro and Denton provided us with Mrs. Toombs's case history. In their detailed case report, they wrote:

> Diane's health, unremarkable until her early twenties, took a dramatic turn for the worse, sending her on a medical roller coaster which nearly culminated in a nervous breakdown. She even had a death wish which caused her to feel guilty because it conflicted with her spiritual values as a Christian. The assistance of M.D.s, chiropractors, psychologists, psychiatrists, and group counseling sessions was all to no avail. After extensive testing, Diane was finally told that her problem was "all in her head."

In a state of exasperation, Mrs. Toombs first consulted Dr. Darbro in the fall of 1983. He put the patient through a full physical examination and a series of diagnostic tests, including answering the yeast-connected illness questionnaire devised by Dr. William Crook. Although that questionnaire is of great significance when the patient scores 160 points or above, Mrs. Toombs's test revealed only 60 subjective points.

However, her physical test was revealing. She displayed a positive Chvostek's sign, the occurrence of facial spasm excited by a slight tap over the facial nerve.

Dr. Darbo explained:

This was indicative of cellular magnesium deficiency, which we have noted in many of our yeast syndrome patients. Indeed, laboratory tests showed Diane to have a low serum magnesium and a low phosphorous level, signifying problems with mineral assimilation. Hair analysis showed further trace mineral difficulties, specifically with transport of calcium and magnesium. Toxic levels of lead and mercury were also present. Food allergy testing demonstrated significant reactivity to corn, wheat, milk, eggs, and more, all of which is indicative of immune system overload. Diane's white blood cells barely moved at all under darkfield microscopic examination, a telltale sign of white blood cell viability problems. The darkfield exam also revealed evidence of cell wall deficient Candida organisms lurking about. [Note that Drs. Darbro and Denton are proponents of Dr. Philip Hoekstra's live blood cell analysis—which has met with much controversy among experts on *C. albicans* and candidiasis— described in Chapter Nine.]

We initiated battle plans by attacking the Candida via Dr. Crook's "caveman diet" for a week, followed by a low carbohydrate diet, vitamin and mineral supplementation, and—our heavy artillery—nystatin. We were disappointed in Diane's lack of progress, and accordingly tried Caprystatin™, then Candistat™. Vitaldophilus™ and Ultradophilus™ [both commercial *L. acidophilus* cultures] were also initiated, all to no avail. Diane not only failed to improve but actually seemed to worsen. She became more environmentally sensitive and had to stop going to church because she couldn't tolerate the outgassing of formaldehyde from a newly installed carpet.

We were perplexed: What to do next?

I began to ask God for wisdom and shortly thereafter attended the November 1985 semi-annual meeting of the American Academy of Medical Preventics, in San Francisco, in which the horrors of mercury amalgams (better known to most of us as "silver dental fillings") were discussed. For some reason Diane came to my mind, and I remembered noting several fillings glistening in her mouth when I'd first examined her.

Could this be the missing connection? Maybe all those other doctors had been correct when they diagnosed her problem as being "all in her head"!

Upon returning to Indianapolis with this thought in mind, Dr. Darbro shared his new information with Dr. Denton and Mrs. Toombs. They decided that removing the "silver"-mercury amalgam fillings was worth a try. After all, nothing else had worked to rid the patient of her candidiasis. A local Indianapolis dentist was found who knew the technique of sequential mercury amalgam dental filling removal as advocated by mercury amalgam specialist Hal Huggins, D.D.S., of Colorado Springs, Colorado. Dr. Huggins is a pioneer in the discovery that mercury used by dentists for filling dental cavities, with the passage of time, escapes from amalgam fillings, new and old, in concentrations considerably exceeding our overly lenient industrial safety limits.[8] The mercury in your dental fillings leaches into the body and is deposited in your kidneys, nerve tissues, brain, bone marrow, endocrine hormone glands, and elsewhere,[9] and damage takes place sufficient to produce subclinical symptoms and to shorten your life.[10]

Dr. Darbro continued the case history of his patient:

Diane's fillings showed extremely high readings of electrical negativity, which means a tremendous amount of mercury was being released from her fillings each time she chewed her food. She was placed on high dosage of vitamin C to chelate out the mercury and her fillings were replaced with suitable nonreactive materials. Within a week she was feeling better. Once again she could go to church, outgassing carpet or not. Three months later she was so remarkably improved both mentally and physically that upon being retested for food allergies we found they had totally disappeared. She just was no longer allergic. Her energy level returned to normal. Thus, once we took care of Diane's "head problems," everything else fell into place.

What's the moral of this story? Now we start by checking for mercury amalgam fillings—finding them in 99.5 percent of all candidiasis patients we examine. We try to interest the patients in getting rid of their "silver"-mercury dental amalgams so that they can rid themselves of this strain on the immune system. We can then expect success in treatment by balancing their body minerals and changing their diets according to laboratory parameters.

In a May 4, 1986, interview, Dr. Denton told us, "I saw Diane Toombs only yesterday. She is just fine. Her husband told me that Diane definitely is better since she's had her amalgams out!" The mercury so suppressed the patient's immune system that candidiasis could retain its hold on her. With the interfering source of immune suppression removed, the yeast syndrome finally responded to treatment and now is gone as well.

MERCURY AMALGAM TOXICITY FROM DENTAL FILLINGS

An article written by Victor Penzer, D.D.S., of Newton Centre, Massachusetts, and reprinted in the *Townsend Letter for Doctors* from the *Journal of the Massachusetts Dental Society*, clarifies the mercury amalgam toxicity issue that has besieged the dental profession since 1833.[11] Dr. Penzer makes plain the significance of mercury deposited in our tissues from mercury amalgamated dental fillings. He says that mercury inhibits enzyme action, disturbs the absorption and utilization of nutrients, and produces electrical currents in the mouth. "Whenever we insert a variety of metals of which amalgam is composed (mercury, silver, tin, zinc, copper, etc.) in a solution of electrolytes, like saliva, we are virtually constructing a galvanic cell." Electrolytic phenomena then occur. These disadvantageous phenomena include electrical currents that interfere with the nervous system, alter the ratios of T-cell lymphocytes so vital for immune defense, stimulate corrosion of dental restorations and other dental structures, cause local irritation, and result in hypersensitivity.[12]

Worse still are the effects for candidiasis victims: mercury leached out of amalgam fillings, when converted to methyl mercury, so disturbs the intestinal flora that *C. albicans* is encouraged to grow. As with Diane Toombs, clinical reports confirm that some patients suffering with disorders of the Candida syndrome fail to get well on the usual antifungal therapy alone. They do, however, recover after the source of mercury intoxication is eliminated.

We strongly advise our readers to discontinue having their teeth filled with silver-mercury amalgams. In 1980, American dentists filled teeth with 200,000 pounds of mercury. Alarmingly, this amount has continued to grow. In 1985 dentists used an estimated 300,000 pounds of the poisonous metal on our teeth, half again the amount used only five years before. If you are committed to wholistic health principles, you might consider having all of your mercury amalgam fillings removed and replaced with porcelain, nonporous resins, or some other suitable material. Ask your candidiasis-conscious physician for a referral to an appropriately trained wholistic dentist.

NOTES

1. A. Liebeskind, "*Candida albicans* as an Allergenic Factor," *Annals of Allergy,* June 1962, 20:394–396.

2. K. Iwata, K. Uchida, H. Endo, M. Okudaira, and Y. Nozu, " 'Canditoxin,' a New Toxic Substance Isolated from a Strain of *Candida albicans,*" *Medical Biology,* 1967, 74:346–350, 351–355, 75:192–195; 1968, 77:151–157, 159–164, 165–169, 171–174; 1971, 82:97–101, 103–108, 109–112; K. Iwata and K. Uchida, "Amino Acid Composition of Canditoxin," *Medical Biology,* 1971, 83:279–281; K. Iwata and K. Uchida, "Denaturation of Canditoxin and Its Relation to Phosphatase Activation," *Medical Biology,* 1971, 83:283–286.

3. K. Iwata, K. Uchida, and M. Okudaira, "Significance of Candidial Toxins in Infection," *Japanese Journal of Medical Mycology,* 1969, 10:95–107; K. Iwata, H. Yamaguchi, Y. Nozu, and K. Uchida, "Influence of Canditoxin on the Metabolism of Cultured Cells," *Medical Biology,* 1972, 85:143–148; K. Iwata, K. Uchida, T. Nagai, T. Ikeda, and M. Okudaira, "Significance of Candidial Toxins in the Pathogenesis of *Candida* Infection," Second International Specialized Symposium on Yeasts, Tokyo, 1972.

4. K. Iwata, "Significance of High-Molecular-Weight Mycotoxins in Infection," *Japanese Journal of Medical Mycology,* 1972,

13:181–186; K. Iwata, "On Mycotoxins, Particularly, High-Molecular-Weight Ones," *Japanese Journal of Medical Mycology*, 1973, 14:117–126; K. Iwata, "Studies on the Mechanism of Fungal Infections," *Japanese Journal of Medical Mycology*, 1975, 16:81–86.

5. K. Iwata, K. Uchida, H. Yamaguchi, and Y. Nozu, "*In Vivo* and *in Vitro* Mechanism of Action of Canditoxin," Proceedings of First Intersectional Congress, *IAMS*, 1975, 4:324–333; K. Iwata and K. Uchida, "Studies on Shock Toxins from *Candida albicans*," Second International Specialized Symposium on Yeasts, Tokyo, 1972.

6. K. Iwata and K. Uchida, "Role of Canditoxin in Experimental *Candida* Infection. Symposium on Toxins," *Journal of Medical Science and Biology*, 1974, 27:130–133; K. Iwata, K. Uchida, and Y. Nozu, "Chemical Analysis of Fatty Granules Produced in the Chick Embryo Cerebellum Cell Culture Under the Influence of Canditoxin," *Medical Biology*, 1971, 83:275–278; K. Iwata, "Toxins Produced by *Candida albicans*," *Contributions to Microbiology and Immunology*, 1977, 4:77–85.

7. M. G. Mustafa, A. D. Hacker, J. J. Ospital, M. Z. Hussain, and S. D. Lee, in S. D. Lee, ed., *Biochemical Effects of Environmental Pollutants*, Ann Arbor, Mich.: Ann Arbor Science, 1975.

8. Hal A. Huggins, *It's All in Your Head*, Colorado Springs, Colo.: Toxic Elements Research Foundation, 1985; S. Ziff, *Silver Dental Fillings: The Toxic Time Bomb*, New York: Aurora Press, 1984.

9. R. Schiel et al., "Studies of the Mercury Content in the Brain and Kidney Related to Number and Condition of Amalgam Fillings," *Medicine and Dental Medicine*, March 12, 1984; M. Nymander, "Report from Karolinska Institute," *Swedish Annual Medical Conference*, Stockholm, November 1984; Report of International Committee—Maximum Allowable Concentrations of Mercury Compounds, *Archives of Environmental Health*, December 19, 1969.

10. T. W. Clarkson, "The Pharmacology of Mercury Compounds," *Annals of the Review of Pharmacology*, 1972, 12:376–406; H. B. Gerstner and J. E. Huff, "Clinical Toxicology of Mercury," *Journal of Toxicology and Environmental Health*, 1977, 2(3):491–526.

11. Victor Penzer, "Amalgam Toxicity: Grand Deception," *Townsend Letter for Doctors*, February–March 1986, 35:58–63.

12. W. Schriever and L. Diamond, "Electromotive Forces and Electric Currents Caused by Metallic Dental Fillings," *Journal of Dental Research*, 1952, 31(2):205–229; J. M. Mumford, "Electrolytic Action in the Mouth and Its Relationship to Pain,"

Journal of Dental Research, 1957, 36:632–640; C. J. Reed and W. Willman, "Galvanism in the Oral Cavity," *Journal of the American Dental Association,* 1940, 27(3):1471–1475; A. A. Guyton, *Textbook of Medical Physiology,* Philadelphia: W. B. Saunders, 1976.

19

Psoriasis and Other Yeast-Connected Skin Troubles

Atopic eczema of the face, neck, and hands was the primary form of generalized, chronic candidiasis manifested by twenty-nine-year-old Jody L. Baccellieri, a registered nurse living in the Portland, Oregon, suburb of Tigard. Atopic eczema was her body's skin manifestation of allergy. Although Mrs. Baccellieri was employed at the University of Oregon Medical School Health Center as a ward nurse, she could find no relief for her discomfort. From age two on, and seemingly with changes in the season—especially at the advent of summer—she agonized with itching skin, superficial inflammation, red rash, small weeping blisters, and crusting scales. Sometimes she experienced thickening, discoloration, or scaling of the skin for no apparent reason. Her condition worsened markedly during both of her pregnancies. Mrs. Baccellieri had grown to accept this skin disorder. When the eczema finally became impossibly irritated, she was forced to seek medical assistance outside the health center.

On October 10, 1983, the nurse brought her complaints to the attention of environmental and preventive medicine specialist T. Daniel Pletsch, M.D., Medical Director of the Riverview Medical Clinic in Vancouver, Washington. Dr.

Pletsch performed a physical examination of the patient, revealing leathery hardening of her skin (lichenification) due to chronic irritation at the front of the neck, the spaces behind both knees, and at areas in front of the elbows. She told a history of suffering with hay fever and mild asthma for the past four years. Premenstrual symptoms had been rather severe during the previous twelve months, she reported. Mrs. Baccellieri also confirmed that she frequently had to take antibiotics for staphylococcus infections. Moreover, she had received several courses of prednisone, a corticosteroid, during preceding years and, in fact, had been taking it constantly for the immediate past six months. Allergy tests that the physician performed on her indicated that she was allergic to five of the six foods tested: corn, milk, eggs, soy, and yeast; only wheat showed a negative result.

Dr. Pletsch started the nurse on two oral Mycostatin™ (nystatin) tablets four times a day, inhalant shots (her seasonal allergic reactions implied inhalant sensitivities), and the elimination (as much as possible) of the foods to which she was allergic. To aid her efforts to follow the Candida control diet, he provided detailed lists of foods to eat and those to avoid.

By January 1984, Jody Baccellieri's eczema was much improved. In fact, she advised the doctor that it was the best it had been in ten years. Her premenstrual syndrome was markedly better, too, even with omitting the prednisone previously prescribed as a PMS remedy.

In our followup telephone interview, Dr. Pletsch added to his initial report:

> Over the next year Jody continued to do quite well. She would have occasional recurrences of the eczema, but this seemed to be related to mold exposure and to some foods, particularly corn, nuts, possibly wheat, and possibly milk. She had increased her nystatin dose to four tablets, four times a day. I prescribed oil of evening primrose empirically [based on prior practical observations as being advantageous]. I find that evening primrose oil is helpful for a lot of skin problems. Gamma-linoleic acid [GLA] and the omega-6 fatty acids in evening primrose oil are excellent as healers of skin

reactions. I also use MaxEPA® with its omega-3 fatty acids, especially eicosapentanoic acid.

Nurse Baccellieri has continued to do well as long as she stays on the antiyeast treatment program and takes her oil of evening primrose food supplement.

Sherry A. Rogers, M.D., who contributed our case report of Eric O'Meara, D.D.S., for Chapter Eighteen, affirms that oil of evening primrose holds great value as a healing agent for skin problems. In *Bestways* magazine, Dr. Rogers writes:

> Efamol™ (oil of evening primrose [distributed as Efamol by Nature's Way Products, Inc. of Springville, Utah, under license from Efmol, Ltd., London, England]) has been found to be important in some, but not all, patients with eczema, PMS, hypertension, obesity, hyperactivity, psoriasis, and chemical sensitivity. In the latter diseases Efamol's gamma-linolenic acid tends to improve the integrity of the cell membrane, thereby making the patient less chemically sensitive. It takes a larger and longer exposure to produce the undesirable symptoms. Because the individual biochemical variables are so great, every chemically sensitive person owes it to herself to evaluate a trial of two months of GLA, one to two capsules three times a day. If there is no improvement, then discontinue it.[1]

SKIN SIGNS OF THE YEAST SYNDROME

Approximately 15 percent of patients with the Candida syndrome have skin lesions of some type.[2] These may consist of multiple, discrete, widely scattered red patches or pimples (2–4 mm in diameter) or larger red nodules (1–2 cm in diameter). The surgical removal of tissue of such lesions and observation of them under the microscope (biopsy) to determine the exact diagnosis often reveals skin layers infiltrated by yeast and pseudomycelial elements. Individuals of either sex, any race, and any age can develop skin signs of the Candida syndrome. Such infections are more likely during pregnancy, premenstrually, in the elderly, in those with debilitating disease such as diabetes or anemia, and in the immunocompromised person. Environmental conditions such as heat, humidity, friction between skin surfaces such as thighs rubbing together, and frequent exposure to water all favor development of candidiasis skin signs and symptoms.

Widespread skin lesions caused by verified *Candida albicans* suggest that the person has a blood-borne infection—Candida septicemia. As such, topical treatment is totally useless. Systemic therapy, as discussed in Section Two of this book, is indicated. Culture of tissue obtained by biopsy may help to confirm the diagnosis of Candida septicemia.[3]

Skin signs of the Candida syndrome take a number of forms: inflammation in the skin folds (Candida intertrigo); rash around the genitals (male balanitis or female vulvitis); diaper rash (diaper dermatitis); inflammation of the nail beds (onychia and paronychia); skin cracking in the corners of the mouth (perleche); athlete's foot (jockopedia); and two more recently discovered to be Candida-connected, oversecretion from the skin's oil glands (seborrheic dermatitis) and psoriasis. We will discuss the last two conditions first, because their relationship to yeast infestation potentially affects about 2 percent of everyone in North America, Europe, Australia, South America, and New Zealand. Asians and Africans seem to have a much lower incidence of psoriasis.

PSORIASIS AND SEBORRHEIC DERMATITIS

Psoriasis is a chronic skin disease that disfigures the faces and bodies of millions of people with its recurrent silvery-red scaly patches. The disease is neither dangerous nor contagious and may appear for the first time during adolescence, then come and go throughout a lifetime. Thomas F. Anderson, M.D., Associate Professor in the Department of Dermatology at the University of Michigan Medical School, Ann Arbor, offers these startling statistics: "If we exclude mild cases, we can conservatively estimate that from 1 percent to 2 percent of the U.S. population suffers from psoriasis. The peak age of onset is between 10 and 30 years."[4]

In presentations that he made to the 1983 and 1985 Yeast–Human Interaction Symposia, E. William Rosenberg, M.D.,

Professor of Dermatology in the Departments of Medicine and Pathology, University of Tennessee College of Medicine in Memphis, expounded on his findings regarding the cause of psoriasis. His conclusion is that an inherited fault in the body's antigen-antibody response to foreign organisms, especially to *C. albicans*, is responsible for many or most cases of psoriasis. Dr. Rosenberg explained,

> We think that psoriasis is a generalized inflammatory disorder initiated by microbial activation of the alternative complement pathway. The visible manifestations of psoriasis on the skin, in this view, occur partly because of microbial activators residing on the skin and partly as a result of the deposition in the skin of microbial products circulating in the bloodstream.

Human leukocyte antigen (HLA) genes have recently been discovered to be a decisive factor in resistance to particular diseases, including psoriasis. When *C. albicans* attempts to invade the body and cause psoriasis, the body cannot resist the assault if the individual's system lacks the HLA genes for producing appropriate defensive antibodies. This genetic disability explains, in part, why psoriasis is one of the diseases that runs in families. The other part is that candidiasis itself is often present in families, too, and makes itself known by bringing on psoriaticlike skin lesions.[5]

The symptomatic silvery-red and itchy psoriasis patches are produced when skin cells multiply about ten times or more faster than they should. The parts of the body most frequently affected are the scalp, knees, elbows, chest, abdomen, palms, and soles of the feet. Dot-shaped red marks may also appear under the fingernails.

Stanley I. Cullen, M.D., Associate Professor of Dermatology in the Department of Medicine at the University of Florida School of Medicine in Gainesville, says: "Seborrheic dermatitis ranges in severity from a mild, scaly, relatively asymptomatic scalp disorder to a severe, markedly pruritic [itchy], recalcitrant dermatitis involving large portions of the cutaneous [skin] surface. Exacerbations and remissions are seen frequently in this condition."[6]

A mild or superficial attack may be limited to the hairline

or eyebrows, or it can cover the outside of the ears, the chest, and the area of the back between the shoulder blades. The skin becomes inflamed and scaly; itching will be mild or severe or may not be present at all. Acute manifestations of seborrheic dermatitis might appear on the face and the neck, and in overweight people they commonly occur in the body folds.

Sometimes seborrheic dermatitis precedes psoriasis. Basically the condition is an excessive discharge of sebum from the oil glands. The excess, called seborrhea, results in an abnormally oily skin.

Seborrheic dermatitis in adults probably represents an inherited disorder of the immune responses, Dr. Rosenberg noted. He believes that *C. albicans* is the responsible organism which produces these outbreaks. He stated, "Seborrheic dermatitis is a common inflammatory condition with both clinical and microscopic similarities to psoriasis."

While Dr. Cullen declares, "The exact cause of seborrheic dermatitis is not known. . . . The role of microorganisms in the etiology [cause] of seborrheic dermatitis is uncertain." Dr. Rosenberg has eliminated the condition in many of his patients by applying antifungal antibiotics—treatment for candidiasis—such as oral and topical ketoconazole, oral nystatin, oral metronidazole, and orally administered cholestyramine. He has also achieved therapeutic effect using anti-Candida drugs for the elimination of psoriasis in several dozen people— research work that stimulated Dr. Trowbridge to begin using this successful approach in his own patients with psoriasis. Dr. Rosenberg reported a 75 percent positive response rate with oral ketoconazole and good results in twelve of fourteen psoriasis patients when they applied topical ketoconazole.

After hearing of the 1982 Yeast–Human Interaction Symposium presentation by Sidney M. Baker, M.D., Medical Director of the Gesell Institute of Human Development in New Haven, Connecticut, in which he told of improvements in psoriasis patients who were prescribed oral nystatin, Dr. Rosenberg launched his own therapeutic trials with the drug. "It is our belief that the long-term control of intestinal yeasts will be of crucial importance in the management of many patients with severe, widespread psoriasis," Dr. Rosenberg boldly claims.

He then tried cholestyramine, an agent that absorbs endotoxin (Canditoxin) and removes it from the gut. Five psoriasis patients found relief from using cholestyramine. Dr. Rosenberg summarized his studies: "It is our present impression that cholestyramine would be of greatest use in cases of generalized pustular psoriasis and in psoriasis in alcohol abusers."

Metronidazole (Flagyl®, made by Searle and Company of San Juan, Puerto Rico, or Protostat®, made by Ortho Pharmaceutical Corporation of Raritan, New Jersey), used for treating trichomonas (trichomonal vaginitis), inflammatory bowel disease, and (by pioneering wholistic physicians) rheumatoid arthritis (following the protocols promulgated by the Rheumatoid Disease Foundation, Route 4, Box 137, Franklin, Tennessee 37064; [615] 646-1030) has now become a useful antipsoriatic agent as well.

Psoriasis should no longer be considerd a skin disorder alone. In many, perhaps a majority, of patients it appears to be the result of the interaction between *C. albicans* and its human host.

CANDIDIASIS DIAPER RASH

When twenty-three-year-old Elsie Burbonsky of Oak Park, Illinois, brought her one-month-old daughter to the pediatrician because of diaper rash, she told the doctor, "I am terribly upset because I think I'm doing a bad job caring for this child. I think I gave her the rash because I recently developed a vaginal discharge that smells fruity."

The young mother was using plasticized and elasticized disposal diapers on the baby. She had been treating the rash with white petroleum jelly and bathing the infant's genital area with a deodorant soap after each urination or stooling.

Aside from the diaper rash, the only other abnormalities the pediatrician observed on physical examination were white, plaquelike lesions on mucous membranes inside the infant's mouth. The doctor realized that Elsie Burbonsky's baby had oral thrush and Candida-connected diaper rash (in England, more elegantly referred to as "napkin dermatitis"). No laboratory studies were needed for further evaluation, since the child's history and physical findings are classic for the diaper dermatitis he had correctly diagnosed.[7]

Three factors contributed to the development of candidiasis diaper rash for this baby:

First, putting an infant in tight, disposable diapers or cloth diapers covered by plastic pants interferes with the normal evaporation of moisture from the skin. The skin is thus kept in a pathologically wet state, making it more susceptible to damage. Maceration (wet soaking with irritation and inflammation) produces an environment that enables bacteria[8] and *C. albicans*[9] to overgrow.

Second, a one-month-old infant is quite active. Therefore, tightly fastened diapers or rubber pants that fit snugly are apt to chafe and irritate as well as macerate the skin. This, coupled with the normal production of ammonia compound in the urine, can produce significant additional inflammation.[10]

Third, the mother of this child probably has vulvovaginal candidiasis so her skin is likely to shed an increased amount of yeast to the infant and onto her diapers during changing. The child possibly has an oral infection due to *C. albicans* as well. The diaper area can readily be coated with yeast. The incidence of *C. albicans* infection is greater in infants with diaper dermatitis than in those without it—so the pediatrician appears correct in assuming that this organism is contributing to the baby's pathological condition.[11]

What should the doctor tell Mrs. Burbonsky about her baby's problem? What steps might he recommend for her to help cure it?

First, a physician considerate of the woman's feelings will assure her that diaper dermatitis is a common difficulty for infants and that its occurrence does not reflect on her competence as a mother. Indeed, he will probably praise her for demonstrating concern by promptly bringing the child for medical treatment.

Second, a physician willing to take the time to provide complete guidelines for managing the skin of the diaper area might offer these:

1. Expose the diaper area to air as much as you can; when this is not possible or convenient, frequent and prompt removal of wet diapers is necessary.

2. Bathing the child with harsh, irritating soaps (such as the deodorant type used by Mrs. Burbonsky) should be avoided. Also avoided should be diaper wipes, rinsing the diaper area with boric acid, or using tightly fitting plasticized or other types of disposable diapers or any rubber pants.

3. A practical course is to bathe the little girl gently with a mild castile soap solution such as Dr. Bronner's™, available from health food stores and some supermarkets. To help maintain a dry environment in the diaper area and minimize friction, apply a lanolin lotion after each washing or rinsing. Washable cloth diapers can be cleaned with this soap, too, then rinsed well and dried without the use of any fabric conditioners in the washer or dryer.

4. Cornstarch is not recommended by many pediatricians for use on baby's bottom, but if powder is applied, cornstarch might be preferable to petroleum-based products, which potentially can cause fluid retention in the skin. Cornstarch is claimed by some physicians to be safer than talc, which can be inhaled by child and mother alike and may lead to lung troubles.[12] The medical profession is divided on the use of baby powders. For example, other physicians believe that pure talcum powder is still among the best of topical treatments. (We suggest that you ask your own doctor's opinion on this.)

Because *C. albicans* is the designated villain in this diaper rash drama, treating the infection with antifungal agents would be appropriate. Here are the treatments that a pediatrician might prescribe:

First, nystatin (Mycostatin™, Nilstat™), 200,000 units (2 ml) orally four times daily for seven to ten days. This medication will help cure oral thrush and decrease the stool counts of *C. albicans*.

Second, when the mother has vulvovaginitis as a manifestation of her own infestation with *C. albicans*, the pediatrician who learns of such a circumstance will likely suggest that she have it treated by her gynecologist or general practitioner. If he instead referred her to a candidiasis-conscious physician, a thorough diagnostic workup might more properly result in Elsie Burbonsky being placed on a complete therapeutic program for full control of the yeast syndrome.

Third, to eradicate yeast infestation from the child's diaper area, the pediatrician might prescribe clotrimazole cream (Lotrimin™, Mycelex™) or miconazole cream (Monistat-7™ or Monistat-Derm™). These topical drugs are potent antifungal agents. The cream is usually prescribed for twice daily application for seven to fourteen days. Other agents used for diaper dermatitis can be associated with undesirable secondary effects. For example, nystatin-gramicidin-triamcinolone cream (Mycolog™) contains ethylenediamine, which sometimes causes contact dermatitis, since reports have been made of acute flareups during treatment in certain individuals.[13] Excessive use of fluorinated topical steroids (cousins to cortisone) may lead to skin atrophy and the development of skin streaks, stripes, or scarlike lines.

CANDIDA INTERTRIGO

The most common and characteristic form of skin candidiasis is Candida intertrigo, which occurs between the buttocks, in the umbilicus, in the skin folds on the inner sides of the upper thighs, in the abdominal crease in obese individuals, in the armpits, in the creases underneath heavy or drooping breasts, in the spaces between the fingers and the toes, and in other places where skin surfaces touch tightly or are subject to heat, moisture, and friction. A disabled, immobile patient may develop Candida intertrigo on his back because of lying on a sweaty sheet. The skin becomes sore, reddened, softened, and denuded, with burning and itching. Compromised in this way, it is vulnerable to infection with *C. albicans*.

Erosio interdigitale blastomycetica is the medical term given to a special variety of Candida intertrigo affecting the interdigital (between the fingers) spaces in persons whose hands are chronically immersed in water, such as dishwashers. The condition seems to favor the third space between the fingers (numbering from the thumb) and spreads to the palm and top of the hand. Paronychia (see below) may follow or be present simultaneously. The finger space itches, sometimes has vesicles (tiny fluid-filled bumps), and is macerated.

Candida perleche (also termed angular stomatitis, or cheilitis), another type of Candida intertrigo, is characterized by bright red erosions and/or fissures (cracks) in the corners of the mouth. Ill-fitting dental plates or toothlessness tends to bring on the condition, apparently by speeding up jawbone resorption (loss of substance through physiological or pathological means). The changing jaw shape leads to creation of an artificial fold at the corners of the mouth, where moisture, food particles, and yeast organisms can accumulate.

ONYCHIA AND PARONYCHIA

Candidiasis involvement of the nail, nailbed, and surrounding soft tissue is a chronic condition afflicting cooks, laundry workers, domestic workers, homemakers (domestic engineers), and others who must frequently immerse their hands in water or use detergents. Having frequent manicures also predisposes you to candidal paronychia by disrupting the normal cuticle. Thumbsucking, cutting the nails incorrectly, and biting the nails also encourage these painful infections.

Paronychia, also referred to as whitlow, is an inflammation around the margin of a finger or toenail, sometimes accompanied by the formation of pus. Onychia is inflammation of the underlying tissue from which the fingernails and toenails are formed. The nails become brittle, ridged, and discolored with yellowish-white patches. The nail plate (growth area) may ultimately be destroyed at its proximal portion, where it first appears from under the flesh.

While paronychia occasionally occurs from a physical injury, the finding of *C. albicans* (by direct microscopic examination of scrapings or by culture) dictates that antiyeast therapy be carried out.

GENITAL CANDIDIASIS

Half of all skin candidiasis conditions affecting the penis and/or vulva are said to be spread by sexual transmission.[14] Details of this sexually transmitted disease problem were presented in Chapter Seventeen.

For a woman, the vulva (outer lips area of the vagina) becomes inflamed. In addition, the skin of the suprapubic and thigh areas, the perineum (space between the vagina and anus) and anal area get bright red. Eroded patches are formed, surrounded by satellite lesions. Painful burning and itching can occur, as well as painful urination. Vulval candidiasis easily spreads to the warm, moist vault of the vagina, to become yeast vulvovaginitis.

For a man, vesicopustules (tiny bumps with fluid and/or pus) begin to form at the glans penis under the foreskin in the uncircumcised. These lesions then coalesce and later rupture, forming shallow, erosive patches. Sexual transmission is probably the major source for the affliction. Because the inner surface of the prepuce (foreskin) provides a warm, moist environment, the Candida infection can thrive there. Spread from here to the scrotal skin is a reliable clinical sign of probable candidiasis, especially when accompanied by itching.

The physician might demonstrate the presence of organisms from affected areas by direct microscopic examination of scrapings or by culture, to rule out clinically similar disorders such as jock itch, contact dermatitis, and pemphigus vulgaris. Treatment of genital candidiasis is described in Chapter Seventeen.

ATHLETE'S FOOT

In August 1962, the American Podiatry Association again presented its two highest research, writing, and exhibits awards, the William J. Stickel Gold Medal and the Hall of Science Silver Medal, to this book's coauthor, Morton Walker, D.P.M., for his investigations into *C. albicans* and other fungal causes of athlete's foot. Dr. Walker investigated the presence of fungal hyphal elements on the feet of 50 patients, then another 38 patients, and finally 325 more. He found that 95 percent of the subjects among these 413 studied had fungal spores on their skin. These dormant spores can become active hyphal elements in dry or macerated scales between the toes, in calluses, in corns, in warts, in detritus of toenails, and in dry flaked keratotic tissue around the borders of the heels.

As chronicled by Dr. Walker's laboratory and clinical research, the following criteria are required for the production of athlete's foot:[15]

1. Hyphae must be in the active phase of growth and reproduction.

2. To produce symptoms, *C. albicans* must have been inoculated by some microtrauma (perhaps by walking barefoot on a locker room floor) in the deeper layers of the skin, where new keratin (a skin protein) is being formed.

3. Moisture must be present; the hyphal elements will not grow in absolute dryness.

The coauthor, a formerly practicing doctor of podiatric medicine, believes:

1. Active growth of the mycelia of yeast is supported by nutrients generated during keratinization (the process in which a portion of skin takes on a protective horny consistency).

2. Eruptions of athlete's foot are allergic manifestations of skin of the feet to Canditoxin.

3. The athlete's foot reaction to Canditoxin is always potentially imminent, because the host person usually has delicately balanced immunity.

4. Preventive measures must be directed at reducing the number of fungus organisms so that a person can more easily resist candidiasis of the feet.

Other factors which influence the onset of athelete's foot are these:

1. Dead keratin in corns, calluses, and toenails tends to encourage *C. albicans* to maintain a host–parasite relationship beneficial to the microorganism.

2. Chronic skin candidiasis may result from foot injury such as irritation caused by shoes, sneakers, boots, or sandals and by lack of drying after bathing.

3. People with toes in close juxtaposition (where they overlap or do not spread apart on standing) can develop athlete's foot faster than others.

4. Warmth, darkness, and moisture, usually present in "modern" closed shoes, predispose the wearer to candidiasis of the feet.

5. Tight shoes that squeeze the toes together predispose the wearer to fungus infection.

6. Maceration from rubbing of moist skin surfaces with or

without sweating increases the alkaline reaction of feet, again predisposing one to athlete's foot.

7. Weak feet that require greater energy and offer earlier fatigue get athlete's foot more quickly than strong ones.

8. Impaired peripheral blood circulation encourages *C. albicans* infection of the feet (and hands).

9. Familial cross-infections are possible but probably not common.

10. In the course of debilitating disease, yeast organisms that are ordinarily innocuous might cause symptoms of athlete's foot.

11. Obesity is a predisposing factor to athlete's foot, perhaps because obese people cannot easily bend to wash their feet, perspiration is greater, and added weight weakens the feet (weakness arises from excess weight actually forcing the foot bones out of normal alignment, often pushing the toes closer together).

12. The sweat of diabetics is a lush moist medium on which fungus thrives.

13. Rheumatoid arthritics and osteoarthritics are predisposed to athlete's foot, possibly because decreased mobility means that toes move less, thus get reduced ventilation and remain fixed in contact together; additionally, those with rheumatoid arthritis have immune system troubles, with a possible defect in defending against yeast-related illness.

14. Of the final 325 people examined by Dr. Walker for athlete's foot, 128 (39 percent) were clinically diagnosed as having it; 112 of these (88 percent) were confirmed cases by laboratory methods; using the 112 laboratory-confirmed patients, a conclusion was drawn that 1 out of every 2.9 people (34 percent) has athlete's foot.

15. Of the 112 laboratory-confirmed cases of athlete's foot, 37 (33 percent) were infected with *C. albicans*. The rest were infected by one of three other fungal organisms: 46 (41 percent) had *Trichophyton mentagrophytes;* 26 (23 percent) were afflicted with *Trichophyton rubrum;* and 13 (12 percent) suffered with *Epidermophyton floccosum*. In ten cultures growing fungi, three (30 percent) showed two different fungus invasions; of the various potential invaders, *C. albicans* was the only fungus overlying the main infecting organism (100 percent).

16. Of the 128 clinically diagnosed athlete's foot patients, 45 (35 percent) were male and 83 (65 percent) were female.

17. Of the 112 laboratory proven fungal invasions, 101 (90 percent) came from sedentary occupations and only 11 (10 percent) were physically active in their full-time jobs.

18. The forty- to fifty-year-old population group has more recurrent attacks of athlete's foot; next in frequency is the ten- to twenty-year-old group; then comes the thirty- to forty-year-old group; the sixty- to seventy-year-old follow with chronic infections, especially of the toenails; the fifty- to sixty-year-olds are next in occurrence; and the zero- to ten-year-olds have a low incidence, probably because of parental supervision over bathing, toenail cutting, and footgear; the seventy- to eighty- and eighty- to ninety-year-olds have chronic fungus infections of the toenails, but there were fewer patients checked in these groups.

19. In order of frequency, fungus infects the toes, the inner border of the foot arch, the metatarsal arch (across the sole of the foot), the outer border of the foot arch, the toenails themselves, the borders of the heel, and the ankle.

20. Athlete's foot from *C. albicans* foments a vicious cycle of signs and symptoms. In the order of their occurrence the difficulties that occur include scaling, itching, maceration, vesicles, burning, inflammation, skin fissures and cracks, peeling, stiffness of the skin, limitation of motion, secondary infection (as from bacteria), toenail involvement, and hard and thickened skin. Dr. Walker recorded that symptoms and signs were recurrent from warm season to warm season in 80 percent of affected patients—thus it is chronic in four out of five infected persons.

STANDARD ACNE TREATMENT ENCOURAGES THE CANDIDA SYNDROME

In one form or another, acne affects 80 percent of all teenagers and young adults who live in industrialized Western countries. Inflammation of the sebaceous (oil) glands just beneath the surface of the skin shows as pimples, blackheads, and whiteheads and, in extreme cases, can result in infected cysts and scarred skin. In severe acne, the skin on the upper body and face may be damaged enough to produce permanent scars. Prompt medical attention to early signs is extremely important. A general practitioner or dermatologist can help prevent bacterial infections that often lead to worsening of the condition or to permanent complications and scars. But to clear the acne bacterial infections, what is a major establishment-type skin treatment? The antibiotic tetracycline!

Sumycin®, Panmycin®, Vibramycin®, and Minocin® are standard antibiotics for acne treatment. Each of these is a member of the tetracycline group of drugs. Their use puts the teenager at risk of acquiring the Candida syndrome—more risk, we believe, than the possible benefits of antibiotic use. If the youth will eat a good diet, seek out the factors which promote improved health, and avoid those factors which interfere with optimal growth and metabolism, he or she will frequently be able to control and overcome the acne condition. Simple measures such as gentle use of a Buf-Puf® cleansing sponge and Dr. Bronner's™ pure castile soap solution are often helpful. Candidiasis-conscious physicians and other alternative health care/preventive medicine practitioners rarely need to employ potentially dangerous drugs when nutritional approaches, including treatment for candidiasis, are often successful in acne therapy and prevention.

A newer treatment for acne, isotretinoin, manufactured in 10mg, 20mg, and 40mg capsules (brand-named Accutane®), has been introduced recently by the Roche Division of Hoffman-La Roche, Inc., of Nutley, New Jersey. The compound interferes with vitamin A metabolism and has been reported to be exceptionally successful. Because of potential liver toxicity and serious birth defects in the babies of pregnant patients, however, use of Accutane® is best reserved for serious cases, especially deeply seated cystic or pustular acne, and careful frequent monitoring by your physician is required. We offer two other concerns to be considered. First, vitamin A is recognized as an important contributor to proper immune system function—the possibility of impaired defenses is a real one. Second, vitamin A has long been recognized as vital to good skin health and integrity. Interruption of vitamin A metabolism might alter normal skin growth, maintenance, and repair.

Still, a lifestyle of fitness and excellent nutrition is not usually the way of life for the average teenager. Antibiotic drugs sometimes become advisable for acne or other pathological conditions. In these cases, the E.R. Squibb & Sons, Inc. (Princeton, New Jersey) pharmaceutical preparation, Mysteclin F®, should be considered, since it contains the anti-Candida drug amphotercin B intelligently combined with tetracycline.

TOPICAL TREATMENT OF SKIN CANDIDIASIS

Removal of any underlying local systemic factors as far as feasible is the most vital step in preventing the development of yeast in the treatment of routine skin candidiasis such as athlete's foot, Candida intertrigo, and diaper dermatitis. Candida intertrigo, for example, may never be brought under control unless heat, humidity, and friction of opposing skin surfaces are countered or eliminated altogether. Obesity may have to be reduced by proper dietary measures in order to remove yeast "breeding grounds" in the skin folds. Endocrine gland factors (described in the next chapter) may have to be treated—for instance, diabetes, hypothyroidism, and pituitary dysfunction should be controlled or reversed. Broad spectrum antibiotics, steroids, and immunosuppressives often need to be discontinued, if possible, as part of the therapeutic approach.

Nonspecific topical preparations of certain types have been used as promoters of a drier skin surface, discouraging the growth of *C. albicans*. Among them are mild bactericidal and fungicidal agents that directly attack microorganisms as well as modify the local environment. Carbol-fuchsin solution (also known as Castellani's paint) is one of these preparations. The formula is 1 percent boric acid, 4.5 percent phenol, 10 percent resorcinol, and 0.3 percent fuchsin in an acetone-alcohol vehicle. Castellani's paint is applied either half- or full-strength, two or three times daily, if active skin infection is present. To help prevent recurrence, carbol-fuchsin solution is sometimes recommended to be painted on once a day. Skin staining resulting from Castellani's paint can be avoided by eliminating the fuchsin.

For treating paronychia, a solution of 2–4 percent thymol,

in either chloroform or absolute alcohol, is prescribed on occasion. However, painting the affected nail plate with this alkyl derivative of phenol can take a long time to resolve nail candidiasis.

For drying chronically moist intertriginous areas, you might try using zinc oxide shake lotion or lanolin. The external application of cornstarch is an old-fashioned home remedy, but carbohydrate in this product can be a nutrient for yeast and we don't favor its use. Except for the dangers inherent with inadvertently inhaling talc, plain unscented talcum powder is acceptable for absorbing excess moisture. Exceptional nutritional products are available from preventive medicine physicians of the wholistic type. Two such items are USF Ointment™ (unsaturated fatty acids) from Standard Process Laboratories of Milwaukee, Wisconsin, and EDAP Dermal Biostimulant™, made by Vitaminerals, Inc., of Glendale, California. Twice daily usage of either topical product is often recommended on affected areas.

Topical antiyeast preparations are classified into polyene antibiotics such as amphotericin B, nystatin, and candicin; imidazol compounds such as clotrimazole, econazole, and miconazole; and miscellaneous agents such as those mentioned already as well as haloprogin, chlordantoin, and iodochlorhydroxyquin. These topical preparations often are applied two to four times a day. Treatment lasts usually three or more weeks. Many physicians advise continuing topical applications for about one month after all lesions disappear to discourage future recurrence. Creams are preferable to ointments, lotions, and solutions, since they are aesthetically more pleasing, do not retain moisture, don't burn or sting on application, and aren't messy and wet. Lotions and solutions sting probably as a result of their alcohol content. They are best applied to the scalp (for local treatment of psoriasis and seborrheic dermatitis) and to the nail areas (for local treatment of onychias and paronychias). Topical treatment of vulvovaginitis may require insertion of vaginal suppositories in addition to creams or nystatin powder (in capsules or as a douche). See the table below for chemical names, trade names, and the form in which the topical products are supplied.

Difficulties with topical preparations include the potential for discoloration, for local irritation, or for allergic sensitization.

TOPICAL THERAPEUTIC AGENTS

CHEMICAL NAME (Generic Chemical)	TRADE NAME (Brand Name)	HOW PRODUCTS ARE SUPPLIED
Amphotericin B	Fungizone	Cream, ointment, lotion
Nystatin	Mycostatin, Nilstat	Cream, ointment, powder, oral suspension, vaginal suppository, oral tablet
	Candex	Lotion
Candicidin	Vanobid	Vaginal ointment, vaginal suppository
Clotrimazole	Lotrimin, Mycelex	Cream, solution, vaginal cream, vaginal suppository, oral troche
Econazole	Spectazole	Cream
Miconazole	Monistat-Derm, Monistat-3, Monistat-7	Cream, lotion, vaginal cream, vaginal suppository
Butoconazole	Femstat	Cream
Sulconazole	Sulcosyn	Cream
Haloprogin	Halotex	Cream, solution
Chlordantoin	Sporostacin	Vaginal cream
Iodochlorhydroxy-quin	Vioform	Cream

(Adapted from Gerald P. Bodey, M.D., and Victor Fainstein, M.D., eds., *Candidiasis* (New York: Raven Press, 1985), p. 238.)

NOTES

1. Sherry A. Rogers, "The Cholesterol Hoax," *Bestways*, July 1985, p. 31.

2. R. M. Soderstrom and E. A. Krull, "Deep Fungal Infections," in J. Callen, ed., *Cutaneous Aspects of Internal Disease*, Chicago: Year Book, 1981, pp. 361–381.

3. G. P. Bodey and M. Luna, "Skin Lesions Associated with

Disseminated Candidiasis," *Journal of the American Medical Association*, 1974, 229:1466–1468.

4. Thomas F. Anderson, "Psoriasis," *Consultant*, March 15, 1985, p. 39.

5. E. W. Rosenberg and P. W. Belew, "Role of Microbial Factors in Psoriasis," in E. M. Farber, A. J. Cox, L. Nall, P. H. Jacobs, eds., *Psoriasis*, New York: Grune & Stratton, 1982, pp. 343–344; E. W. Rosenberg and P. W. Belew, "Microbial Factors in Psoriasis," *Archives of Dermatology*, 1982, 118:143–144.

6. Stanley I. Cullen, "Understanding and Treating Seborrheic Dermatitis," *Hospital Medicine*, January 1985, p. 226.

7. Fredric D. Burg and Paul J. Honig, "Diaper Rash," *Drug Therapy*, January 1984, pp. 140–142.

8. J. J. Leyden and A. M. Kligman, "The Role of Microorganisms in Diaper Dermatitis," *Archives of Dermatology*, 1978, 114:56–59.

9. L. F. Montes, R. F. Pittillo, et al., "Microbial Flora in Infants' Skin: Comparison of Types of Microorganisms Between Normal Skin and Diaper Dermatitis," *Archives of Dermatology*, 1971, 103:640–648.

10. J. J. Leyden, S. Katz, R. Stewart, et al., "Urinary Ammonia and Ammonia-producing Microorganisms in Infants with and without Diaper Dermatitis," *Archives of Dermatology*, 1971, 113:640–648.

11. P. N. Dixon and M. P. Warin-English, "Role of *Candida albicans* Infection in Napkin Rashes," *British Medical Journal*, 1981, 2:23–27.

12. H. G. Mofenson, J. Greensher, A. DiTommasso, et al., "Baby Powder—a Hazard," *Journal of Pediatrics*, 1981, 68:265–266.

13. A. A. Fisher, F. Pascher, and N. B. Kanof, "Allergic Contact Dermatitis Due to Ingredients of Vehicles," *Archives of Dermatology*, 1971, 104:286–290.

14. R. N. Thin, M. Leighton, and M. J. Dixom, "How Often Is Genital Yeast Infection Sexually Transmitted?" *British Medical Journal*, 1977, 2:93–94.

15. Morton Walker, "A Chronical of Tinea Pedis and Chloroxylenol for Control of Tinea Pedis," *Journal of the American Podiatry Association*, September 1962, 52:737–745.

20

Candida Exhaustion of the Endocrine System

In 1972 a twenty-two-year-old registered nurse, Carol Bostelman of Allentown, Pennsylvania, consulted local physician Arthur L. Koch, D.O., to find help with her endocrine system imbalance. She sought relief from severe menstrual cramps, endometriosis, blockage of both fallopian tubes (passageways on either side of the uterus, through which the egg is conveyed from the ovary to the uterine cavity), genitourinary tract disorders, and discomforts relating to her gastrointestinal tract. These major health disturbances for the young woman had not been aided by the several physicians she previously consulted.

Her disorders continued and she became pregnant in the middle of 1973, delivering the child early in 1974. Following childbirth and at her own request, Mrs. Bostelman was prescribed birth control pills. She continued to suffer a variety of minor difficulties, including premenstrual syndrome (PMS), easy bruising, and recurrent sore throats and bacterial infections. Dr. Koch now realizes that yeast infestation may have been Mrs. Bostelman's main underlying pathology back then, but twelve years ago few physicians other than discoverer Orian Truss recognized the Candida syndrome as a clinical entity that mimics many different disorders.

In 1976 Mrs. Bostelman developed a nondescript body rash that seemed related to a fungal infection. Dr. Koch prescribed antifungal treatment that worked. The rash cleared. Then the patient again began to develop endocrine system trouble. She experienced severe PMS, including very sore and swollen breasts, nausea, headaches, frequent bloating, and missed menstrual periods. This whole PMS complex of symptoms caused her absolute daily misery.

New York City gynecologist Sherwin A. Kaufman, M.D., says that PMS is not normal, even though it affects at least 60 percent of all women to some extent.[1] Its persistence represents a dysfunction of the endocrine glands—endocrinopathy. PMS symptoms begin from two weeks to the day before menstruation. Discomforts often include one or more of the following: nonspecific feelings of depression, fatigue, sleeplessness, irritability, anxiety, restlessness, emotional outbursts, anger, mood changes, lack of concentration, impaired judgment; outbreaks of acne; headache and backache; nausea, constipation, or diarrhea; a tight or swollen feeling in the pelvic area and legs; breast tenderness and swelling; a bloated or puffy feeling in the abdomen (some women temporarily gain several pounds from fluid retention); increased thirst; and an increase or decrease in sexual desire. Such generalizations about symptoms don't necessarily indicate premenstrual syndrome. But if you go for a minimum of a week each month with virtually no symptoms, chances are that you indeed experience PMS-related hormone problems.

The next two years brought a worsening of PMS for Mrs. Bostelman. Gastrointestinal complaints also developed, associated with the stress of her father developing multiple sclerosis. Laboratory test results indicated that she had hypocalcemia (too little calcium in the blood). Diagnostic tests for gallbladder and digestive functions showed no clearcut source for her discomforts. In fact, repeated diagnostic X-ray examinations revealed no abnormalities at all, and it began to look as though Mrs. Bostelman's diverse symptoms were "all in her head."

Soon she developed an irritable bowel syndrome (sometimes referred to as colitis or spastic colon), known today as often connected to the Candida syndrome. At that time this underlying yeast condition remained unidentified to all but a handful of physicians. Taking "the Pill" was part of this patient's daily regimen, further worsening her polysystemic chronic candidiasis problems.

In April 1981, Mrs. Bostelman sought medical assistance at the emergency room of the local hospital because of a sudden and disabling lower abdominal pain. She was admitted and underwent an exploratory operation (laparotomy) into the abdominal cavity. Clinical diagnoses at operation were pelvic endometriosis with a cyst, and bilateral tubal occlusion (blockage) along with multiple adhesions (sticking together of organs that normally slide freely past each other). After her hospitalization, the patient consulted a gynecologist for treatment of her endometriosis. She also returned to Dr. Koch, but only for treatment of an iron deficiency anemia.

Treatment of her endometriosis by the gynecologist was a failure, so thirty-one-year-old Carol Bostelman followed the path needlessly taken by so many women: she wound up with a hysterectomy—the surgical removal of her uterus. Out of an estimated 2 million *un*necessary operations performed in the United States each year (a conservative figure, according to Sidney Wolfe, M.D., of Ralph Nader's Health Research Group), hysterectomy is at the top of the list. Lately, gynecological surgeons have abandoned the question of "necessary" and "unnecessary" operations and have endorsed hysterectomy for the sole purpose of sterilization. They've even changed the procedure's name and currently advise women regarding "hysterilizations."[2] Whatever you call it, cutting out the uterus is nothing more than a fancy Band-Aid—and a potentially dangerous one at that.

Being without a uterus may rid a woman of many symptoms of PMS. When the ovaries are removed as well—so-called surgical menopause—the body is exposed to a variety of other disorders associated with endocrinopathies. For instance, Mrs. Bostelman's weight ballooned from 107 to 128 pounds. Feeling sluggish and bloated, and developing a constant low back pain, she feared that symptoms of PMS had returned, although she had been told this would not occur. As will happen, she was involved in a motor vehicle accident that worsened her back problem. Her complexion developed acne-type eruptions, and she noted a great deal of discomfort from a vulvovaginal yeast infection.

Finally, in 1982, Carol Bostelman elected to put herself, once again, under the complete medical supervision of Dr. Koch. Arthur L. Koch, D.O., is in general wholistic medical practice, employing health care alternatives such as chelation therapy and nutritional approaches. Dr. Koch prides himself on watching for preventive medicine advances that drift out of the medical mainstream. In July 1982 he attended the first Yeast–Human Interaction Symposium and returned with striking new knowledge to assist Mrs. Bostelman with her longstanding health troubles. Piecing her health history together, he saw that she fit into the yeast syndrome.

In a written report followed by our extensive telephone interview on February 21, 1986, Dr. Koch advised:

Reevaluation of the patient's condition from the time I have known her until the present was done. I started her on a low carbohydrate diet and had her read the book, *The Yeast Connection*. She returned several days later wanting to start the antiyeast therapy, for candidiasis was her underlying problem as it always had been. After I started her on the Candida control diet and 500,000 units of nystatin four times a day, the patient quickly reported having no more headaches. She acquired more energy than she knew what to do with and became the envy of all of her nurse co-workers. Her weight, when last I saw her in my office in November 1985, had reduced to 112 pounds, and she was progressing satisfactorily. Her complexion cleared, energy levels were at a new high, and she enjoyed an uplifted outlook on life.

This has been one of the most dramatic improvements I've ever had in treating the yeast syndrome. There have been many others, but the things that makes this case outstanding is that Carol Bostelman is a registered nurse and well informed as to what might be the orthodox medical treatment—which does not work for her. Today, Carol looks about fifteen years younger than her true age [thirty-six years]; she has the nicest complexion you've ever seen; her energy level is off the top of the wall; the bunch of registered nurses with whom she works just don't have the ability to keep up with her. Carol's candidiasis is completely cleared up. She keeps referring patients to me for treatment of the Candida syndrome.

CANDIDA EXHAUSTION OF THE ENDOCRINE SYSTEM

The Candida syndrome is more noticeable in women than in men, probably as a result of yeast upsetting the more complex and fragile female hormone cycle. Scientific reports, as described in the December 1985 Yeast–Human Interaction Symposium research presentation of David Feldman, M.D. (see Chapter Five), indicate that *Candida albicans* can bind to adrenal steroids, apparently producing adrenal insufficiency. The Candida organism competes for adrenal hormones with the normal cells of a candidiasis patient.

Yeast-related illness also shows up in the disorders of gonads, thyroid, parathyroid, and other endocrine organs. Addressing the subject of thyroid insufficiency associated with Candida infestation, endocrinologist Phyllis Saifer, M.D., M.P.H., of San Francisco, current secretary of the American Academy of Environmental Medicine, alerts her colleagues to a unique medical situation. She cautions that the really difficult to manage yeast syndrome patient often has thyroid trouble, ovarian trouble, both, or some other manifestation of endocrine system exhaustion. For instance, Dr. Saifer stated during a conference held at Brigham Young University in September 1982,

Many patients with environmental illness, in particular those with yeast-connected problems, appear to have thyroiditis. Yet, the physical examination of the thyroid often shows no irregularities and routine T-3, T-4, and thyroid stimulating hormone [TSH] blood studies may all be entirely normal. Precise diagnosis is often difficult, although measurement of T-lymphocyte cells may help. I suspect thyroiditis in the difficult to manage brittle patient with symptoms of fatigue, depression, chilling, constipation, irregular menses, and other associated symptoms.

Such glandular dysfunction as Dr. Saifer described usually responds well to anti-Candida therapy. Some of the treatment involves taking raw glandular extracts, garlic and onions (see Chapter Eleven), mini-dose candidiasis immunotherapy with TCE (Trichophyton/Candida/Epidermophyton) vaccine (see Chapter Twelve), and use of nystatin by ingesting, enema instilling, snizzling, or sniffing (see Chapter Ten), plus a Candida control diet that eliminates grains, chocolate, honey, and fruit (see the whole of Section Three on the four-phase Celebration of Healthy Eating program). The administration of prescription thyroid products is sometimes needed as well.

Candida exhaustion of the endocrine system is not a single disease, but rather the result of differing predisposing aberrations in the victim's immune system—ranging from subtle to life-threatening.[3] Patients with Candida endocrinopathies are prone to develop various disabilities, such as:[4]

1. hypothyroidism, subnormal activity of the thyroid gland, bringing about mental and physical slowing, undue sensitivity to cold, reduced pulse rate, increased weight gain, and coarsening of the skin

2. thyroiditis, inflammation of the thyroid gland with an abnormal immune response in which lymphocytes invade the tissues of this endocrine gland (examples of specific disorders are Hashimoto's disease and Grave's disease)

3. hypoadrenalism, inadequate secretion of the adrenal glands, characterized by low blood pressure, depression, loss of strength, physical exhaustion, and low metabolism

4. diabetes mellitus, an endocrine disease in which carbohydrate metabolism goes awry, with resulting high blood sugars and inability to tolerate usual dietary loads of sugars or starches

5. hypoparathyroidism, inadequate function of the parathyroid glands, causing a fall in the blood concentration of calcium and, rarely, muscle spasms (called tetany)

6. pernicious anemia, a disorder that involves a failure of secretion of "instrinsic factor" (produced in the stomach to enable absorption of vitamin B_{12} from the small bowel) resulting in defective production of red blood cells

7. hepatitis, inflammation of the liver, frequently due to a virus infection because of immunodeficiency

8. alopecia, loss of hair from areas where it normally grows

9. vitiligo, a condition in which areas of skin lose their pigment and become whiter than surrounding skin.

During her presentation on Candida endocrinopathies at the 1985 Yeast–Human Interaction Symposium, Dr. Saifer included these nine endocrinopathies mentioned above and added seventeen more to the list. They are a group of disorders arising from autoimmune dysregulation associated with the Candida syndrome. Dr. Saifer explained that the above conditions, together with the autoimmune endocrinopathies to follow, comprise the "APICH syndrome." The acronym, APICH, stands for *a*utoimmune *p*olyendocrinopathy *i*mmune-dysregulation *c*andidosis (the condition of having Candida infestation) *h*ypersensitivity syndrome. The complete medical term is a mouthful, and that's why she abbreviates it to APICH. Dr. Saifer added to the exhaustion diseases or symptom complexes of the autoimmune endocrine system that potentially affect candidiasis victims. They are the following (not listed in the order of their frequency of occurrence):

10. premenstrual syndrome (PMS)

11. Addison's disease, a syndrome due to inadequate secretion of corticosteroid hormones by the adrenal glands, bringing on weakness, darker pigmentation of the skin, loss of energy, and low blood pressure

12. oöphoritis (also called ovaritis), an inflammation of one or both ovaries, either on their surfaces or within, possibly resulting from fallopian tube infection or blockage; next to thyroiditis, oöauphoritis is the most common endocrinopathy tied to the Candida syndrome

13. myasthenia gravis, a chronic disease marked by abnormal fatigue and weakness of selected muscles, associated with impaired ability of the neurotransmitter acetylcholine to induce muscular contraction, producing temporary paralysis, drooping of the upper eyelid, and double vision

14. pemphigus, a skin disease marked by successive outbreaks of blisters

15. allergic rhinitis, inflammation of the mucous membrane of the nose from allergy, often causing nasal congestion, nasal drainage, or postnasal drainage

16. schizophrenia, severe mental illness characterized by a disintegration of the thinking or emotional processes, loss of contact with reality, and emotional unresponsiveness (see Chapter Seventeen)

17. autism, a severe (psychiatric) disorder of childhood seen as inability to communicate by speech or to form abstract concepts, repetitive and limited patterns of behavior, and obsessive resistance to small changes in familiar surroundings (see Chapter Seventeen)

18. sprue, deficient absorption of food due to disease of the small intestine

19. celiac disease (nontropical sprue), sensitivity of the intestinal lining to the protein gliadin, which is contained in gluten in the germ of wheat, oats, and rye, with resulting atrophy of the digestive and absorptive cells of the intestine

20. idiopathic thrombocytopenic purpura, a deficiency of blood platelets apparently caused by autoantibodies destroying them, of unknown origin and producing purple skin rashes that are actually bruises

21. testiculitis, inflammation of the testicles (a disease similar to oöphoritis in women)

22. pituitary deficiency with amenorrhea, the absence or unexpected stopping of menstrual periods because of underfunction of the pituitary gland

23. systemic lupus erythematosis, a chronic inflammatory disease of connective tissues, affecting the skin and blood vessels and various internal organs, sometimes showing as a red scaly rash on the face that looks like a mask across the nose and cheeks, arthritis, and progressive damage to the kidneys (see the case of Juliana Picola in Chapter Twenty-One)

24. rheumatoid arthritis, the second most common rheumatic disease, involving acute and persisting inflammation of the joints

25. Sjögren's syndrome, extreme dryness of the mucous membranes of the mouth and eyes, often seen in menopausal women, associated with rheumatoid arthritis, Raynaud's phenomenon (decreased circulation in the fingers), and/or dental caries, and can be characterized by purpuric (bruiselike) spots on the face and decreased function of the salivary glands and tear ducts—often with the need to use artificial tear drops to keep the eyeballs moist (see the case of Judy Rosenfeld described in Chapter Twenty-One)

26. Goodpasture's syndrome, an uncommon hypersensitivity disorder of unknown cause, manifested by lung hemorrhage (bleeding) with severe and progressive inflammation of the kidney tubules, eventually leading to kidney failure.

"All of the above twenty-six conditions of APICH syndrome are autoimmune diseases in which antibodies to 'self' can be demonstrated," Dr. Saifer said. They are systemic autoimmune problems, and a distinct relationship to the Candida syndrome appears likely.

PATIENT HEALTH HISTORY IN THE APICH SYNDROME

"Family history in APICH syndrome is very important, giving the doctor the greatest clue as to whether he/she is dealing with more than candidosis [candidiasis] alone. The APICH diseases are definitely inherited and favor the females." Dr. Saifer added,

> Most of these families have health histories of various disturbances, such as hypo- and hyperthyroid disorders, "nervous breakdowns" (from undiagnosed thyroid disease), rheumatoid arthritis, "female problems," allergies such as hay fever, eczema, and asthma, drug sensitivities, alcoholism, cancer, pernicious anemia, diabetes mellitus, and a history of female reproductive and endocrine disorders from the use of the drug DES [diethylstilbesterol].

The patient with APICH syndrome related to the yeast syndrome will frequently report a long history of symptoms going back to childhood or a family history of problems. In addition to (or instead of) the above-mentioned endocrinopathy symptoms, signs, diseases, and syndromes, one or more of the following disorders will be included:

1. infantile colic, especially associated with intake of milk or other dairy products

2. childhood allergies, often with respiratory infections leading to the overuse of antibiotics

3. unexpected exacerbation of allergies at puberty

4. onset of fatigue or emotional disorders at puberty

5. irregular menses, beginning at puberty and possibly continuing to adulthood

6. postpartum depression with fatigue (this is a physical endocrine dysfunction and should not be considered a psychological phenomenon as it erroneously is characterized by most obstetricians and family physicians)

7. actual nervous breakdown or severe anxiety-stress syndromes with marked impairment of coping abilities

8. fibrocystic breast dysplasia

9. endometriosis

10. mitral valve prolapse, often with magnesium mineral deficiency that goes unrecognized by the traditional-thinking cardiologist, internist, or general physician

11. premenstrual syndrome (peaking in women at the age group of thirty-five to forty-five)

12. intolerance to oral contraceptives or other steroids (with the woman experiencing a lot of side effects)

13. increasingly severe food and/or chemical sensitivities (apparently associated with the use of chemicals in housecleaning, gardening, office building exposures or in fabrics, carpets, or wallcoverings)

14. thyroiditis (which turns up most often in Candida exhaustion of the patient's endocrine system), the incidence among women being ten times that of men

15. oöphoritis (the second most frequent occurrence in endocrine exhaustion from the Candida syndrome), producing ovarian difficulty in becoming pregnant—effectively an infertility situation.

During his lecture at the 1985 San Francisco Yeast–Human Interaction Symposium, immunopathologist Edward Winger, M.D., of Oakland, California, said that ovarian disorders are seen in 75 percent of the patients with chronic vaginal candidiasis. Such yeast vaginitis creates hormone dysfunctions that get in the way of fertility. Clinical ecologist Lawrence D. Dickey, M.D., of Fort Collins, Colorado, past president of the American Academy of Environmental Medicine, repeatedly speaks of clinical ecologists being able to help infertile couples establish a pregnancy just by starting the woman (or both of them) on the antiyeast program. Ovarian disorders frequently diminish a woman's sex drive as well.

Dr. Winger endorsed Dr. Saifer's description of the APICH syndrome evolving from the yeast syndrome. There appears to be a triad of disorders, he explained, consisting of, first, candidiasis, second, autoimmune antibody production, and third, endocrinopathy—together, an expression of the APICH syndrome. Laboratory diagnosis of this triad or of the APICH syndrome itself is aided by the antiovarian antibody test developed by Dr. Winger. Presence of any ovarian antibodies in the blood is abnormal. In addition, laboratory testing performed six days premenstrually should turn up estrogen blood levels below 50 picograms per milliliter (pg/ml) and progesterone blood levels should be higher than 1,500 nanograms per milliliter (ng/ml). Variations from these expected blood levels—either elevated estrogen level or decreased progesterone level—are abnormal. Abnormal levels of these hormones tend to be present with suppressed ovarian function.

Treatment to aid in controlling the APICH syndrome disorders is prescribed by candidiasis-conscious wholistic medical practitioners: excellent nutrition, dietary supplements, immune system stimulation, environmental control, stress reduction, correction of chronic underlying infection, supportive psychotherapy, and surgery, if necessary.

IATROGENIC ENDOCRINOPATHY VIEWED BY CLARISSA CANDIDA

Dr. Saifer says, "There seem to be two subgroups of candidiasis patients, the acquired and the genetically predisposed." In this chapter we have just learned about the genetically predisposed victims of the Candida syndrome who have arrived at endocrine system exhaustion. Eventually they appear to develop one or more of the antoimmune endocrinopathies of the APICH syndrome. They are extremely ill people who become exceedingly difficult to turn toward health for even the most candidiasis-informed physicians. A long history of serious disorders distinguishes these unfortunates from the far larger group of acquired candidiasis patients.

"The acquired group appears to have iatrogenic [doctor-caused] disease resulting from the use of oral contraceptives or oral antibiotics prescribed long-term for conditions such as acne. These acquired candidiasis patients usually have enjoyed good health and are free of allergic, metabolic, and endocrine disorders," explained Dr. Saifer. But then they change as the result of no treatment or incorrect treatment administered by physicians uninformed or misinformed about the Candida syndrome. Individual patients in the acquired candidiasis group can be shaped into becoming victims of the APICH syndrome by iatrogenic endocrinopathy. Iatrogenic endocrinopathy is the term for a condition of endocrine exhaustion associated with deep infestation of *C. albicans,* seemingly resulting as either an unforeseen or inevitable side effect of treatment administered or prescribed by a physician. If you check back with Clarissa Candida in Chapter Two, you may recognize that the yeast's universe, our friend Jane, was suffering from polyendocrinopathies. When and how did these manifestations of the APICH syndrome come on the unlucky woman? It started when Jane was beset by vulvovaginal candidiasis. Let's have Clarissa Candida tell you the method of her mischief:

Remember me, reader? Let me update you: I'm now living in another woman's body. Jane is dead! My relatives recycled her.

Just before Jane died, I was moved to some other universe on the head of her husband's penis. The condition that he had for a while (with me as the fomentor) was balanitis, inflammation of the glans penis underneath his foreskin. He ignored the redness and swelling I caused and then I jumped off when the man planted me into the dark, warm, moist cavity of another vagina . . . a place that I love to be.

To me, a human being is merely a variety of changing cells supporting two constant populations of memory cells, the brain's neurons and the universe's defensive cells comprising the immune system. Many of the defense cells have been referred to by this book's authors as "lymphocytes" or specialized "T- and B-cells." I remember when Jane was the only universe for me and my grand-aunt, Connie Candida. We were searching for a new toehold further within Jane's vagina. Along came one of Jane's immune system defense patrols. It consisted of a big macrophage (a large scavenger cell), some monocytes (white blood cells that ingest foreign particles), a few T-lymphocytes (killer and control cells), and a lonely B-lymphocyte (antibody producer, which normally is found in the lymph nodes).

They spotted me, Aunt Connie and the rest of her Candida brood. The patrol members had a quick conference and then came around to check microorganism identifications (IDs). Of course, as an ID, each *C. albicans* held up surface antigens and masked its true identity. The macrophage, monocytes, T-lymphocytes, and B-lymphocyte were completely fooled. The macrophage said, "They look okay to me. They've been here for years, some since birth, passed the test with other patrols earlier on, so I guess it's all right for them to stay." The others agreed and the patrol left us yeasts in peace.

A day later, for some dumb reason Jane swallowed a double dose of birth control pills. Aunt Connie's crowd and I moved in to cover the whole inner chamber and outer lips of her lower orifice. Half a million new yeast organisms grew, over 7,000 Candida colonies per gram of vaginal discharge. That's a lot! When Jane had sexual relations with her husband that particular night, penile penetration felt as if she were being stabbed with a hot poker.

We were thriving and expanding. The next time her immune defense patrol came around, all they saw was a massive sea of yeasts. One of Jane's monocytes was heard to say to a lymphocyte, "Balls afire! We're in a pickle! Let's get out of here before they get us!" So you see, Jane's defensive white blood cell mechanisms are either fooled by our disguises or made quite afraid by our overwhelming numbers.

Fortunately for Aunt Connie Candida, me, and all of our strain, Jane returned once again to her establishment-type, conventionally practicing gynecologist, one who follows organized medicine's drug-prescribing party line. Listening rather hurriedly to her complaints, the gynecologist took a look, and said, "Well, that's still yeast. We've tried before to control it but none of the medicines have worked well with you. You'll just have to live with it!"

Aunt Connie heard Jane protest, "But, doctor, I can't take it. This is interfering with my love life. Every time I try to have sex, it hurts."

The doctor replied, "Just drink a martini or two beforehand."

Jane said, "I've tried that. Neither martinis nor whiskey sours are any good. I still feel pain."

So the doctor paused a moment and came up with the standard pat answer. He said quickly, "We'll just have to try again with a different antibiotic. There's lots of 'em!" Then he left the examination room.

Hah! To be candid, I was able to work on exhausting Jane's endocrine systems from then on. . . . It was the beginning of her end.

NOTES

1. Sherwin A. Kaufman, *Sexual Sabotage*, New York: Macmillan, 1981, p. 50.

2. Deborah Larned, "The Epidemic in Unnecessary Hysterectomy," in Claudia Dreifus, ed., *Seizing Our Bodies*, New York: Vintage Books, 1979, p. 195.

3. T. L. Ray and K. D. Wuepper, "Recent Advances in Cutaneous Candidiasis," *International Journal of Dermatology*, 1978, 17:683–690.

4. J. Dolen, S. K. Varma, and M. A. South, "Chronic Mucocutaneous Candidiasis-Endocrinopathies," *Cutis*, 1981, 28:592–605; N. Howaritz, J. L. Nordlund, A. B. Lerner, and J. Bystryn, "Autoantibodies to Melanocytes: Occurrence in Patients with Vitiligo and Chronic Mucocutaneous Candidiasis," *Archives of Dermatology*, 1981, 117:705–708.

21

Major Illnesses Related to the Yeast Syndrome

A board-certified rheumatologist practicing in Lancaster, Pennsylvania, made the diagnosis of systemic lupus erythematosus (SLE) as the source of symptoms for Juliana Picola, a forty-one-year-old schoolteacher living in the nearby coal-region town of Wiconisco, Pennsylvania. Mrs. Picola was experiencing disabling pain in her lim' s, shoulders, and back. She worked every day but felt exhausted by 6 PM, having no energy left for any other tasks. For two years, she had suffered with these distressing symptoms.

SLE (also called just "lupus") is a bizarre disease somewhat related to rheumatoid arthritis that attacks various parts of the body. Among Americans, about 50,000 new cases turn up each year, chiefly in women of childbearing age. SLE belongs to a group of autoimmune diseases in which the body's own tissues are attacked by the very cells whose normal function is to fight off foreign invasion—elements of the immune system we have already discussed at length. The symptoms and severity of lupus vary considerably from person to person and from time to time during its course. Earliest indications may be severe pains in the joints, intermittent fever, or profound fatigue. Also present could be a characteristic butterfly-shaped reddened rash spreading across the nose and the cheeks. Diagnostic blood tests help confirm the presence of the disease.

On April 2, 1985, Mrs. Picola consulted wholistic osteopathic physician Harold C. Walmer, D.O., of Elizabethtown, Pennsylvania. In practice for thirty-five years, Dr. Walmer utilizes a variety of complementary medicine techniques, including sclerotherapy, medical acupuncture, chelation therapy, osteopathic manipulation, nutrition, and wholistic preventive medicine. As part of his examination of the patient, Dr. Walmer found that she possessed two characteristics that could be complicating her major illness. Mrs. Picola had the yeast syndrome and also had numerous silver-mercury amalgam dental fillings in her mouth.

During our March 1986 interview, Dr. Walmer described his health care procedure with Mrs. Picola:

> You are aware of the big controversy raging among health professionals about the slow mercury intoxication of people who have these amalgam fillings in their teeth. It's my impression that such dental patients do develop infections and/or allergies of the head, neck, and chest directly due to immune system suppression by mercury vapors escaping from their metallic fillings. The infection cause being unknown, such patients often are treated by their doctors with antibiotics. They later get more infections and are again treated with more antibiotics—and on and on. Each time the person chews on his amalgams, a tiny amount of mercury vaporizes; it's inhaled, and gets into the respiratory system, the brain, the internal organs, and travels throughout the body. Immune system suppression from mercury toxicity allows abundant *Candida albicans* overgrowth, thus bringing on the Candida syndrome.
>
> Prior to the onset of her systemic lupus erythematosus, Juliana Picola had a great deal of dental work done including the insertion of metal crowns on top of her mercury amalgam fillings. I tested Mrs. Picola with the dermatron [an electronic instrument that determines the status of acupuncture meridians] and learned that there was disturbance of the lymphatic distribution in her mouth. I was able to neutralize the high readings with

homeopathic remedies. The rheumatologist's previous diagnostic tests had reported that her antinuclear antibodies (ANAs) were elevated to 1:80. By September 1985, after she had her mercury deposits removed in the sequence that they were first put in, dental fillings replaced by nonmetallic composites, her ANA dropped markedly to stop the exhaustion of her adrenals.

In addition, I treated Mrs. Picola's candidiasis with nystatin, Vitaldophilus™ (a culture of *Lactobacillus acidophilus*), Kyolic™, Immunase™ (an enzyme product with nutrients added to the formula), calcium and magnesium, the Candida control diet, and electrical acupuncture. By May 28, 1985 [in just seven weeks] the patient reported that she was feeling really well. She was getting less tired and pain was diminished, especially in her back. In June 1985 improvement continued. In July 1985 her hands still felt stiff but aching had gone away. When she went off the antiyeast diet, achiness returned.

During the fall of 1985, I treated vaginitis for her with Orithrush™ douche concentrate. She had resumed anti-Candida treatment faithfully. When she entered my practice in April 1985 her Y-score [yeast diagnostic questionnaire score] was elevated to 167 [almost a sure sign that the patient had candidiasis]. I checked her again in November 1985, and the Y-score had improved down to 107. On December 5 she reported feeling wonderful. By February 2, 1986, her ANA test was negative. The immune system had restored itself. Today, March 15, 1986, her systemic lupus erythematosus symptoms have completely disappeared. I just spoke with Mrs. Picola, and she is anxious to let your readers know how imperative it is to have silver-mercury dental amalgams removed and candidiasis treated for the relief of major illnesses.

A GROWING CONCERN
FOR PEOPLE WITH MAJOR ILLNESSES

In addition to systemic lupus erythematosus, the yeast syndrome has been part of pathology in patients with diabetes mellitus, inflammation of the pancreas (pancreatitis), cirrhosis of the liver (hepatic cirrhosis), inflammation of the liver from virus infection or amoebic dysentery (hepatitis), multiple sclerosis, urea and other nitrogenous waste compounds in the blood (uremia), inflammatory disease of the gastrointestinal tract, aplastic anemia, severe trauma, severe anxiety-stress syndromes, and cancer. People who have undergone organ transplants or are victims of malignant diseases of the blood (the blood dyscrasias) such as leukemia are especially likely to suffer with yeast-related illnesses.[1]

Incidences of the Candida syndrome complicating a major illness are increasing steadily. For example, in the period 1954–1958, the National Cancer Institute advises that candidiasis was found in 7 percent of cases of acute leukemia. But in the period 1959–1964, the prevalence rose to 20 percent.[2] From 1972 to 1975, presence of the Candida syndrome jumped again to 33 percent in those affected with leukemia.[3]

As strongly implied in the last chapter by endocrinologist Phyllis Saifer, M.D., all indications point to yeast infestation being a disease resulting from medical progress. For instance, 28 percent of patients who receive bone marrow transplants suffer with some form of candidiasis.[4] It was a common finding in the early experience of surgical specialists performing kidney transplantation.[5] Also candidiasis is frequently diagnosed in premature infants and newborns.[6] A postulated mechanism in these infested infants is that organisms in the vagina can penetrate the intact or ruptured fetal membranes and infect the amniotic fluid. The fetus then swallows and aspirates the infected fluid, resulting in infection of the gastrointestinal tract and lungs. Also suspected is that the fungus crosses the placenta and causes widespread involvement of the infant's viscera.

Candidiasis also strikes at surgical patients. A study of surgical cases conducted between 1960 and 1970 turned up 49 percent who had polysystemic chronic candidiasis develop. Startlingly, more than half the infections occurred during the last two years of the study period![7] The frequency of the candidemia (*C. albicans* infection in the blood) in patients with burn wounds has increased substantially, ever since bacterial wound infections have been successfully controlled. In one study, only 2 percent of burn patients had candidemia between 1959 and 1969, compared to 14 percent between 1970 and 1971.[8]

In the Bahamas, a symposium entitled, "Candidiasis: A Growing Concern," sponsored by the Miles Pharmaceuticals Division of Miles Laboratories, Inc., West Haven, Connecticut, was held on November 26, 1983. The symposium's chairman, Gerald P. Bodey, M.D., Professor of Medicine and Chief of the Section of Infectious Diseases, Department of Internal Medicine, the University of Texas, M. D. Anderson Hospital and Tumor Institute in Houston, Texas, explained that candidiasis is an increasing threat to all patients with malignant diseases. Those with blood-related cancers such as leukemia and those undergoing cancer chemotherapy are especially at risk, owing to injury to their immune defense systems.

THE YEAST SYNDROME IN LEUKEMIA VICTIMS

Dr. Bodey explained to his audience of physicians who attend major illnesses:

We reviewed our population of patients with acute leukemia who were undergoing initial remission-induction chemotherapy in order to determine the cause of remission failures [the patients who died]. Fifty-eight percent of the patients did achieve a complete remission, but among the 102 failures we found that 71 percent failed because they died of an infectious complication during the initial remission-induction period. What was distressing from this information was that 40 percent of the patient population showed fungal infection as the cause of death. One of the changes that has occurred in recent years is that fungal infections are occurring early on in patients with acute leukemia, whereas in the past these infections tended to be a terminal event.

In the 1980s, about 40 percent of all cancer patients become infected with fungus, most of it coming from *C. albicans*. Other Candida species that infest cancer patients, but to a lesser extent, are *C. tropicalis*, *C. pseudotropicalis*, *C. guilliermondi*, *C. krusei*, *C. parapsilosis*, and *C. stellatoidea*.

FACTORS PREDISPOSING CANCER PATIENTS TO THE CANDIDA SYNDROME

A number of malignancies are associated with the Candida syndrome. Victims of these conjoined diseases show similar factors predisposing them to both. In the following paragraphs, the order of their frequency is numbered and the designated factors encouraging the development of candidiasis are bold printed.

Dr. Boley claims, (1) "**Neutropenia** is probably the most important factor, since the majority of these infections do occur in patients with hematological malignancies who are neutropenic." Neutropenia is a decrease in the number of neutrophils (defender white blood cells) in the circulation. The result for the patient is an increased susceptibility to fungal infections. Dr. Bodey affirms, "Even in the solid tumor population [cancers other than those of blood circulation cells], a substantial number of fungal infections are occurring in patients who have neutropenia as a consequence of intensive myelosuppressive [white blood cell–depressing] chemotherapy."

(2) "**Gastrointestinal ulceration** occurs with many antitumor agents [cancer chemotherapy drugs], which then permits colonization and invasion into the tissues and subsequent hematogenous dissemination [candidiasis spreading in the blood to all parts of the body]," Dr. Bodey said.

"There have been several recent reports in the literature of the increasing frequency of Candida infection in patients who have undergone (3) **extensive surgical procedures** for malignant disease."

(4) "**Intravenous hyperalimenation** is clearly an important factor," he continued. Intravenous hyperalimentation is the direct feeding of nutritional components (vitamins, minerals, amino acids, fats, and sugars) into the bloodstream through a tube placed into the patient's vein, the amounts given being

far in excess of those that can be provided by a usual arm "IV" for a hospitalized patient. The feeding of nutrients in this way permits "total" replacement of nutritional needs at a steady slow rate and minimizes overloading of the kidneys. Hospital personnel are now seeing a substantial number of patients with fungus in the blood (fungemia) as a consequence of hyperalimentation technology that uses long intravenous catheters and hypertonic (concentrated) glucose solutions.

(5) **Tissue damage** is also a problem in all types of fungal infections, at least in those caused by Candida and Aspergillus [another fungus]. Here," said Dr. Bodey, "the sites of infection are frequently areas that have been previously infected with bacterial pathogens. Of course, the administration of antibiotics facilitates colonization of the GI tract [by fungi] as a consequence of alterations in the flora, and this may tip the balance in favor of fungal organisms, particularly C. albicans.

"Another factor is (6) **hyperglycemia,** which may be induced as a consequence of the administration of adrenal corticosteroids or, of course, in elderly patients who have a fairly high frequency of diabetes with hyperglycemia." Hyperglycemia is excess glucose (sugar) in the bloodstream. As noted by Dr. Bodey, it may occur in a variety of diseases, the most significant being diabetes mellitus, in which insufficient insulin in the blood is often also accompanied by excessive intake of carbohydrates (sugars and starches). Untreated, hyperglycemia may eventually progress to diabetic coma. High blood sugar readily supports the growth of yeast in and on body tissues. The combination of neutropenia and hyperglycemia particularly predisposes a person to the acquisition of a fungal infection.

Above all other factors, however, (7) **impaired cellular immunity** is the main problem that makes cancer patients highly susceptible to developing the yeast syndrome.

YEAST SYNDROME
MANIFESTATIONS IN CANCER PATIENTS

Cancer patients who simultaneously suffer with *C. albicans* overgrowth manifest a variety of separate disorders. "First, there is oropharyngeal candidiasis [thrush in the mouth and throat]," Dr. Bodey said, "which is fairly common. It is a consequence in part of chemotherapeutic agents [cancer-killing drugs] that cause denudation of the buccal mucosa [membrane linings of the inner cheeks]."

Candida endophthalmitis, inflammation confined to the back chamber of the eye (located behind the lens), may be caused by the yeast organism.

Dr. Bodey said, "Another syndrome is Candida myositis, and this occurs most frequently in patients with leukemia. Patients have fairly intense myalgia [muscle aches and pains]. Usually, they will also have the typical skin rash associated with candidiasis, and the organism can frequently be detected [in the tissues] if a muscle biopsy is obtained. The neutropenic patient who has persistent fever and complains of muscle pain should be investigated for Candida infection. . . . Almost any organ can be involved in disseminated candidiasis [the most invasive and most serious manifestation of the Candida syndrome]. . . . A characteristic skin lesion has multiple nontender, pinkish-purplish subcutaneous [under the skin surface] nodules. The vast majority of these patients will have positive blood cultures [for *C. albicans*] as well. The lesions may be discrete or confluent. In some instances they may be so diffuse and numerous that it looks like an acute allergic reaction."

In treatment, Dr. Bodey advised that the important factor for survival of a cancer patient with coexisting Candida syndrome is the presence or absence of neutropenia. The cure rate is less than 5 percent in neutropenic patients. Amphotericin B is usually used, giving a 32 percent survival rate for those who do not also have neutropenia. Intravenous miconazole is sometimes used, with a reported 10 percent survival rate. Cancer and candidiasis are a deadly combination.

SERIOUS CANDIDA ILLNESS
IN THE GASTROINTESTINAL TRACT

Paula Cassini, a twenty-nine-year-old housewife living in Hoboken, New Jersey, first visited Milan J. Packovich, M.D., of Paramus, New Jersey, in March 1985. Mrs. Cassini complained of chronic ulcerative colitis, inflammation, and deep erosions in the colon (large intestine) and rectum. A progressive disease often resistant to treatment, ulcerative colitis may occur in childhood or in old age. Characteristically it develops in young people, with 75 percent of all cases beginning before age forty. More women are afflicted than men, and evidence indicates that ulcerative colitis is probably a genetic disorder.

Current research is establishing a causal relationship between an aberration in the immune process and development of this disease. Since it varies in intensity from person to person and over time in the same person, accurate diagnosis must be based on meticulous and detailed history taking and examinations, so that other possible conditions are ruled out. Typical manifestations include diarrhea and bleeding, which may alternate with constipation in the early stages of the illness. Over time, diarrhea becomes the main symptom, with as many as twenty bowel movements in twenty-four hours, interrupting sleep patterns and creating constant fatigue in the victim. Abdominal tenderness, cramps, weight loss, progressive anemia, and dehydration severe enough to require intravenous replacement of vital body fluids may necessitate hospitalization. The condition can deteriorate into colonic cancer.

Standard treatment for ulcerative colitis, as administered by establishment-type physicians, consists of bed rest, a high protein/low roughage diet, blood transfusion when anemia is present, fluid replacement, antibiotics to control secondary bacterial infection, retention enemas containing corticosteroids (cortisone), large doses of corticosteroids by mouth or by rectal suppositories, and psychiatric therapy to sustain the patient through the depression that is often associated with this devastating chronic disease. Surgical removal of the affected part of the bowel is not an uncommon procedure for extreme cases of ulcerative colitis. After surgery, previously unaffected segments of intestine can develop the full-blown condition, often resulting in a perpetual treatment program.

Paula Cassini wanted no more establishment-type treatment for her bowel problem. For nearly two years, her treatment included 100 mg daily of the corticosteroid prednisone and 1,500 mg daily of the immunosuppressant azulfidine. She had developed the typical "moon face" appearance associated with chronic steroid use. Now Mrs. Cassini was looking for alternative treatments. Her diagnosis had been made by a board-certified gastroenterologist in September 1983, after he performed a colonoscopy (visual examination of the large bowel through a tube inserted into the rectum).

At the time of her initial evaluation by Dr. Packovich on March 22, 1985, she related a past history including typical disorders associated with the Candida syndrome. Mrs. Cassini had experienced recurrent vaginal infections, painful menstrual periods at age sixteen, marked constipation during her high school years, headaches of undetermined cause striking repeatedly since she was about twenty-one years old, and hives presently occurring (thought by her dermatologist to be from allergies to tea, tomatoes, and Swiss cheese). The patient's father had been a chronic cigarette smoker; her mother raised a large number of plants in the family home. Mrs. Cassini also admitted to having premenstrual tension with irritable personality changes. Her home, she noted, was very damp—including a basement with creeping mildew.

She said that ulcerative colitis resulted in four bloody loose bowel movements daily, plus more frequent blood mucus without stool. The additional combination of fatigue, a lack of sex drive, dry skin, and loss of scalp hair had her feeling quite depressed. Mrs. Cassini's basal body temperatures were recorded by Dr. Packovich to be below an acceptable level. She was frankly worried.

In addition to eliciting details of this patient's history of precursors for candidiasis, the internist performed a thorough physical examination, ordered laboratory tests, and gave her a yeast questionnaire. She proved to have mild anemia and a raging case of the yeast syndrome, both complicating her major illness. Dr. Packovich placed Mrs. Cassini on an intensive therapeutic regimen against yeast, including a low sugar, milk-free diet low in yeast foods. He prescribed cod liver oil, safflower oil, calcium orotate, magnesium orotate, oral yeast-free vitamin-mineral-trace element compound, and oral nystatin. Intravenous infusions of vitamins, minerals, and trace elements were offered as well. Biocatalytic water was advised for her to drink, and the doctor discontinued the patient's use of prednisone and azulfidine.

By July 30, 1985, just four months later, Mrs. Cassini reported having only two bowel movements a day, with no further diarrhea or bloody mucus. Trace amounts of red blood were seen intermittently on the formed stool. She described herself as having much more energy and physical endurance.

On September 15, 1985, Paula Cassini appeared at Dr. Packovich's Medical Nutrition Center looking attractive and healthy and describing herself as feeling "great." She was full of energy, and her laboratory blood counts showed no more evidence of anemia. She told of enjoying one well-formed bowel movement a day, without any blood or bloody mucus. Treatment of the yeast syndrome helped to clear her ulcerative colitis completely.

When the small bowel is involved with candidiasis, radiographic examination may reveal thickened mucosal folds in the duodenal and jejunal portions. Dilation might be present in the jejunal loops, that two-fifths of the small intestine connecting the duodenum to the ileum. White patches can be seen through an endoscope in the entire duodenum, giving the mucosal lining a speckled pattern.[9]

The most common symptom attributed to large bowel candidiasis is diarrhea. Other symptoms include flatulence (excessive gas), abdominal pain, rectal bleeding, and an itchy anus. In many patients, intestinal candidiasis is characterized by intermittent, watery, explosive diarrhea without blood or mucus. As many as eight to ten stools can be counted each day, sometimes for periods of several weeks. A fast and practical way to establish the presence of excessive numbers of Candida organisms in this situation is by direct microscopic examination of a small amount of stool suspended in salt water or iodine. Most often, the diagnosis of candidiasis in patients with protracted diarrhea will be based on detection of budding yeast and mycelial forms in the stool and on the therapeutic response of the patient to oral nystatin.[10] A study of fifty adults who had recurrent diarrhea and a variety of GI symptoms indicated that all of them had a heavy growth of *C. albicans* in the stool.[11]

Jerry S. Trier, M.D., Director of the Division of Gastroenterology at Brigham and Women's Hospital in Boston, told candidiasis symposium participants in the Bahamas,

The organs that are attacked most frequently in the GI tract are the esophagus, and, increasingly, the stomach. Recent studies in peptic ulcer disease indicate that gastric ulcers are frequently invaded by Candida organisms. It is not surprising that candidiasis is a common infection of the GI tract, since the prevalence of Candida in the oral flora exceeds 50 percent. There's an 80 percent prevalence of Candida organisms in routine stool cultures.

Dr. Trier also said that the most common clinical symptom of candidiasis of the throat is a burning sensation or pain felt below the breastbone when food or fluid is swallowed, particularly hot drinks or alcohol. This symptom is termed esophagitis. Patients with esophageal candidiasis can also have a rather constant nagging retrosternal pain (aching behind the breastbone) or back pain. "A complication of esophageal candidiasis that may develop is significant and sometimes massive upper GI bleeding from esophageal erosions," he cautioned.

"Denture sore mouth occurs in as high as 65 percent of geriatric wearers of full upper dentures," said Samuel Dreizen, M.D., Professor and Chairman of the Department of Oral Oncology at the University of Texas Health Science Center at Houston. Thus, chronic atrophic oral candidiasis hits people who require false teeth. "It is marked by chronic redness and swelling of that part of the palatal [roof of the mouth] mucosa that comes into contact with the prosthetic appliance," Dr. Dreizen explained. "It is usually symptomless. *C. albicans* can be cultured from both the involved mucosa and the inner lining of the denture. Denture stomatitis [inflammation of the mucous lining of the mouth] responds to antifungal therapy combined with correction of the physical factors by mechanically relieving the denture sore spots, and with hygienic procedures that are designed to disinfect the denture of yeast."

FUNGUS INFECTION OF THE EYES

Homemaker Judith (Judy) L. Rosenfeld, forty-one years old, of East Aurora, New York, told Sherry Rogers, M.D., of Syracuse, "I can stand the twenty-eight years of my suffering with rheumatoid arthritis, but I cannot tolerate anymore the Sjögren's syndrome that I've had for the last three years. My eyes are so dry I have to use liquid tears every fifteen minutes. I don't dare go out of the house, because I look so dreadful with my constantly cracked, dry lips."

"Her tongue did look like that of a cadaver," agreed Dr. Rogers. "She was extremely dry. Judy was forced to drop artificial tears into her eyes about twenty-five times a day. In the middle of talking face to face with someone, she would have to stop and put in eyedrops. It was embarrassing for her. Not doing so, however, would have her eyelids stick shut. It was nystatin that totally reversed her Sjögren's syndrome."

Sjögren's syndrome, often associated with rheumatoid arthritis, is a dryness of mucous membrane linings of the mouth and other areas. Even worse, there can be decreased function of the lachrymal glands, located above the outer corner of each eye. These glands secrete tears through six or more little tubes which wash dust and dirt from the eyes. The tears also contain the enzyme lysozyme, a substance that combats bacteria. In Sjögren's syndrome, the lachrymal ducts can become obstructed by a swelling in the corner of the eye, which also contains pus when infected.

Judy Rosenfeld revealed her case history in a letter. She wrote:

> I have rheumatoid arthritis and Sjögren's syndrome. After going to a few doctors and then to a rheumatologist and an ophthalmologist, both of these specialists said they could do nothing for my eyes. I found Dr. Rogers through a magazine article that she wrote on clinical ecology and environmental illness. After testing me, Dr. Rogers turned up *C. albicans* as one of my high reactions. We decided I could try some nystatin and see what it would do. With my first dose, within the hour I noticed a different feeling of a slight moistness in my mouth. As I continued

to take the nystatin I was able to dramatically reduce the use of artificial tears. Plus my dry mouth was very much improved. I have been able to get a job and go to school activities with my children and live a better quality of life. I can't consider myself healed or cured, but I have a better knowledge of keeping on an even keel with my arthritis. I do use eye drops a few times a day, but the nystatin has been a real Godsend.

"As good as it was for her to reduce her need for artificial tears as an eye lubricant, Judy Rosenfeld, even with her acute rheumatoid arthritis, had absolutely no pain for the first time in twenty-eight years," reported Dr. Rogers. "No pain medication was required once we had tested her to the yeast, molds, and foods to which she was sensitive. Remember that I mentioned the most severely affected people with candidiasis do not merely have the Candida syndrome. Instead, they have candidiasis as one of many aspects of the total body burden that has made them victims of the twentieth century disease, environmental illness or EI [see Chapter Eighteen]."

C. albicans may also be the culprit in uveitis. Uveitis is an inflammation of any part of the vascular and muscular middle layer of the eyeball known as the uveal tract. This uvea is formed by the iris, the ciliary body, and the choroid. Yeast organisms can especially inflame the colored vascular layer of the eye. The causes of posterior uveitis, confined to the choroid, are different from anterior uveitis, a painful condition confined to the iris and ciliary body. All types may lead to visual impairment, and uveitis is an important cause of blindness. In most cases the disease appears to originate in the uveal tract itself, but it can occur in other parts of the eye, particularly the cornea and sclera.

Uveitis is a severe and frequently chronic condition, for which medical therapy is often inadequate. Treatment consists of drugs that suppress the inflammation combined with measures to relieve the discomfort along with more specific drug treatment if a particular cause of the uveitis is found. Drugs are usually given as drops, injections, or tablets, and often in combination. Investigators have recently looked at food allergy as a possible cause in some cases. Now it appears that chronic candidiasis may be involved.

Twenty-one patients with uveitis of unknown cause (six acute, fifteen chronic) were studied. A positive intradermal test to Candida extract occurred within fifteen minutes in twelve of the twenty-one patients. All patients had a strong delayed skin response forty-eight to seventy-two hours after testing.

Eleven of the uveitis patients had a systemic reaction to Candida extract. An eye reaction was observed fifteen days later in nineteen of the patients, either after they were tested intradermally or after they were injected subcutaneously with Candida extract, or both. Of this group, ten worsened for two to three days and nine improved.

A control group of patients with uveitis of unknown cause did not show any eye reactions to candidiasis testing.

Sixteen of twenty-one patients treated six months with antifungal therapy and/or Candida desensitization showed improved vision and/or decreased eye inflammation. None of the patients studied had skin or eye reactions to other antigens.

This detailed study suggests that certain cases of uveitis may result from an interaction between *C. albicans*, the immune system, and the uveal tract. The high response rate in the study to antifungal therapy and Candida desensitization suggests a new cause, and, similarly, a new approach needs to be considered for difficult-to-treat eye diseases.[12]

MULTIPLE SCLEROSIS REDUCTION
FROM CANDIDIASIS TREATMENT

A bookkeeper for her husband's automotive repair shop, thirty-seven-year-old Carol Wilson of Carey, Ohio, has multiple sclerosis (MS). She had been examined by a board-certified neurologist in 1983. His impression was that MS explained Mrs. Wilson's various symptoms—reduced muscle coordination for fine movements, double vision, tremors, slightly slurred speech, and some other physical signs. For confirmation, he referred her in October 1984 to the Ohio State University College of Medicine at Columbus. The neurologist's judgment proved to be correct. University physicians told the patient that she would "continue to get worse gradually and slowly."

"Carol was highly skeptical of physicians when she came to see me in January 1985," said L. Terry Chappell, M.D., of Bluffton, Ohio, "because she felt very discouraged by what they told her. She did come at the recommendation of David Myers, R.Ph., a pharmacist in her town of Carey. I examined her. It was evident to me that the patient needed a nutritional program."

Multiple sclerosis is an incurable and eventually crippling disease of the central nervous system. Practically unknown in tropical countries, it is widely prevalent in temperate climates, where its chief victims are between the ages of twenty and forty. MS is almost never seen to commence in anyone over fifty years old. Some medical experts believe that the disease is caused by a slow-acting virus to which the victim has faulty immunity responses.

Hardened patches—called plaques—developed in a random pattern in MS scatter throughout the brain and spinal cord. These patches interfere with function along the affected parts of the nervous system. Symptoms vary widely from case to case and from time to time in the same patient. One of the first indications of the disease is double vision or loss of some part of the visual field. Tremors may affect small muscle coordination, making sewing or writing impossible; speech can become slurred; clumsiness of movement, intermittent loss of bladder control, tingling sensations in various parts of the body, and partial paralysis may occur. The disease is chronic and sometimes seriously disabling, although it is practically never fatal. Correct diagnosis requires the expertise of a neurologist, since the symptoms can easily be attributed to other conditions. The maintenance of good health and resistance to infection is important since MS is aggravated by other illnesses.

MS patients commonly have other complicating symptoms, and this was the case for Carol Wilson. Dr. Chappell explained about the patient's candidiasis complication in his November 1985 written report to us:

The Y-score on her yeast questionnaire was 273 [normal is 60 or below]. Her multiple complaints included a lack of energy, pain and swelling in her joints, weakness, diarrhea, bloating, and constipation at times. She had erratic vision, dizziness, irritability, vaginitis with discharge, premenstrual syndrome, and profuse allergy-like symptoms.

In February 1985, I began Carol on a complete food supplement program and started her also on the Serodex homeopathic solution at the 6X dilution. Most of her symptoms were markedly improved when she was halfway through her treatment. By the time she finished the Serodex at the end of three months, she was so much better. For instance, whereas before Carol was homebound with an inability even to do her daily tasks around the house, now she could resume working.

Although she still retained some elements of tiredness, she was tremendously improved with increased energy. Her allergy symptoms improved. Her digestion got better with a more regular bowel pattern. She continued to have some dizziness. Her thinking patterns, however, were much better with a more retentive memory and no feelings of "spaciness." Her depression lifted and the numbness and tingling she had felt in her extremities went away. The vaginal discharge was considerably lessened as were debilitating premenstrual symptoms that she had complained about. Her vision was still somewhat erratic, but she noticed a big improvement with that as well.

She did have a brief flareup of symptoms when she ran out of Serodex, and I continued her on a maintenance of a 500X concentration of ten drops a day with further resolution of the worst of her symptoms. They got better steadily. Carol also was treated for hypoglycemia, and aged liquid garlic extract has been added to her nutritional program.

On May 1, 1986, when we checked on Carol Wilson's progress with Dr. Chappell, he told us that she was still in fine shape and wanted us to share her candidiasis–multiple sclerosis success story with others.

CANDIDIASIS AS A CONTRIBUTOR
TO ACQUIRED IMMUNE DEFICIENCY SYNDROME

Many health problems involving acquired immune deficiency syndrome may be recognized as extensions of signs and symptoms seen in the person who suffers with polysystemic chronic candidiasis. "The first signs of AIDS can be so innocuous they might be overlooked," wrote Robin Henig in the *New York Times Magazine*. They are:

- low-grade, persistent fever
- night sweats
- dry coughs that are not related to a cold or to smoking
- shortness of breath with minor exertion
- loss of weight that is not related to dieting or increase in physical activity
- blurred vision
- persistent and severe headaches
- swollen lymph nodes in the neck or under the arms that are not linked to a transient infection of known origin
- creamy-white patches on the tongue
- persistent or recurrent itching around the anus
- diarrhea, bloody stools, or gastrointestinal upset that does not go away
- cuts and infections that do not heal as quickly as usual
- skin rashes or discolorations that refuse to disappear and may get larger
- Kaposi's sarcoma: recently appearing purple, blue, or pink spots or hard nodules on top of or beneath the skin that do not go away, may increase in size, and can't be written off as bruises, blood blisters, insect bites, or pimples.

"Sometimes the patient is troubled by a common infection that he cannot shake—most typically shingles or oral thrush (a yeast infection of the mouth and throat)," continued Henig. "Abdominal cramps may also occur. Because AIDS can begin so benignly, homosexual men in apparent good health are flocking to clinics and doctors' offices to see whether they have a hidden case of AIDS."[13]

One of the most significant scientific studies relating to AIDS ever published failed to win broad attention by the American orthodox medical community. It is an investigation of the frequency with which unexplained oral candidiasis has been associated with later development of unequivocal acquired immune deficiency syndrome. The research was published in *The New England Journal of Medicine*.

Twenty-two previously healthy white adults with Candida infection of the mouth that had appeared for no apparent reason also had various signs and symptoms of immunodeficiency—which put them at risk to contract AIDS if exposed. They were compared with twenty similar patients, also with signs and symptoms of immunodeficiency that potentially had them at risk to get AIDS, but this control group of twenty did not have oral candidiasis (thrush). All were intravenous drug abusers, homosexual or bisexual men, or both. Eventually thirteen of the twenty-two patients having thrush (59 percent) acquired a major opportunistic infection or Kaposi's sarcoma within an average period of three months. None of the twenty control patients came down with any infection or cancer, and they were followed for up to twenty-one months. Moreover, fifteen of the twenty-two patients with oral candidiasis showed a slightly higher T-suppressor cell ratio, and twelve of these fifteen (80 percent) later developed AIDS.

The six medical investigators summarized the findings of their prospective study: "We conclude that in patients at high risk for AIDS, the presence of unexplained oral candidiasis predicts the development of serious opportunistic infections more than 50 percent of the time. Whether the remainder will have AIDS is not yet known."[14]

From this study we learn that the Candida syndrome is at least a reflection of an immunosuppressed status—perhaps even a major contributor to immune compromise. It could well be a critical factor pushing people toward contracting immune deficiency diseases.

A combined group of Los Angeles medical research teams reported in *The New England Journal of Medicine* that they "treated several young, previously healthy, homosexual men for multiple episodes of *Pneumocystis carinii* pneumonia, extensive mucosal candidiasis, and severe viral infections. The clinical manifestations and studies of cellular immune function in these patients indicated a similar severe acquired T-cell defect." The common characteristic of these patients was that they suffered "in the pathogenesis of the immunocompromised state" and that all of them simultaneously had candidiasis infections of the mouth. The seven medical scientists added, "This syndrome represents a potentially transmissible immune deficiency [AIDS]."[15]

FREE RADICAL PATHOLOGY PRODUCED BY CANDIDIASIS

Candidiasis is well known for its occurrence with a variety of disorders.[16,17] While the cause and effect relationship of *C. albicans* in these many conditions is just becoming clear, the organism has been confirmed as responsible in problems as simple as annoying minor infections accompanying certain diseases to major serious illnesses.[18] Early in 1986, Stephen A. Levine, Ph.D., Director of Research of the Allergy Research Group and Nutri-Cology, Inc., of San Leandro, California, expounded on his concepts relating to the role of *C. albicans* in the production of free radical pathology.

A free radical is a reactive atom or molecule with an unpaired electron in its orbit. This loose electron is free to clash with an "electron-rich" (fully paired) molecule floating nearby, for instance within your body cells. In the process of clashing, the free radical produces an oxidation effect which is often dramatically destructive (causing pathology) at a molecular level. Free radical pathology over time produces numerous increasing damaging effects to cellular structures, inside cells, between cells, and by cells (such as with cancer). Often free radical effects are the precursors to disabling cellular strains or stresses, including those from chemical, physical, emotional, thermal, and other types of internal and external environmental stressors. Typical disease states to which free radicals contribute are cataracts, cirrhosis, diabetes, allergies, arthritis, heart attack, hardening of the arteries, emphysema, infections, and much more. Free radical pathology, in fact, enters into every type of cellular dysfunction of the human body.

In his ground-breaking book, *Antioxidant Adaptation: Its Role in Free Radical Pathology*, Dr. Levine presents "Ten Postulates of Free Radical Pathology and Antioxidant Adaptation." In summary, he says:

1. Ecological illness is a disease manifestation of free radical oxidant overload.

2. Acute and chronic hypersensitivity reactions are sequelae of the immune response system.

3. The various stressors involving oxygen exchange bring on acute or chronic inflammatory and degenerative disorders.

4. Antioxidant adaptability allows a person to tolerate oxidative stress.

5. Nutritional antioxidant therapy (especially with selenium) restores the free radical counteractant enzyme, glutathione peroxidase.

6. Antioxidant nutrients such as vitamins A, C, E, beta-carotene, selenium, and zinc are immune stimulants and anticarcinogens.

7. Immune dysfunction may arise from inflammatory prostaglandins (physiologically active compounds formed from essential fatty acids), which are present in ecologically ill people.

8. Emotional stress is physically destructive to the body by oxidation of catechol hormones (such as epinephrine, the stress hormone) to free radical derivatives.

9. Free radical pathology underlies the development of cancer, cardiovascular disease, and other degenerative diseases by electrochemical phenomena.

10. *C. albicans* exacerbates free radical oxidative stress by stimulating more inflammatory prostaglandins, which, in turn, suppress immunity.[19]

In *The Yeast Syndrome*, Dr. Levine's tenth postulate concerns us most, although all of them enter into the production of tissue destruction and disease itself. During our interview, Dr. Levine focused on iodine deficiency, apparently common in candidiasis victims, and explained that they "may become selectively sensitive to yeast infections due to inactivity of the myeloperoxidase enzyme, which uses iodine in cell-mediated immune function." Free radicals can have good or bad effects for the body. In this case, free radicals generated by action of the myeloperoxidase enzyme are utilized to fight off yeast and are part of the cellular antiyeast free radical artillery.

Also, selenium deficiency in the candidiasis patient may cause a predisposition to yeast infection. Phagocytes (the devouring kind of white blood cell) require selenium for the absorption and removal of bad free radicals. "The cell," Dr. Levine explained, "generates antioxidant protection intracellularly [inside itself] against the back diffusion of hydrogen peroxide formed from free radicals. The primary killing of yeast is accomplished by the immune capacity of the host cells. The simple attachment of the yeast hyphae activates the oxidative metabolism of the phagocytes, which sets the defense action into motion."

C. albicans generates large quantities of acetaldehyde when in a low oxygen environment. Low oxygen results from any chronically inflamed tissues. Acetaldehyde, containing only one carbon more than formaldehyde used to preserve biological specimens for decades, is damaging to host cells by free radical and peroxidative mechanisms. When yeast cells are limited in oxygen supply they also are more resistant to immune defenses. Thus a decrease in cellular oxygen supply is a major contributing factor to candidiasis susceptibility.

At the annual meeting of the Infectious Disease Society for Obstetrics and Gynecology in 1985, a report was offered that cellular immunity to Candida was markedly reduced in those women who had been diagnosed with candidiasis because of the inflammatory mediator substance, prostaglandin E_2. PGE_2 interferes with a cell's ability to kill the yeast. Excessive free radical damage to macrophages, which produce the PGE_2, causes activation and release of the substance. In simple terms, Dr. Levine clarified: "Chronic inflammation associated with the yeast syndrome leads to immune suppression by overstimulating macrophage to produce inflammatory prostaglandin E_2. It is likely that excessive free radical damage to macrophage cell membranes causes the activation of the inflammation substance."

NOTES

1. B. Barrett, W. Volwiler, W.M.M. Kirby, and C. R. Jensen, "Fatal Systemic Moniliasis Following Pancreatitis," *Archives of Internal Medicine,* 1957, 99:209–213; D. L. Dennis, C. G. Peterson, and W. S. Fletcher, "Candida Septicemia in the Severely Traumatized Patient," *Journal of Trauma,* 1968, 8:177–186; D. B. Louria, D. P. Stiff, and B. Bennett, "Disseminated Moniliasis

in the Adult," *Medicine*, 1962, 41:307–333; V.K.G. Pillay, D. M. Wilson, T. S. Ing, and R. M. Kark, "Fungus Infection in Steroid-Treated Systemic Lupus Erythematosus," *Journal of the American Medical Association*, 1968, 205:261–265; D. R. Triger, D. N. Slater, J. R. Goepel, and J.C.E. Underwood, "Systemic Candidiasis Complicating Acute Hepatic Failure in Patients Treated with Cimetidine," *Lancet*, 1981, 2:837–838.

2. G. P. Bodey, "Fungal Infections Complicating Acute Leukemia," *Journal of Chronic Diseases*, 1966, 19:667–687.

3. R. L. Myerowitz, G. J. Pazin, and C. M. Allen, "Disseminated Candidiasis. Changes in Incidence, Underlying Diseases and Pathology," *American Journal of Clinical Pathology*, 1977, 68:29–38.

4. G. R. Sandford, W. G. Merz, J. R. Wingard, P. Charache, R. Saral, "The Value of Fungal Surveillance Cultures as Predictors of Systemic Fungal Infections," *Journal of Infectious Diseases*, 1980, 142:503–509; D. W. Winston, R. P. Gale, D. V. Meyer, L. S. Young, and UCLA Bone Marrow Transplant Team, "Infectious Complications of Human Bone Marrow Transplantation," *Journal of Clinical Investigation*, 1979, 58:1–31.

5. D. Rifkin, T. L. Marchioro, S. A. Schneck, and R. B. Hill, Jr., "Systemic Fungal Infections Complicating Renal Transplantation and Immunosuppressive Therapy. Clinical, Microbiologic, Neurologic, and Pathologic Features," *American Journal of Medicine*, 1967, 43:28–38.

6. H. R. Hill, T. G. Mitchell, J. M. Matsen, and P. G. Quie, "Recovery from Disseminated Candidiasis in a Premature Neonate," *Pediatrics*, 1974, 53:748–752; M. A. Keller, B. B. Sellers, Jr., M. E. Melish, G. W. Kaplan, K. E. Miller, and S. A. Mendoza, "Systemic Candidiasis in Infants. A Case Presentation and Literature Review," *American Journal of Diseases in Children*, 1977, 131:1260–1263.

7. J. D. Gaines and J. S. Remington, "Disseminated Candidiasis in the Surgical Patient," *Surgery*, 1972, 72:730–736.

8. K. E. Richards, C. L. Pierson, L. Bucciarelli, and I. Feller, "Monilia Sepsis in the Surgical Patient," *Surgical Clinics of North America*, 1972, 52:1399–1406.

9. S. N. Joshi, P. J. Garvin, and Y. C. Sunwoo, "Candidiasis of the Duodenum and Jejunum," *Gastroenterology*, 1981, 80:829–833.

10. J. G. Kane, J. H. Chretien, and V. F. Caragus, "Diarrhea Caused by Candida," *Lancet*, 1976, 1:335–336.

11. P. A. Kantrowitz, D. J. Fleischli, and W. T. Butler, "Successful Treatment of Chronic Esophageal Moniliasis with a Viscous Suspension of Nystatin," *Gastroenterology*, 1969, 57:424.

12. E. Bloch-Michel and J. C. Timsit, "Uveitis with Allergy to Candidin," *Ophthalmologica*, 1985, 195:102.

13. Robin Marantz Henig, "AIDS—A New Disease's Deadly Odyssey," *New York Times Magazine*, February 6, 1983, p. 28.

14. Robert S. Klein, Carol A. Harris, Catherine Butkus Small, Bernice Moll, Martin Lesser, and Gerald H. Friedland, "Oral Candidiasis in High-Risk Patients as the Initial Manifestation of the Acquired Immunodeficiency Syndrome," *New England Journal of Medicine*, August 9, 1984, p. 354.

15. Michael S. Gottlieb, Robert Schroff, Howard M. Schanker, Joel D. Weisman, Peng Thim Fan, Robert A. Wolf, and Andrew Saxon, "*Pneumocystis carini* Pneumonia and Mucosal Candidiasis in Previously Healthy Homosexual Men," *New England Journal of Medicine*, December 10, 1985.

16. S. Castells, S. Fikrig, S. Inamdar, and E. Ortil, "Familial Moniliasis, Defective Delayed Hypersensitivity, and Adrenocorticotropic Hormone Deficiency," *Journal of Pediatrics*, 1971, 79:72–79; C. E. Sonck and O. Somersalo, "The Yeast Flora of the Anogenital Region in Diabetic Girls," *Archives of Dermatology*, 1963, 88:846–852.

17. H. L. Winner, "General Features of *Candida* Infection," p. 6–12, in H. I. Winner and R. Hurley, eds., *Symposium on Candida Infection*, Edinburgh: Livingstone, 1963.

18. G. Holti, "*Candida* Allergy," in H. I. Winner and R. Hurley, eds., *Symposium on Candida Infection*, Edinburgh: Livingstone, 1963; O. Neufeld and W. L. Wallbank, "Case of *Candida* Asthma and Its Management," *Michigan State Medical Society*, 1952, 51:1419–1420.

19. Stephen A. Levine and Parris M. Kidd, *Antioxidant Adaptation: Its Role in Free Radical Pathology*, San Leandro, Calif.: Biocurrents Division, Allergy Research Group, 1985, pp. x–xi.

22

Answers to Common Questions About The Yeast Syndrome

THE CANDIDA CONTROL DIET

Q. Why can't I have fruit on the Candida control diet?
A. We want to minimize the sugars that yeasts can find inside your body. Yeasts feed on sugars, including those found in fruits, and one way to limit their growth is to starve them.

Additionally, many fruits are loaded with yeasts. A good example is stomping on grapes to make wine. Yeasts live on the outside skin of grapes, and winemakers put these yeasts in contact with sugar inside the grapes simply by crushing the fruit. Yeast fermentation then happily takes place.

In heavy doses, natural fruit sugar is bad for you but good for the spread of your candidiasis.

One of the indices that measure how well you are doing much later in treatment is adding fruits to your anti-Candida diet. This addition is accomplished gradually, in phases three and four of the four-phase Celebration of Healthy Eating (CHE) program. If you notice no resumption of candidiasis symptoms, consider this a sign that your immune defense system is rebuilding as desired.

Q. Why can I have lemons and limes but not other citrus?
A. Lemons and limes do not tend to have as much sugar content. Lemon and lime acids seem to have a purging or purifying effect on the body. We encourage you to squeeze them (fresh) onto your vegetables or into your purified water or herb tea for flavoring.

Q. What is the timing for each phase of the 4-phase CHE?
A. Most adults must stay on phase one, a really restrictive diet of meat/eggs/vegetables/yogurt (the MEVY diet), for three to four weeks. Phase two, a moderately restrictive diet, might be necessary for three to four months. Phase three, the gradual return toward a normal healthy eating program, lasts for six to twenty-four months (or longer). Phase four, basically unrestricted eating (limiting processed foods), is continued indefinitely.

Q. How long do I have to stay on this antiyeast diet?
A. As long as you have the yeast syndrome. Children between the ages of one month and five years often return to healthy eating in a few months. Older people need to remain on the program longer. In the teen years, candidiasis patients must stay on it a year or so. Adults progress through their 4-phase CHE for periods as long as required to have them feeling a full sense of wellness. For the young, the Candida control diet requires less time because they are actively remodeling and enlarging their internal components. Adults take longer because they are only gradually replacing parts as they wear out.

Q. May I eat anything else except what is on my lists?
A. No. Eating foods other than those on your 4-phase CHE lists can prolong the length of time it takes for you to get well. The phase dietary lists define what is best for your biochemical system presently affected by the Candida syndrome. The major role played by the physician in designing a yeast-related illness treatment program that is best for you is to learn how and with what you want to cheat in your eating— then to adapt your dietary therapy to best meet your health and social needs. Changes can be made, but you have to help your physician by advising him in detail about your personal desires. For example, if you crave chocolate just before your

menses, don't give into the cravings. Advise your physician, who then might suspect a copper nutritional deficiency. If this is correct, a copper supplement may quickly rid you of your cravings for chocolate.

Q. May I eat potatoes?
A. Yes. Potatoes are part of the phase-2 CHE. But eat potatoes and similar foods in moderation, because they are starches. Molecules of starches can be visualized simply as hundreds or thousands of sugars holding hands in a long chain.

Q. How often may I eat popcorn and potatoes?
A. We recommend that you can add popcorn as a snack in phase-2 CHE. One-half to one cup of popped corn twice a day is a reasonable amount. Try to add only a little butter and almost no salt. Potatoes also are part of phase-2 eating, but serving them every day is not a good idea because of the starch load they offer. People with arthritis and candidiasis probably should avoid the nightshade family of plant foods (of which the potato is a member), because many people report worsening of arthritis symptoms when eating these foods.

Q. Why can I eat some beans and not others?
A. You should not add beans or other foods until you are advised to do so by your physician. The 4-phase CHE program adds foods in a logical progression, minimizing your chances of "backsliding" on your journey to better health.

Q. Why can't I have milk products?
A. Milk itself is forbidden but milk products are allowed. Human milk is good for infants. Cow's milk is good for calves. Milk from sources other than women is not suitable for humans, and milk is not needed after infancy. Milk contains a variety of substances probably harmful to those beyond infancy, since it has been tentatively linked to health disorders such as arthritis. Milk is not the excellent source of calcium it is touted to be by the milk industry. Cow's milk has a poor balance of proteins and an even worse balance of fats. We urge you to avoid homogenized and pasteurized milk, which may contribute to heart disease. Milk products such as yogurt, kefir, and cheese, on the other hand, have more beneficial components. These are acceptable, cheese being somewhat less so than yogurt.

Q. Do I have to eat yogurt?
A. No, but you will feel better if you do. Yogurt has been processed by Lactobacillus bacteria, so it no longer resembles milk. This processing turns yogurt into an easily usable food for your body, since the bacteria adds vitamins, proteins, and other advantageous nutrients. The yogurt germs present can take up residence in your gut and discourage the growth of yeast. Taking *Lactobacillus acidophilus* live cultures alone probably is not as effective for nutritional healing as taking actual live cultured yogurt. You deserve to get the B vitamins, proteins, organic acids, extra calcium, and other nutrients available from yogurt. Most people who "stick with it" for four short weeks find that they notice measurable benefits from this pleasant addition to their diet.

Q How much yogurt should I eat each day?
A. About three cups daily—or whatever quantity feels comfortable.

Q. How am I going to eat yogurt when I don't like its taste?
A. Take a quantity of plain yogurt, mix it with an equal amount of ice, drop in a raw egg, add a dash of vanilla or other food flavoring, and blenderize it. The subsequent yogurt drink is delicious. After you eat yogurt daily for a month or so, you will be surprised with how pleasant you find its taste.

Q. Is yogurt with fruit as beneficial as plain yogurt?
A. No. Fruited yogurt can be laced with yeast, not to mention the sugars present that can feed your existing internal yeast. Furthermore, commercially prepared fruited yogurt is often highly sugared and treated with other chemicals.

Q. May I eat nuts?
A. Yes, but we push nuts over to phases three and four because they somewhat encourage yeast growth and have a higher allergy-causing potential.

Q. Can I drink anything besides water?
A. Yes. Besides pure spring water, mineral water, and other bottled waters, you can drink herbal teas without caffeine. When you feel absolutely forced, you may take decaffeinated coffee or tea. On occasion, you can drink the nonsugared

Kool-Aid®-type drinks containing artificial sweeteners. Be cautioned, however, because our opinion is that they are not appropriate as beverages for anyone since they contain additives (colorings and flavorings) that have toxic and carcinogenic (cancer-causing) potential. Do not drink soft drinks—even diet soft drinks—since they provide too much phosphorus. They also perpetuate the addicting taste of sweetness. Avoid reinforcing a sweet tooth developed earlier in life. Remember, primitive man drank only water. Disregard the enticements offered by the cola manufacturers, who would addict you to their sweet-tasting products.

Q. May I eat salt and pepper?
A. Yes. But limit your salt intake. Sea salt is better to take, since it offers trace minerals. We recommend the substitution of herbs, such as Mrs. Dash™, in place of salt. Add a special taste with parsley, herbs, and spices—experiment with your taste buds.

Q. May I have butter?
A. Yes! Butter is real food, but don't eat too much of it. Avoid spreading or melting margarine on your food. Margarine's unnatural formula is akin to that of axle-grease. The body does not know how to handle this unnatural compound, so it "shelves" margarine and free radical pathology results, possibly contributing to atherosclerosis (fatty hardening of blood vessel walls).

Q. How may I add foods back into my menu plan when I have finished the restrictive meat/eggs/vegetables/yogurt (MEVY) diet?
A. Combined with your personal physician's advice, the 4-phase CHE offers specific directions.

Q. What spices should I avoid?
A. None. Some candidiasis-conscious physicians do offer specific guidelines to avoid certain herbs and spices; Dr. Trowbridge has not found this restriction to be necessary.

Q. May I eat potato chips from the health food store?
A. No. Chips are fried, and we are dead set against fried foods, except perhaps those prepared in a wok. The oils used for frying foods break down and produce peroxidation prod-

ucts that you eat. Peroxidation products trigger free radical production inside your body—aging and degenerative chemistry in the cells are the result. Fried foods from fast food establishments, for instance, are nothing more than attractively packaged cancer and heart disease. Multiple recyclings of the oil used to cook commercial fried foods (such as French fries, hamburgers, and fried fish) allow rancidity to develop quickly. Rancid food is poisonous to your health, but the fast food establishments usually disguise rancid-tasting food with seasonings such as catsup, salt, mustard, onions, garlic, and other spices in their "secret sauce" formulas. Beware, eating most of the food products served in fast food restaurants brings you a little closer to death.

Q. How much should I eat on the 4-phase CHE program?
A. As much as you are able. There is no quantity limitation. Most of the time we find that people don't eat enough. You will discover that eating large quantities of vegetables provides much bulk and not much substance. Consequently, if you weigh too much, you tend to lose weight on the 4-phase CHE program, without worrying at all about counting calories.

Q. Will I lose weight on the Candida control diet?
A. If you are overweight, yes, pounds will roll off. If you are underweight, it's likely that pounds will be added. In other words, the 4-phase CHE tends to normalize your body's weight. Our anti-Candida eating program becomes a rebalancing of your entire body processes, including the metabolism that stabilizes your weight.

Q. Would my pretreatment weight gain be a by-product of the Candida syndrome?
A. Yes. Candidiasis disrupts the sugar-handling, fat-handling, and protein metabolism of your body. Food cravings and food allergies contribute to excessive intake of foods that often increase your weight.

Q. May I chew sugarless gum?
A. There is no good reason to chew any gum. Chewing gum appears to increase the rate at which mercury leaves your silver-mercury amalgam dental fillings and enters your body to poison you.

Q. Why do people with the yeast syndrome crave sweets?
A. Yeasts feed on sugar and probably are demanding more carbohydrate. Your enzyme systems may be malfunctioning by not sending sugar breakdown products into the Krebs citric acid cycle. When you thus fail to receive as much energy from the sugar in your foods, you are driven to consume more energy-forming foods. Hypoglycemia, which can be associated with the Candida syndrome, will also give you a craving for sweets.

Q. During my battle with yeast, why have I craved salt?
A. You may be suffering with adrenal stress from exhaustion with the war on yeast. Perhaps your need is for specific vitamin and mineral supplementation to support adrenal exhaustion. Other stress-related factors might be present as well.

Q. Can the yeast syndrome be controlled with diet only?
A. In some cases, yes. However, the majority of patients require medication. The mainstay of treatment first is diet, second is nutritional supplementation, third is medication, and fourth is nutritional supplements (such as caprylic acid) that act like medication. Combinations of these determine how quickly you get well—they are used in accordance with your various candidiasis disorders. No one treatment program is correct for all people.

NUTRITIONAL SUPPLEMENTS

Q. Do I have to take nutritional supplementation forever?
A. No. Pills supplying nutrients are merely substitutes for bushels full of foods that you might have to eat to get the dosage of nutrients you require in your state of illness. Nutritional supplements are concentrated food components for quick use by the body. Remember, however, that you might need months or years for the nutritional supplements to help replace cellular components assaulted by toxins. After you have rebuilt defective "people-parts," you won't need much extra supplementation.

Q. Why must I take food supplements at all?
A. Canditoxin appears to interfere with a number of body biochemical functions. Nutritional supplements help to re-

place body deficits that manifest themselves as fatigue, malaise, lethargy, and other symptoms. Metabolic reactions aided by replacement nutrition (such as essential fatty acids, vitamin B_6, and reduced magnesium blood levels) can help you feel better early in the treatment program.

MEDICATIONS

Q. Into what liquid or food should I mix my nystatin to make it more palatable?
A. Yogurt, water, or anything else, but nothing sweet.

Q. Is nystatin the only medication that I can take to control yeast infestation?
A. No. Ketoconazole is used for many patients. Several other prescription agents are available for internal, topical, oral, and vaginal application. Moreover, nutrients that act like medications, such as the short chain fatty acids, garlic, taheebo tea, acidophilus, homeopathic remedies, and others can help do a good job of controlling candidiasis.

Q. Is it okay for me to take Nizoral™ and nystatin together?
A. Yes. This might be required in order to return you to health. But Nizoral™ (ketoconazole) usage must be checked by monthly liver studies (blood testing). Abnormally high liver function studies may be reflecting the acetaldehyde hypothesis proposed by Dr. C. Orian Truss, with acetaldehyde produced in the gut by *C. albicans* being absorbed and causing liver toxicity. This is one explanation for some patients who start a treatment program with elevated liver function tests that return to normal after taking nystatin and/or ketoconazole or other antiyeast agents.

Q. Is there one certain way to kill yeast infections?
A. Yes, sterilizing you completely with intensive medications would kill off all yeast microorganisms, but that method is not practical. Treatment is not directed at killing every Candida organism. Rather, the effort is to place your body in proper balance—an equilibration—with its microorganisms, so that *C. albicans* returns to its usual commensalism—living in harmony with your body as its universe.

"DIE-OFF" OR THE HERXHEIMER REACTION

Q. Why do I feel so tired if this antiyeast therapy program is supposed to make me feel better?
A. There are four possible reasons. First, you are performing metabolic rearrangements within your body—a very expensive effort requiring lots of energy. Less energy becomes available for you to focus outwardly, and additional nutritional supplements might be needed.

Second, until your body systems catch up, they are still liable to the yeast toxins being released, causing "die-off," or the Herxheimer reaction. As you take sledgehammer types of medication, your yeasts break open and release poisons that make you feel miserable.

Third, you may be eating insufficiently. Some people cut down drastically on their food intake, and the Candida control diet is nutritionally limited. Phase-1 CHE is not a good diet to stay on for a very long time because you won't get everything that you need.

Fourth, you may be hypoglycemic—a victim of low blood sugar. Going for long periods between meals without eating may have you feel worse—hypoglycemia requires that you eat small meals or snacks often. The phase-1 CHE program prevents you from getting the extra starch that in the past might have carried you through low blood sugar cycles.

Q. How long should the "die-off" period last?
A. From a few days to a few weeks. Most people can expect to experience some part of the Herxheimer reaction. Those who adhere strictly to the antiyeast program frequently have "die-off" that disappears in three, four, or five days. Those not following the antiyeast program as directed or having a tremendous yeast burden might well stay in a "die-off" cycle for a longer time. A number of manipulations of your therapeutic program by your physician can help get you out of this "die-off" phase.

Q. I feel as if I have flu symptoms. Could this be the Herxheimer "die-off" reaction, or am I sick?
A. If you have just started the antiyeast program, just made a change in it, or are suddenly adhering rigidly to it, you probably are experiencing "die-off." If none of these conditions

prevail but you unexpectedly feel sick, you probably have the flu or some similar illness. Proper diagnosis requires an appropriate health history and physical examination.

Q. Why am I feeling badly only three days after starting treatment for the yeast syndrome?
A. Taking treatment against the Candida syndrome has you going through lots of withdrawals: sugar withdrawal, food allergy-addiction withdrawal, and yeast "die-off," in which Candida organisms break open and release their toxic cell contents. You can help reduce your discomfort by drinking large amounts of fluids (especially purified water), taking more yogurt, eating more roughage such as crunchy vegetables, and using detoxifying enemas.

GENERAL

Q. How old does a person have to be to be affected by the yeast syndrome?
A. One needs only to be alive. Newborns frequently become infected with *C. albicans* as they come down the birth canal or while they are being cared for by their mothers or older siblings. While the oldest people do get yeast infestations, they rarely experience truly severe symptoms of candidiasis. Older adults grew up in an era when we did not have high tech antibiotics, cortisone, birth control pills, and fast foods. As a consequence, they are less often and less severely afflicted with Candida-connected illnesses.

Q. Is there a test for the yeast syndrome?
A. Yes. A few years ago there was none, but now there are several, including detailed questionnaires and various laboratory tests, such as the anti-Candida antibody test. The laboratory tests look for your reactivity to specific antigens against which you have previously directed antibodies.

Q. While taking treatment for candidiasis, should I get allergy testing or just continue with my allergy shots?
A. If you are diagnosed as having the Candida syndrome, it's less likely that you'll require allergy testing or allergy injections until after yeast disorders have been substantially con-

trolled. Allergies tend to correct themselves when you get rid of candidiasis. But we are not suggesting that you should stop your allergy injections, since they won't do you any harm or interfere with antiyeast therapy. Some people require a comprehensive allergy evaluation and intensive allergy treatment program in order to make progress with their candidiasis treatment.

Q. Is candidiasis a sexually transmitted disease—can my sexual partner and I pass yeast to each other?
A. Although not strictly categorized as an STD (sexually transmitted disease), yes, candidiasis can be spread that way. Women frequently have vulvovaginal yeast that can be asymptomatic (no discharge, itching, or burning). Men who are uncircumcised can have balanitis (candidiasis under the foreskin). By engaging in sexual intercourse, a man may inject the vagina with yeast. Also a yeast-infected vagina might seed a man's foreskin.

Some men complain of a burning feeling on the penis following sex. They are probably reacting to the yeast toxins (Canditoxin) present in their partner's vagina. Women seem to tolerate such sensitivity as part of living, apparently accepting discomforts more readily than do men. In fact, it's common for women to run to the same gynecologists for five years or more with the same vaginal discharge. That is noble fidelity to their doctors. When you acquire a car that's a "lemon," don't you turn it back in? Why not hold the same standard for a doctor whose lemonlike care is less than complete?

Q. How might all symptoms of illness that I have be related to the yeast syndrome?
A. Not every disorder is yeast-related, but many are. That is due to the system set up by *C. albicans*. The organism gives off toxins that float around the body and produce dysfunction wherever they lodge. For instance, the Canditoxin interrupts vitamin B_6 metabolism, and every cell depends upon vitamin B_6. Canditoxin interrupts the delta-6 desaturase enzyme pathway for long chain fatty acids, used by cells for making local hormones called prostaglandins. Canditoxin interrupts acetyl-Co-A function, stopping sugar from being processed in the most efficient manner—and virtually all cells depend on this

pathway. Many more metabolic processes are interfered with by Candida toxins. Every cell depends on these basic systems, and *C. albicans* is able to bring about disruption in them. The organism and its products are a source of global effects in the microorganism's universe, the human body. (Incidentally, pets and other animals can suffer with chronic candidiasis, just as humans do.)

Q. What makes yeast such a potent troublemaker for me?
A. Yeast is not the primary reason for your yeast-connected illness. Rather, the source really is your immune defense system, which has malfunctioned sufficiently to allow yeast overgrowth. If your immunity were stronger, you would have killed off excess *C. albicans* and the organism would not have overgrown. You would then have no problem today. Therapy must therefore be directed at holding yeast growth down while nutritional supplements, diet, and lifestyle changes encourage the healing of your altered metabolic processes and immune defense systems.

Q. How can yeast infections cause headaches and dizziness?
A. Headaches and dizziness are merely symptoms. Symptoms—the various indications of illness—manifest themselves according to the part of the body affected. Headache is possibly the most common affliction of man. In the United States alone about a billion dollars are spent yearly on medication for relief of this disorder. Dizziness, or vertigo, is a disorientation in space due to disturbance of the balancing mechanism. Both symptoms can indicate that your brain is affected by Canditoxin that has passed through the blood-brain barrier and is interrupting functioning of the mind. This helps to explain why a person suffering with the Candida syndrome can also experience depression, anxiety, difficulty in concentrating, loss of memory, mood changes, headache, dizziness, and other mind/brain symptoms.

Q. Why do antibiotics bring on yeast infections?
A. The prescribed antibiotic does not distinguish good germs from bad. Rather it kills any bacteria. Without friendly bacteria in your gut to keep down yeast growth, the balance is upset and yeast flourish where they should not. That balance is critical to keeping the host–parasite relationship in equilibrium.

Q. What are the most common yeast-related illness symptoms?
A. Poor memory, feelings of unreality, irritability, headache, inability to concentrate, continual tiredness, lethargy, depression, drowsiness, muscle weakness, numbness/tingling, uncoordination, vulvovaginitis, urinary infections, urinary system disorders, oral thrush, bloating, constipation, diarrhea, abdominal pain, heartburn, gas, indigestion, diaper rash, athlete's foot, jock itch, skin eruptions, psoriasis, nasal congestion, sore throats, persistent coughs, blurred vision, fluid in ears, earaches, allergies, asthma, acne, prostatitis, premenstrual syndrome, joint swellings, and joint pains.

Q. How is the yeast syndrome connected to chronic sinus and ear infections?
A. The problem starts with your immune system suppression. The immune system does not work well to defend you from sinus cavity and ear infections. Mucous membranes of the sinuses and ears appear to harbor yeast organisms quite readily in their exudates. Yeasts cause membrane swelling and mucous blockage. Bacterial infection develops in the blocked area. Subsequent treatment with antibiotic prescriptions stops any friendly bacterial organisms from interfering with more yeast growth. The fungi supersede bacteria and become the dominant organisms on these mucous membranes.

Q. What are the main predisposing causes of the yeast syndrome?
A. There are four: (1) the overuse of antibiotics as prescriptions and as additives in meat and poultry; (2) the use of hormonal medications such as corticosteroids and birth control pills; (3) poor dietary habits, especially excessive intake of sugars, starches, and fried foods; and (4) general nutritional deficiencies. All of these suppress your immune defense system and foster *C. albicans* overgrowth.

Q. Does candidiasis primarily affect women, or do men get it, too?
A. The yeast syndrome mainly occurs in women—about 60 percent of the cases; 20 percent of candidiasis cases are in men; the remaining 20 percent are in children—evenly distributed between boys and girls. Women have more places to hide yeast; they go to doctors more often, thus receiving

more medications that encourage yeast overgrowth. Unproven is the speculation that women have more nutritional deficiencies because of providing nutritional building blocks to the fetus and through nursing, setting the stage for weakened immune system function. Children have candidiasis problems that simply go unrecognized for years, just as they do in adults.

Q. Are some age groups more susceptible to the yeast syndrome?
A. In the mid-1980s, the most susceptible group seems to be those in their forties and younger because they are the ones most exposed to antibiotics, cortisone, birth control pills, and fast food eating as a way of life. Sulfa drugs were developed in 1933 in Germany, and penicillin was first produced around 1940 in England. They were used in the military during World War II and became widely available to the public in the late 1940s. (Most antibiotics used today were developed in the 1960s.) Younger people have received antibiotics periodically for most of their lives. Those aged fifty and above frequently have escaped being saturated with antibiotics that predispose people to the Candida syndrome. Scores on the yeast questionnaires need to be supported by clinical evaluation, positive laboratory test results, and therapeutic trials for yeast infection.

Q. How may my yeast infection be diagnosed?
A. Your history of disorders is taken, a yeast questionnaire is given to you to answer, a physical evaluation of your health status is made by the doctor, laboratory testing is carried out, and a therapeutic trial is undertaken.

Q. Is the yeast syndrome an illness in itself, or does it generate from another illness?
A. Candidiasis can be an illness in itself, but that is rare because the immune system usually keeps yeast in good control. Yeast infection flares when an imbalance occurs in the immune system or when a change takes place in the other natural host factors such as reduction in the friendly bacteria of the gut. Yeast are opportunistic organisms, generally overgrowing when the conditions are right in your body.

Q. What illnesses in the past have failed to be recognized as yeast-related?
A. Psychiatric symptoms of various types such as schizophrenia and depression; esophagitis supposedly from hiatal hernia; chronic urinary tract infection (cystitis); chronic bowel distress such as colitis; skin eruptions as from psoriasis; and many more. The list grows longer each month. Fortunately for the medical consumer, candidiasis-conscious physicians are learning now to control and even cure disease problems that still baffle even the best of establishment-type doctors. Perhaps this obsolescence of drug-oriented conventional therapies is why treatment for the Candida syndrome has drawn such a vehement reaction from the traditionally practicing medical community. The allopathic establishment types must now go back to the classroom and lecture hall to relearn some medicine. That often is a reason for traditionalist health professionals to withhold their approval of wholistic medical approaches.

Q. Is the yeast syndrome ever cured?
A. Yes! Cures are often established. Certainly control of the condition is commonplace, usually without the patient having to remain on a strict diet or an anti-Candida medication.

Q. I have been taking treatment for the yeast syndrome, but I'm not getting better. What must I do? What should my doctor do?
A. First, have a serious talk with your physician to make sure that he understands what your health problems presently are, what they have been since the beginning, and how they have or have not changed. Speak to him of how you have improved and how you have not. Describe in what way some problems have leveled off in their improvement, what new problems have arisen, and the progress you have made.

Second, determine whether you have stayed faithful to the therapeutic program, adhered to the dietary measures, taken the advised nutritional supplements, taken the prescribed medications, and made no unusual omissions or additions, such as over-the-counter medications or supplemental nutrients.

Third, look at how you've complied with all testing procedures that your physician has recommended. If he has suggested further testing, be sure you have gone through a tubeless gastric analysis (Heidelberg testing), hair mineral analysis, yeast antibody studies, cultures, blood tests, allergy tests, or whatever else, so that all factors can be properly and fairly evaluated. Since you are not feeling better, your physician must determine whether other tests need to be performed. If so, be certain to have them, in order to help your physician get a handle on the remaining problems.

Fourth, discuss with your physician potential changes in treatment that might be the next appropriate steps. For instance, if only nystatin has been used, could ketoconazole be substituted or added? Maybe short chain fatty acids could be prescribed? What about adding to your nutritional supplements—or increasing dosages? In other words, allow your physician an opportunity to alter his approach or treatment philosophy as circumstances change.

Good medical practice for coping with treatment failure at this point might dictate attempting some rather unusual methods. You and your doctor might consider, for example, immunotherapy or more exotic nutritionals such as *pau d'arco* herbal tea or high doses of liquid aged garlic extract.

Then there are nonspecific techniques sometimes helpful for candidiasis: supplementing with naturally potent and balanced live green foods like wheat grass juice, powder, or tablets or green barley powder. We have not previously mentioned the cereal grasses, but they do provide concentrated live food packages of vitamins, minerals, enzymes, amino acids, chlorophyll, and numerous unknown nutrients. David Darbro, M.D., of Indianapolis, Indiana, is investigating and using barley green powder as an immune system enhancer. Derived from the juice of young barley leaves, it is supercharged with nutrition and energy.

Responding to the above discussions, your physician's next step in dealing with your continued inability to get better is likely to be a search for occult infections. Not infrequently, a focal infection in a tooth prevents improvement in persistent yeast vaginitis or other disorders of the Candida syndrome. Remember that your doctor is treating only a portion of the iceberg of systemic involvement. What's not seen or unknown "below the surface" could be exceedingly important.

Protozoan infections could be part of your complication.

Warren M. Levin, M.D., of New York City advises us that he has found intestinal parasites in his chronic candidiasis patients. In an explanatory letter, Dr. Levin writes:

With the cooperation of a specialist in parasitology, Louis Parrish, M. D., of New York City, I have been finding an extraordinary incidence of *Entameba histolytica* and *Giardia lamblia* in the careful rectal swabbing of candidiasis patients. Immediate examination of the specimen turns up the parasites. These protozoa organisms encourage the growth of *C. albicans* and vice versa. The elimination of all of the offending organisms, together with attention to the mercury amalgam problem, has improved our treatment success rate significantly.

The time has come to undertake full investigations for allergy-related troubles. Don't expect merely some standard allergy "scratch" or "patch" tests. Instead, insist that your physician make use of the full complement of clinical ecology tests, such as serial dilution endpoint titration, provocative neutralization testing, or similar techniques that have a proven track record for symptom relief. Try the cytotoxic food allergy test or the more recently derived IgG food allergy testing (which measures the level of IgG antibody you have directed at food antigens). Amino acid profiles on your urine might also be helpful. Investigate blood, urine, and hair element testing for physiological mineral levels (such as mercury toxicity from dental fillings), pathological mineral levels, and the intricate metabolism of both mineral types.

If you still feel no improvement with disorders of the Candida syndrome, discuss with your physician the possibility that an undiagnosed standard disease is the source of symptoms. Tests for such diseases will be required, often including hospitalization. For example, if gut absorption problems are suspected, here are some of the tests that could be done: six-hour glucose tolerance tests with sugar levels every half-hour; lactose tolerance test; xylose tolerance test; small bowel X-rays; and small bowel endoscopy with biopsy.

Immune competency tests might be needed to determine that all facets of your defense system are present and are capable of normal function.

There may be an endocrinopathy present, and a full scale of screens for hormones might be advised to establish that each of the endocrine systems is operating correctly.

Talk with your physician about some of the more esoteric possibilities such as heavy metal poisoning, toxic chemicals in your drinking water, or toxic exposures at work or at home. Specific tests have been developed, including CPST for pesticides, CPhST for phenols, GVST for solvents, PAHST for herbicides, PCBs for PCBs, VBST™ for volatile brominates, HSST™ for hydrocarbon solvents, and OPPST for organophosphate pesticides, all available through John L. Laseter, Ph.D., Chief Scientist at Enviro•Health Systems, Richardson, Texas 75081; (800)558-0069, or (214)234-5577.

Finally, free radical toxicity might be the best explanation for the health problems that you are having. High-dose antioxidant nutritional therapy or intravenous chelation therapy may be required.

Getting better with your health difficulties ultimately becomes your personal responsibility. Physicians and health educators can give you the keys to unlock illness puzzles, but you must put them into the locks and turn them. If you are failing to improve despite the best efforts put forth by you and your physician, by all means ask for referral to another wholistic-minded physician, whose slightly different insights might hold the promise of resolving the Candida syndrome for you.

Q. Where do doctors get training in immunology related to yeast infestation problems?
A. Some training is given in medical school. A small proportion of premedical students get to do research in immunology and microbiology. Study of the immune system has recently gained in popularity as a result of immune diseases like AIDS becoming prevalent in our society. The prior and forthcoming yeast–human interaction conferences are the prime sources where physicians receive information about disorders connected with candidiasis. In the beginning of investigation and treatment of the Candida syndrome, physicians from many parts of the United States journeyed to the Birmingham, Alabama, office of C. Orian Truss, M.D.,

to observe and learn. Also, doctors can consult the footnotes and bibliographic references presented in this book. Other than these sources, there is no formal training on the Candida syndrome.

Appendix I

Suggested Readings

· **Baker, Sherry.** "An Epidemic in Disguise." *Omni Magazine*, March 1985.

Baker, Sidney M. "The Yeast Problem." *Gesell Institute Newsletter* 2, no. 5, December, 1982.

Battista, Al. "You Can Stop Fungus Infections." *Health Express Magazine*, August, 1983.

Chaitow, Leon. *Candida albicans: Could Yeast Be Your Problem?* New York: Thorsons, 1985.

Connolly, Pat, and Associates. *The Candida albicans Yeast-Free Cookbook.* La Mesa, Calif.: Price Pottenger Nutrition Foundation, 1984.

Crook, William G. *The Yeast Connection: A Medical Breakthrough.* 2nd ed., Jackson, Tenn.: Professional Books, 1984.

Crook, William G. *Yeasts and How They Can Make You Sick.* Jackson, Tenn.: Professional Books, 1984.

Faelten, Sharon, and the Editors of Prevention™ Magazine. *The Allergy Self-Help Book.* Emmaus, Penn.: Rodale Press, 1983.

Forman, Robert. *How to Control Your Allergies.* New York: Larchmont Books, 1979.

Fredericks, Carlton. "The Yeast Is Yet To Come." *Let's Live Magazine*, August, 1984.

Golos, Natalie, and James A. O'Shea. *Environmental Medicine: How To Diagnose and Manage Allergies.* New Canaan, Conn.: Keats, 1986.

Golos, Natalie, and Frances Golos Golbitz, with Frances Spatz Leighton. *Coping with Your Allergies*. New York: Simon & Schuster, 1979.

Hagglund, Howard E. *Why Do I Feel So Bad (When the Doctor Says I'm O.K.)?* 2nd ed. Oklahoma City: IED Press, 1984.

Hagglund, Howard E., and Marsha Ferrier. *Help! I Feel Awful! P.C.C. or Allergies Could Be Causing Your Problems*. Norman, Okla.: HEH Medical, 1985.

Hoffer, Abram, and Morton Walker. *Orthomolecular Nutrition*. New Canaan, Conn.: Keats, 1978.

Kupsinel, Roy. *The Fungus Among Us*. Oviedo, Fla.: Health Consciousness Magazine, 1984.

Lorenzani, Shirley S. *Candida: A Twentieth Century Disease*. New Canaan, Conn.: Keats, 1986.

Lorenzani, Shirley S. *"Candida albicans:* Is This Strain of Yeast Friend or Foe?" *Let's Live Magazine*, April, 1983.

Mandell, Marshall, and Lynne Waller Scanlon. *Dr. Mandell's 5-Day Allergy Relief System*. New York: Crowell, 1979.

Randolph, Theron G., and Ralph W. Moss. *An Alternative Approach to Allergies*. New York: Bantam Books, 1980.

Rapp, Doris J. *Allergies and Your Family*. New York: Sterling, 1982.

Rockwell, Sally. *Coping with Candida Cookbook*. Seattle: Diet Design by Rockwell, 1984.

Rose, Elizabeth. *Lady of Gray*. Santa Monica, Calif.: Butterfly, 1985.

Russell-Manning, Betsy. *Candida, Silver (Mercury) Fillings, and the Immune System*. San Francisco: Greensward Press, 1985.

Sheinkin, David, Michael Schachter, and Richard Hutton. *The Food Connection*. New York: Bobbs-Merrill, 1979.

Truss, C. Orian. *The Missing Diagnosis*. Birmingham, Ala.: The Author (P.O. Box 26508), 1983.

Wade, Carlson. *Nutrition and Your Immune System*. New Canaan, Conn.: Keats, 1986.

Walker, Morton, and Joan Walker. *Sexual Nutrition: The Lovers' Diet*. New York: Zebra Books, 1984.

Wunderlich, Ray C., Jr., and Dwight K. Kalita. *Candida albicans: How To Fight an Exploding Epidemic of Yeast-Related Diseases*. New Canaan, Conn.: Keats, 1984.

Zamm, Alfred V., with Robert Gannon. *Why Your House May Endanger Your Health*. New York: Simon & Schuster, 1980.

Appendix II

Organizations and Support Groups Providing Further Information on the Yeast Syndrome

American Academy of Environmental Medicine, 2005 Franklin Street, #490, Denver, CO 80205, or P.O. Box 16106, Denver, CO 80216.

Candida Research and Information Foundation, 31111 Palomares Road, Castro Valley, CA 94552, President Gail Nielsen.

Candida Study Group, Price-Pottinger Foundation, P.O. Box 2614, La Mesa, CA 92041, Moderated by John Jaeckle.

Critical Illness Research Foundation, Inc., 2614 Highland Avenue, Birmingham, AL 35206.

Environmental Health Association, 3609 Folsom Boulevard, Sacramento, CA 95816.

HEAL, 505 North Lakeshore Drive, #6506, Chicago, IL 60611, or P.O. Box 1369, Evanston, IL 60204.

Huxley Institute for Biosocial Research, 900 North Federal Highway, #330, Boca Raton, FL 33432.

International Health Foundation, Inc., P.O. Box 1000HF, Jackson, TN 38302.

Linus Pauling Institute of Science and Medicine, 440 Page Mill Road, Palo Alto, CA 94306.

Price-Pottenger Nutrition Foundation, 5871 El Cajon Boulevard, San Diego, CA 92115.

Appendix III

Selected Bibliography for Health Professionals

MEDICAL BOOKS

Bodey, Gerald P., and Victor Fainstein. *Candidiasis.* New York: Raven Press, 1985.

Dadd, D. L., and A. S. Levin. *A Consumer Guide for the Chemically Sensitive.* San Francisco: Non-Toxic Lifestyles, 1982.

Levin, A. S., and M. Zellerback. *Type 1/Type 2 Allergy Relief System.* Los Angeles: J.P. Tarcher, 1983.

Levine, Stephen A., with Parris M. Kidd. *Antioxidant Adaptation: Its Role in Free Radical Pathology.* San Leandro, Calif.: Biocurrents Division, Allergy Research Group, 1985.

Odds, F. C. *Candida and Candidosis.* Baltimore: University Park Press, 1979.

Rippon, John W. *Medical Mycology: The Pathogenic Fungi and the Pathogenic Actinomycetes.* 2nd ed. Philadelphia: Saunders, 1982.

Winner, H. I., and Rosalinde Hurley. *Candida Albicans.* Boston: Little, Brown, 1964.

CLINICAL AND LABORATORY JOURNAL ARTICLES

Cardiac

Benack, B. T., et al. "Subacute Bacterial Endocarditis Due to *Streptococcus viridans* and *Candida albicans*." *St. Vincent's Hosp. Med. Bull.* 196, 4:2–4.

Henderson, J., and **J. F. Nickerson**. "Bacterial Endocarditis with *Candida albicans* Superinfection." *Can. Med. Assoc. J.* 1964, 90:452–458.

Ihde, D. C. "Cardiac Candidiasis in Cancer Patients." *Cancer* 1978, 41:2364–2371.

Koelle, W. A., and **B. H. Pastor**. "*Candida albicans* Endocarditis after Aortic Valvulotomy." *New Engl. J. Med.* 1956, 255:997–999.

Persellin, R. H., et al. "Fungal Endocarditis Following Cardiac Surgery." *Ann. Internal Med.* 1961, 54:127–134.

Prinsloo, J. G., et al. "*Candida albicans* Endocarditis. Case Successfully Treated with Amphotericin B." *Am. J. Dis. Child.* 1966, 111:446–447.

Central Nervous System

Delvita, V. T., et al. "Candida Meningitis." *Arch. Internal Med.* 1966, 117:527–535.

Cutaneous

Hansen, R. C., et al. "Candida Breast Lesions Associated with Infantile Thrush—an Unrecognized Nursing Problem." *Clin. Res.* 1977, 25:178A.

Jahn, C. L., and **J. D. Cherry**. "Congenital Cutaneous Candidiasis." *Pediatrics* 1964, 33:440–441.

Kam, L. A., and **G. P. Giacoia**. "Congenital Cutaneous Candidiasis." *Am. J. Dis. Child.* 1975, 129:1215–1218.

Orbach, E. J. "*Candida albicans*, a Contributing Cause of Torpid Vascular Ulcers of the Lower Extremities." *Angiology* 1965, 16:664–672.

Reiss, F. "Milestones in Dermatology: XV. Candidiasis in Dermatology." *Excerpta Med. Sec. XIII* 1956, 10:93–94.

Esophageal

Dutta, S. K., et al. "Immunological Studies in Acute Pseudomembranous Esophageal Candidiasis." *Gastroenterol.* 1978, 75:292–296.

Dutta, S. K., et al. "Reversible Specific Cellular Immunity Defect in Esophageal Candidiasis." *Gastroenterol*. 1977, 72:1054.

Hachiya, K. A., et al. "Candida Esophagitis Following Antibiotic Usage." *Pediatr. Infect. Dis*. 1982, 3:168–170.

Kobayashi, R. H., et al. "Candida Esophagitis and Laryngitis in Patients with Chronic Mucocutaneous Candidiasis." *Clin. Res*. 1979, 27:114A.

Lallemant, Y., and R. Natali. "Esophagitis from *Candida albicans*." *Ann. Oto-Laryngol*. 1963, 80:826–828.

Mathieson, R., and S. K. Dutta. "Candida Esophagitis." *Dig. Dis. Sci*. 1983, 28(4):365–370.

Wickremesinghe, P. C., et al. "Candida Esophagitis." *Gastroenterol*. 1974, 66:829.

Gastrointestinal

Garagusi, F. V., et al. "Diarrhoea Caused by Candida." *Lancet* 1976, 1:697–698.

Gillespie, P. E., et al. "Gastric Candidiasis." *Med. J. Australia* 1978, 1:228–229.

Johnson, D. E., et al. "Candida Peritonitis in the Newborn Infant." *J. Pediat*. 1980, 97:298–300.

Moreton, J. R., and D. G. Friend. "Iatrogenic Diseases of the Gastrointestinal Tract." *Postgrad. Med*. 1959, 26:14–27.

Smith, E. R., et al. "Antibiotic-Induced Diarrhoea." *Drugs* 1975, 10:329–332.

Thomas, E., and K. R. Reedy. "Nonhealing Duodenal Ulceration Due to Candida." *J. Clin. Gastroenterol*. 1983, 5(1):55–58.

Weinstein, L. "The Impact of Antibiotics on the Gastrointestinal Tract." *Am. J. Gastroenterol*. 1958, 30:61–67.

General

Awachat, A. K. "Candidiasis." *Antiseptic* 1961, 58:43–50.

Drummond, M. "Clinical and Therapeutic Aspects of *Candida albicans*." *Irish J. Med. Sci*. 1956, 6:415–416.

Fujii, R., et al. "Studies on the Candida Infections in Childhood." *J. Antibiotics* (Japan). 1958, 11:40–44.

Guerrero, R. M., et al. "Candidiasis in Filipino Children." *J. Philippine Med. Assoc*. 1957, 33:271–279.

Shepherd, M. G. "Candidiasis: An Infectious Disease of Increasing Importance." *N.A. Dent. J*. 1982, 78(353):89–93.

Sohn, C. A., et al. "Candidiasis: Pharmacologic Management." *Female Patient* 1983, 8:54–55, 59–60.

Mucocutaneous Candidiasis

Chapper, R. R., et al. "Mucocutaneous Candidiasis or Mucocutaneous Microbiosis." *J. Am. Med. Assoc.* 1978, 239:428–429.

Mackie, R. M. "Mucocutaneous Candidiasis Responsive to Transfer Factor Therapy." *J. Roy. Soc. Med.* 1979, 72:926–927.

Meade, R. H. "Treatment of Chronic Mucocutaneous Candidiasis." *Ann. Internal Med.* 1977, 86:314–315.

Sam, W. M., Jr. "Chronic Mucocutaneous Candidiasis. Immunologic Studies of Three Generations of a Single Family." *Am. J. Med.* 1979, 67:948–959.

Simon, M. R., et al. "Chronic Mucocutaneous Candidiasis/CMC/Clinically Exacerbated by Type I Hypersensitivity." *J. Allergy Clin. Immunol.* 1978, 61:187.

Ocular

Ainley, R., and **B. Smith.** "Fungal Flora of the Conjuctival Sac in Healthy and Diseased Eyes." *Brit. J. Ophthalmol.* 1965, 49:505–515.

Almeda, E. M. "Trends in the Management of Uveitis." *Philippine J. Surg.* 1965, 228–230.

Corcelle, L. "Keratitis Due to *Candida albicans.*" *Bull. Soc. Franc. Ophthalmol.* 1975, 87:618–620.

Suie, T., and **W. H. Havener.** "Mycology of the Eye: A Review." *A. J. Ophthalmol.* 1963, 56:63–77.

Onychial

Esteeves, J. "Pathogenesis and Treatment of Chronic Paronychia." *Dermatologica* 1959, 119:229–238.

Opportunistic

Burchard, K. W., et al. "Fungal Sepsis in Surgical Patients." *Arch. Surg.* 1983, 118(2):217–221.

Hahn, D., et al. "Infection in Acute Leukemia Patients Receiving Oral Nonabsorbable Antibiotics." *Antimicrobial Agents Chemother.* 1978, 13:958–964.

Negroni, R. "Therapy of Opportunistic Mycoses." *Dermatologica* 1979, 159(1):223–232.

Procknow, J. J. "Treatment of Opportunistic Fungus Infections." *Lab. Invest.* 1962, 11:1217–1230.

Salli, I., and **R. Hand.** "Invasive Fungal Infection in the Immunosuppressed Host." *Intern. J. Clin. Pharmacol. Biopharm.* 1975, 11:267–276.

Oral

Barclay, J. K. "Pharmacology and Therapeutics in Oral Medicine." *Curr. Ther.* 1975, 16:65–66, 69–71, 73, 77.

Epstein, J. B., et al. "Oral Candidiasis: Effects of Antifungal Therapy Upon Clinical Signs and Symptoms, Salivary Antibody, and Mucosal Adherence of *Candida albicans.*" *Oral Surg.* 1981, 51(1):32–36.

Holbrook, W. P., et al. "Sensitivity of *Candida albicans* from Patients with Chronic Oral Candidiasis." *Postgrad. Med. J.* 1979, 55:692–694.

Varkey, B. "Oral Antifungal Therapy. Current Status of Ketoconazole." *Postgrad. Med.* 1983, 73(1):52–53.

Oropharyngeal

Tytgat, G. N., et al. "A Case of Chronic Oropharyngo-esophageal Candidiasis with Immunological Deficiency. Successful Treatment with Miconazole." *Gastroenterol.* 1977, 72:536–540.

Otolaryngeal

Haberman, R. S., et al. "Candida Epiglottitis." *Arch. Otolaryngol.* 1983, 109:770–771.

Smyth, G. D. "Fungal Infection in Otology." *Brit. J. Dermatol.* 1964, 76:425–428.

Pulmonary

Branscomb, B. V., et al. "Fungal Infections of the Lungs." *Am. Rev. Resp. Dis.* 1963, 87:784–787.

Franck, W. A., et al. "Candidiasis and Sarcoidosis." *N.Y. State J. Med.* 1977, 77:122–124.

Pearl, M. A., and H. Sidransky. "Fungus Infections of the Lung in Patients Treated with Corticosteroids and Antibiotics." *Bull. Tulane Univ. Med. Fac.* 1959, 19:34–42.

Rosenbaum, R. B., et al. "*Candida albicans* Pneumonia. Diagnosis by Pulmonary Aspiration, Recovery Without Treatment." *Am. Rev. Resp. Dis.* 1974, 109:373–378.

Systemic, Generalized, Candidemia, Septicemia

Kressel, B., et al. "Early Clinical Recognition of Disseminated Candidiasis by Muscle and Skin Biopsy." *Ann. Internal Med.* 1978, 138:429–433.

Warren, R. C., et al. "Diagnosis of Invasive Candidosis by Enzyme Immunoassay of Serum Antigen." *Brit. Med. J.* 1977, 1:1183–1185.

Urinary

Bridet, J., et al. "Treatment of Urogenital Syndromes Due to *Trichomonas vaginalis* and *Candida albicans*. A Rapid and Efficient Treatment." *Clin. Trials J.* 1978, 15:151–159.

Fisher, J., et al. "Fungus Balls of the Urinary Tract." *Clin. Res.* 1977, 25:28A.

Kennelly, B. M. "*Candida albicans* Cystitis Cured by Nystatin Bladder Instillations." *S. African Med. J.* 1965, 39:414–417.

Vulvovaginal

Balsdon, M. J., and **S. V. Drew.** "Practical Management of Vaginal Discharge." *Update* 1983, 27:1299–1312.

Blight, W. J. "Acute Allergic Vaginitis Caused by *Candida albicans*." *Can. Fam. Physician* 1984, 30:449, 451–452.

Canby, J. P. "Vaginal Discharge in Children: A Practical Approach to Therapy." *J. Med. Assoc. Georgia* 1965, 54:367–369.

Cassar, N. L. "High Potency Nystatin Cream in the Treatment of Vulvovaginal Candidiasis." *Curr. Ther. Res.* 1983, 34:305–310.

Drake, S. M., et al. "Vaginal pH and Microflora Related to Yeast Infections and Treatment." *Br. J. Vener. Dis.* 1980, 56(2):107–110.

Evans, T. N. "Sexually Transmissible Diseases." *Am. J. Obstet. Gynecol.* 1976, 125:116–133.

Felman, Y. M., and **J. A. Nikitas.** "Genital Candidiasis." *Cutis* 1983, 31(4):369, 372–374, 377.

Friedrich, E. G., Jr. "Vaginitis." *Amer. Fam. Physician* 1983, 28(5):238–242.

Mackenzie Fiddes, T. "Effective Treatment of Vaginal Discharge and Nonspecific Urethritis in the Female." *Curr. Ther.* 1979, 20(6):59–63.

Masterton, G., et al. "Vaginal Candidosis." *Brit. Med. J.* 1976, 1:712–713.

McNelis, D., et al. "Treatment of Vulvovaginal Candidiasis in Pregnancy. A Comparative Study." *Obstet. Gynecol.* 1977, 50:674–678.

Miles, M. R., L. Olsen, and **A. Rogers.** "Recurrent Vaginal Candidiasis: Importance of an Intestinal Reservoir." *J. Am. Med. Assoc.* 1977, 238(17):1836–1837.

Milne, J. D., and **D. W. Warnock.** "Effect of Simultaneous Oral and Vaginal Teatment on the Rate of Cure and Relapse in Vaginal Candidosis." *Brit. J. Vener. Dis.* 1979, 55:362–365.

Van Slyke, K. K., et al. "Treatment of Vulvovaginal Candidiasis with Boric Acid Powder." *Am. J. Obstet. Gynecol.* 1981, 15/141(2):145–148.

Wilcox, R. R. "How Suitable Are Available Pharmaceuticals for the Treatment of Sexually Transmitted Diseases? Conditions Presenting as Genital Discharges." *Br. J. Vener. Dis.* 1977, 53/5:314–323.

Wholistic Medicine

Barnes, J. L., et al. "Host-Parasite Interactions in the Pathogenesis of Experimental Renal Candidiasis." *Lab. Invest.* 1983, 49(4):460.

Cooper, M. D., and R. H. Buckley. "Development Immunology and the Immunodeficiency Diseases." *J. Am. Med. Assoc.* 1982, 248(20):2658–2669.

Crook, W. G. "Adolescent Behavior." *Clinical Pediatrics* 1982, 21(8):501.

Crook, W. G. "The Coming Revolution in Medicine." *J. Tennessee Med. Assoc.* 1983, 76(3):145–149.

Crook, W. G. "PMS and Yeasts: An Etiologic Connection?" *Hospital Practice* 1983, 18(9):21.

Crook, W. G. "Yeast-Connected Immune System Disorders: A Common and Usually Unrecognized Cause of Chronic Illness." *J. Holistic Med.* Fall 1983.

Furman, R. M., and D. G. Ahearn. "*Candida ciferri* and *Candida chropterorum* Isolated from Clinical Specimens." *J. Clin. Micro.* 1983, 18(5):1252.

Galland, Leo. "Nutritional Implications of Mitral Valve Prolapse." *J. Am. Col. Nut.* 1983, 2:3.

Gresham, G. A., and C. H. Whittle. "Studies of the Invasive Mycelial Form of *Candida albicans.*" *Sabouraudia* 1962, 1:30.

Iwata, K. "A Review of the Literature on Drunken Symptoms Due to Yeasts in the Gastrointestinal Tract." In *Yeasts and Yeast-like Microorganisms in Medical Science.* Proceedings of the Second International Specialized Symposium on Yeasts. Tokyo: University of Tokyo Press, 1974, pp. 260–268.

Lawton, A. R., and M. D. Cooper. "Immune Deficiency Diseases." In *Harrison's Principles in Internal Medicine.* Edited by Thorn and Adams. New York: McGraw-Hill, 1976, pp. 402–409.

Levin, A. S., et al. "Tumor Specific Transfer Factor Therapy in Osteogenic Sarcoma." *Immmunotherapy in Cancer.* Proceedings of ITR, Chicago, 1975.

Reingerz, E. L., et al. "Abnormalities of T-Cell Maturation and Regulation in Human Beings with Immunodeficiency Disorders." *J. Clin. Invest.* 1981, 68:699–705.

Appendix IV

Directory of Physicians Who Offer Treatment for the Yeast Syndrome

This listing, alphabetical by state, then country, has been gathered from several sources: personal communication with individual physicians furnishing patient histories; Roy Kupsinel, M.D., editor/publisher of the holistic magazine, *Health Consciousness* (P.O. Box 550, Oviedo, FL 32765), who has been compiling such a list for a few years; attendees at the 1982 and 1983 Yeast–Human Interaction Symposiums (the 1985 list of attendees was not made available); and responses to questionnaires mailed to physician-members of the American Academy of Environmental Medicine and the American Academy of Medical Preventics.

Physicians who wish to be listed in future editions of this book are invited to contact the authors through the publisher.

ALABAMA

Biomed Associates, P.C., 759 Valley Street, Birmingham, AL 35226; (205) 823-6180.

Genie Brannon, M.D., 107 Medical Arts Building, Anniston, AL 36201; (205) 236-0375.

Wade Brannon, M.D., 107 Medical Arts Building, Anniston, AL 36201; (205) 236-0375.

Andrew M. Brown, M.D., 515 South Third Street, Gadsden, AL 35901; (205) 547-4971.

Max Cooper, M.D., 224 Tumor Institute, University Station, Birmingham, AL 35294; (205) 322-7125.

L. Clark Granvlee, Jr., M.D., P.O. Box 55148, Birmingham, AL 35255; (205) 328-3000.

Joseph B. Miller, M.D., 5901 Airport Boulevard, Mobile, AL 36608; (205) 342-8540.

William S. Moughon, Jr., M.D., 1900 Fourteenth Avenue South, Birmingham, AL 35205; (205) 933-2875.

Guss J. Prosch, Jr., M.D., 759 Valley Street, Birmingham, AL 35226; (205) 823-6180.

William J. Robertson, M.D., St. Vincent's Professional Building, 2660 Tenth Avenue South, Birmingham, AL 35202; (205) 933-8141.

C. Orian Truss, M.D., 2614 Highland Avenue, Birmingham, AL 35202-1799; (205) 328-6481.

Christopher Truss, M.D., 332 Park Avenue, Birmingham, AL 35226; (205) 823-3742.

ALASKA

F. Russell Manuel, M.D., M.Sc., 4200 Lake Otis Parkway, Suite 304, Anchorage, AK 99508; (907) 562-7070.

Robert Jay Rowen, M.D., Omni Medical Center, 615 East Eighty-second Street, Suite 300, Anchorage, AK 99518; (907) 344-7775.

ARIZONA

Lloyd D. Arnold, D.O., 4025 West Bell Road, Suite 3, Phoenix, AZ 85023; (602) 939-8916.

Emmanuel G. Barnet, M.D., 550 West Thomas Road, Phoenix, AZ 85013; (602) 264-7957.

ARKANSAS

Rosemary C. Brandt, M.D., 500 South University, Suite 808, Little Rock, AR 72205; (501) 664-3010.

Harold Hedges, M.D., 424 North University, Little Rock, AR 72205; (501) 664-4810.

Maurice L. Stephens, M.D., Route 5, Box 168, Mena, AR 71953; (501) 394-6300.

Aubrey Worrell, Jr., M.D., 3900 Hickory Street, Pine Bluff, AR 71603; (501) 535-8200.

CALIFORNIA

American Biologics-Mexico, S.A. Hospital, 1180 Walnut Avenue, Chula Vista, CA 92011; (619) 429-8200.

Laszlo I. Belenyessy, M.D., 2901 Wilshire Boulevard, Suite 435, Santa Monica, CA 90403; (213) 828-4480.

Marc D. Braunstein, D.O., 24953 Paseo De Valencia, Suite 17C, Laguna Hills, CA 92653; (714) 583-0760.

Floyd H. Brigham, M.D., P.O. Box 1228, 18661 Highway 120, Groveland, CA 95321; (209) 962-7121.

Donald G. Cameron, M.D., 13227 Wolf Road, Grass Valley, CA 95949; (916) 268-0181.

H. Richard Casdorph, M.D., Ph.D. 23121 Verdugo Dr., Suite 204, Laguna Hills CA 92653; (714) 583-7666.

Robert F. Cathcart III, M.D., 127 Second Street, Los Altos, CA 94022; (415) 949-2822.

T. Dosumu-Johnson, M.D., Alvarado Medical Center, 6505 Alvarado Road, Suite 207, San Diego, CA 92120; (619) 583-4664.

Larry Eckstein, M.D., 1437 Seventh Street, Suite 301, Santa Monica, CA 90401; (213) 458-8020.

Charles G. Gabelman, M.D., 24953 Pasco de Valencia, Suite 16-C, Laguna Hills, CA 92653; (714) 859-9851.

Jane R. Gard, M.D., Human Environmental Medicine, Inc., 6505 Alvarado Road, Suite 101, San Diego, CA 92120; (619) 583-5865.

Garry F. Gordon, M.D., Preventive Medical Clinic, 1816 Tribute Road, Sacramento, CA 95815; (916) 925-7811.

Robert Harmon, M.D., 43-576 Washington Street, Palm Desert, CA 92260; (619) 345-2696.

Robert Haskell, M.D., 12 Aqua Vista Drive, San Rafael, CA 94901; (415) 668-1300.

John A. Henderson, M.D., A.P.C., 2055 Third Ave., San Diego, CA 92101; (619) 239-7747.

C. Fred Hering III, M.D., 212-A West Foothill Boulevard, Monrovia, CA 91016; (818) 357-2226.

H. J. Hoegerman, M.D., 101 West Arrellaga Street, Santa Barbara, CA 93101; (805) 963-1824.

M. Jahangiri, M.D., 2156 Santa Fe, Los Angeles, CA 90058; (213) 587-3218.

Zane R. Kime, M.D., M.S., 1212 High Street, Suite 204, Auburn, CA 95603; (916) 823-3421.

Esther M. Kirk, M.D., 10921 Wilshire Boulevard, Suite 706, West Los Angeles, CA 90024; (213) 208-5543.

A. Leonard Klepp, M.D., Inc. 16311 Ventura Blvd., Suite 725, Encino, CA 91436; (818) 981-5511.

Alan S. Levin, M.D., Levin Clinical Laboratories, 450 Sutter, Suite 1138, San Francisco, CA 94108; (415) 922-1444.

Emil Levin, M.D., 450 S. Beverly Drive, Beverly Hills, CA 90210; (213) 556-2091.

Cathie-Ann Lippman, M.D., 292 S. La Cienega Blvd., Suite 202-204, Beverly Hills, CA 90211; (213) 659-9187.

Claude J. Marquette, M.D., 525 South Drive, Suite 115, Mountain View, CA 94040; (415) 964-6700.

Marian C. Maynard, M.D., 1844 San Miguel Drive, Suite 3048, Walnut Creek, CA 94596; (415) 933-2405.

Barnard McGinity, M.D., 694J Fair Oaks Boulevard, Carmichael, CA 98605; (916) 485-4556.

John D. Michael, M.D., 6536 Telegraph Ave., #A-201, Oakland, CA 94609 One block from Berkeley; (415) 547-8111.

Charles Moss, M.D., 8950 Villa La Jolla Drive, Suite 2162, La Jolla, CA 92037; (619) 453-1314.

Kurt C. Olson, M.D., 21700 West Golden Triangle Road, Suite 101, Saugus, CA 91350; (805) 259-3220.

Sunil P. Perera, M.D., 404 Sunrise Avenue, Roseville, CA 95678; (916) 782-7758.

Robert J. Peterson, D.O., 8041 Newman Ave., Suite 100, Huntington Beach, CA 92647.

Marvin M. Portner, M.D., 910 Via De La Paz, #102, Pacific Palisades, CA 90272; (213) 454-3100 or 454-6226.

James E. Privitera, M.D., 105 Grand View, Covina, CA 91723; (213) 966-1618.

Donald E. Reiner, M.D., 1414 D South Miller Street, Santa Maria, CA 93454; (805) 925-0961.

Michael E. Rosenbaum, M.D., 232 E. Blithedale, Mill Valley, CA 94941; (415) 383-1262.

Phyllis Saifer, M.D., 3031 Telegraph Avenue, Suite 213, Berkeley, CA 94705; (415) 849-3346.

W. J. Sayer, M.D., F.A.C.A., F.A.A.A., Diplomate American Board of Allergy & Clinical Immunology, 145 North California Ave., Palo Alto, CA 94301-3911; (415) 321-3361.

Frank A. Shallenberger, M.D., 3144 Buskirk, Walnut Creek, CA 94523; (415) 938-0238, (415) 938-0271.

Murray Susser, M.D., 2730 Wilshire Boulevard, #110, Santa Monica, CA 90403; (213) 453-4424.

Lawrence H. Taylor, M.D., 2313 El Cajon Boulevard, San Diego, CA 92104; (619) 296-6208 or 296-6209.

Richard J. Trevino, M.D., 280 North Jackson Avenue, San Jose, CA 95116; (408) 926-5300.

Ronald Wempen, M.D., 3620 S. Bristol Street, Suite 306, Santa Ana, CA 92704; (714) 546-4325.

Edward E. Winger, M.D., 400 Twenty-Ninth Street, Oakland, CA 94609; (415) 839-6477.

COLORADO

Mabel Brelje, M.D., Villa Clinic, P.C., 3222 South Vance Street, Lakewood, CO 80227; (303) 986-6446.

Lawrence D. Dickey, M.D., 109 West Olive Street, Fort Collins, CO 80524; (303) 482-6001.

William E. Doell, D.O., 7777 West Thirty-eighth Avenue, Suite A124, Wheatridge, CO 80033; (303) 422-0585.

J. R. Fish, M.D., F.A.C.S., 3030 North Hancock Ave., Colorado Springs, CO 80907.

Kendall Gerdes, M.D., 1617 Vine Street, Denver, CO 80206; (303) 377-8837.

Rob W. Krakovitz, M.D., P.O. Box 9618, Aspen, CO 81612; (303) 925-8762.

Diane McHose, D.O., 17111 South Golden Road, Golden, CO 80401; (303) 278-0764.

Nicholas G. Nonas, M.D., 950 East Harvard, Suite 450, Denver, CO 80210; (303) 722-7534.

Francis Waickman, M.D., 109 West Olive Street, Fort Collins, CO 80524; (303) 923-4879.

CONNECTICUT

Sidney McDonald Baker, M.D., Gesell Institute of Human Development, 310 Prospect Street, New Haven, CT 06511; (203) 776-8125.

Alan M. Dattner, M.D., Route L, Box 69, North Grosvenordale, CT 06255; (203) 923-9596.

Marshall Mandell, M.D., Alan Mandell Center for Bio-Ecologic Diseases, 3 Brush Street, Norwalk, CT 06850; (203) 838-4706.

Robert McLellan, M.D., Gesell Institute of Human Development, 310 Prospect Street, New Haven, CT 06511; (203) 776-8125.

Warren R. Pistey, M.D., Bridgeport Hospital, Department of Pathology, 267 Grant Street, Bridgeport, CT 06602; (203) 384-3000.

DELAWARE

Jerry Groll, M.D., 421 Savannah Road, Lewes, DE 19958; (302) 645-2833

DISTRICT OF COLUMBIA

George H. Mitchell, M.D., P.C., Metropolitan Medical Center, Suite 404, 2112 F Street, N.W., Washington, D.C. 20037; (202) 429-9456.

FLORIDA

Ervin Barr, D.O., 2350 West Oakland Park Boulevard, Fort Lauderdale, FL 33331; (305) 731-8080.

Stanley J. Cannon, M.D., Galloway Plaza, 9805 Southwest 87th Avenue, Miami, FL 33176; (305) 279-3020.

Donald J. Carrow, M.D., The Largo Center for Preventive and General Medicine, 1501 South Belcher Road, Largo, FL 33541; (813) 536-3531.

Martin Dayton, M.D., D.O., 18600 Collins Avenue, Miami, FL 33160; (305) 931-8484.

Hobart Feldman, M.D., 16800 Northwest Second Avenue, Suite 301, North Miami Beach, FL 33169; (305) 652-1062.

Joel Friedman, M.D., 218 N.W. Second Avenue, Gainesville, FL 32601; (904) 377-0015.

T. Friedmann, M.D., 600 Bird Bay Drive, Venice, FL 33595; (813) 484-2455.

J. Gordon Godorov, D.O., Holistic Lifestyle Center, 9055 Southwest Eighty-seventh Avenue, Suite 307, Miami, FL 33176; (305) 595-0671.

Howard Herring, M.D., Medical Center Clinic, 8333 North Davis Highway, P.O. Box 151, Pensacola, FL 32591; (904) 478-4121.

Roy Kupsinel, M.D., Lost Horizon Health Awareness Center, Shangri-La Lane, Box 550, Oviedo, FL 32765; (303) 365-6681.

Life Care Center, 76 East McNab Road, Pompano Beach, FL 33060; (305) 786-0370.

Alfred S. Massam, M.D., F.A.A.F.P., P.O. Box 1328, Wauchula, FL 33873; (813) 773-6668.

Herbert Pardell, D.O., Preventive Medical Center of Hollywood, 1818 East Sheridan Street, Hollywood, FL 33020; (305) 922-7333.

Dan C. Roehm, M.D., 3400 Park Central Blvd. North, Suite 34, Pompano Beach, FL 33064; (305) 977-3700.

Robert J. Rogers, M.D., Rogers Clinic of Preventive Medicine, Affiliate of Health World International, Inc., 15 West Avenue B, Melbourne, FL 32901; (305) 723-2360.

I. Randall Ross, M.D., 375 South Courtenay Parkway, Merritt Island, FL 32952; (305) 453-3420.

Robert R. Roth, M.D., 811 S.E. 13th Avenue, Deerfield Beach, FL 33441; (305) 426-8532.

Richard J. Sabates, M.D., Preventive Medical Center of Hollywood, 1818 East Sheridan Street, Hollywood, FL 33020; (305) 922-7333.

Joya Lynn Schoen, M.D., P.A., 1900 North Orange Avenue, Orlando, FL 32804; (305) 898-2951.

Forrest E. Smith, D.O., Vero Beach Medical Clinic, Inc., 1408 Sixteenth Street, Vero Beach, FL 32960; (305) 567-4115.

Robert Stroud, M.D., 570 Memorial Circle, Ormond Beach, FL 32074; (904) 677-3642.

Glen Wagner, M.D., 121 Sixth Avenue, Indialantic, FL 32903; (305) 723-5915.

Ray C. Wunderlich, Jr., M.D., 666 Sixth Street South, St. Petersburg, FL 33701; (813) 822-3612.

Chin Yong Cho, M.D., Chin Yong Lee, M.D., 4301 Thirty-second Street West, Suite C20, Bradenton, FL 33505; (813) 753-6188, (813) 756-8833 (service).

GEORGIA

William C. Douglass, M.D., 2470 Windy Hill Road, Suite 440, Marietta, GA 30067-8603; (404) 953-0710.

James L. Fletcher, Jr., M.D., Medical College of Georgia, Department of Family Medicine, Augusta, GA 30909; (404) 828-4577.

J. Gilbert Foster, Jr., M.D., 435 King Road, N.W., Atlanta, GA 30342; (404) 261-3197.

Milton Fried, M.D., Milton Fried Medical Clinic, P.C., 4426 Tilly Mill Road, Atlanta, GA 30360; (404) 451-4857.

Melvin Haysman, M.D., 5105 Paulsen Street, Suite 133, Savannah, GA 31405; (912) 355-5410.

Marcia Franklin, M.D., Wildwood Sanitarium and Hospital, Wildwood, GA 30757; (404) 820-1493.

A. ʼSteve Orr, M.D., 490 Peachtree Street, Suite 374-C, Atlanta, GA 30308; (404) 688-7793.

Young S. Shin, M.D., 1135 Hudson Bridge Road, Stockbridge (Atlanta), GA 30281; (404) 474-3666.

Robert M. Webster, M.D., Route 1, Box 72-C, Fairburn, GA 30213; (404) 766-0239.

IDAHO

Charles T. McGee, M.D., 1717 Lincoln Way, Suite 108, Coeur d'Alene, ID 83814; (208) 664-1478.

ILLINOIS

Paul J. Dunn, M.D., 715 Lake Street, Oak Park, IL 60301; (312) 383-3800.

Stephen K. Elsasser, D.O., Family Practice Center of Metamora, 205 South Engelwood Drive, Metamora, IL 61548; (309) 367-2321.

Robert C. Filice, M.D., 24 West 500 Maple Avenue, Suite 216, Naperville, IL 60540; (312) 369-1220.

James H. Johnson, M.D., 251 East Chicago Avenue, Suite 626, Chicago, IL 60611; (312) 943-5405.

Robert Marshall, M.D., 505 North Lakeshore Drive, Suite 6506, Chicago, IL 60611; (312) 828-9480.

Gary O'Berg, M.D., 4911 Route 31, Crystall Lake, IL 60014; (815) 455-1990.

Theron Randolph, M.D., 505 North Lakeshore Drive, Suite 6506, Chicago, IL 60611; (312) 828-9480.

George E. Shambaugh, Jr., M.D., Shambaugh Hearing and Allergy Institute, 40 South Clay, Hinsdale, IL 60521; (312) 887-1130.

Robert S. Waters, M.D., 739 Roosevelt Road, Building 8, #314, Glen Ellyn, IL 60137; (708) 790-8100.

INDIANA

David A. Darbro, M.D., Family Health Care Center, 2124 East Hanna Avenue, Indianapolis, IN 46227; (317) 787-7221.

Sandra C. Denton, M.D., Family Health Care Center, 2124 East Hanna Avenue, Indianapolis, IN 46227; (317) 787-7221.

James K. Hill, M.D., 8801 North Meridian Street, Indianapolis, IN 46260; (317) 846-7342.

John F. O'Brian, M.D., 3217 Lake Avenue, Fort Wayne, IN 46805; (219) 422-9471.

IOWA

Vernon P. Varner, M.D., 328 East Washington Street, Suite 200, Iowa City, IA 52240; (319) 337-6483.

KANSAS

Stevens B. Acker, M.D., 1100 North St. Francis, Suite 400, Wichita, KS 67214; (316) 263-7002.

Charles T. Hinshaw, M.D., 5101 Kings Row, Wichita, KS 67208; (316) 682-0460.

Hugh D. Riordan, M.D., The Olive W. Garvey Center for the Improvement of Human Functioning, Inc., 3100 N. Hillside Ave., Wichita, KS 67219; (316) 682-3100.

KENTUCKY

Kirk D. Morgan, M.D., 9105 U.S. 42, Prospect, KY 40059; (502) 228-0156, also 3101 Breckenridge Lane, Louisville, KY 40220; (502) 459-0315.

Walt Stoll, M.D., 1412 North Broadway, Lexington, KY 40505; (606) 233-4273.

LOUISIANA

James Foster, M.D., 100 Smart Place, Slidell, LA 70458; (504) 649-3483, 1-(800)-232-3438.

MARYLAND

James H. Brodsky, M.D., 4701 Willard Avenue, Suite 224, Chevy Chase, MD 20815; (301) 652-6760.

MASSACHUSETTS

Carol Englender, M.D., 1340 Centre Street, Newton Centre, MA 02159; (617) 965-7770.

J. Aaron Herschfus, M.D., 64 S. Main Street, P.O. Box 336, Sharon, MA 02067; (617) 784-2082.

Jeanne Therese Hubbuch, M.D., 33 Ashcroft Street, Jamaica Plain, MA 02130; (617) 661-6225.

Michael Janson, M.D., 2557 Massachusetts Avenue, Cambridge, MA 02140; (617) 661-6225.

Joseph P. Keenan, M.D., 75 Springfield Road, Westfield, MA 01085; (413) 568-2304.

Edgar S. Miller, D.O., 131 Sudbury Road, Concord, MA 01742; (617) 369-6030.

James O'Shea, M.D., Doctors Medical Center, 50 Prospect Street, Lawrence, MA 01841; (617) 683-2632.

Robert E. Rechtschaffen, M.D., 21 Everett Avenue, Belchertown, MA 01007; (413) 323-7212.

Richard B. Yules, M.D., Haelen Medical Center, 475 Pleasant Street, Worcester, MA 01609; (617) 791-6305.

MICHIGAN

Grant R. Born, D.O., 2687 Forty-fourth Street, S.E., Grand Rapids, MI 49508; (616) 455-3550.

Harry R. Butler, M.D., 1821 King Road, Trenton, MI 48183; (313) 676-2800.

Cornelius F. Derrick, M.D., 1821 King Road, Trenton, MI 48183; (313) 675-0678.

Larry E. Hearin, M.D., 2900 East Grand River Avenue, Howell, MI 48843; (517) 546-7920.

Doyle B. Hill, D.O. 2520 North Euclid Avenue, Bay City, MI 48706; (517) 686-5200.

Doyle B. Hill, D.O. 907 Cass Avenue, Bay City, MI 48706; (517) 879-5111.

Eugene Homelster, M.D., 12925 Pennsylvania, Riverview, MI 48192; (313) 284-8819.

J. M. Nutt, D.O., 420 South Lafayette, Greenville, MI 48838; (616) 691-7468.

Paul A. Parente, D.O., 29538 Orchard Lake Road, Farmington Hills, MI 48018; (313) 626-7544.

Paul A. Parente, D.O., 30275 Thirteen Mile Road, Farmington Hills, MI 48018; (313) 626-9690.

Albert J. Scarchilli, D.O., 29538 Orchard Lake Road, Farmington Hills, MI 48018; (313) 626-6544.

Albert Scarchilli, D.O., 30257 Thirteen Mile Road, Farmington Hills, MI 48018; (313) 626-9690.

Richard E. Tapert, D.O., 15850 East Warren, Detroit, MI 48224; (313) 885-5405.

Robert G. Thomas, M.D., Three Oaks Medical Center, 21 North Elm Street, Three Oaks, MI 49128; (616) 756-9531.

Jerry A. Walker, D.O., 5681 South Beech Daly, Dearborn Heights, MI 48125; (313) 292-9550.

MINNESOTA

Harold A. Johnson, Ph.D., N.D., 1517 E. Lake Street, Minneapolis, MN 55407; (612) 920-2942.

Pamela A. Morford, M.D., 2545 Chicago Avenue South, Suite #515, Minneapolis, MN 55404; (612) 683-5250.

Keith Sehnert, M.D., 4210 Fremont Avenue South, Minneapolis, MN 55409; (612) 824-5134.

MISSISSIPPI

Robert T. Cates, M.D., Cates Medical & Nutrition Clinic, 12 Professional Parkway, Ridgeland, MS 39157; (601) 856-6000.

Thomas S. Glasgow, M.D., 2161 S. Lamar Blvd., Oxford, MS 38655; (601) 234-1791.

Pravinchandra P. Patel, M.D., P.O. Drawer DD, Coldwater, MS 38618-0924; (601) 736-2376.

MISSOURI

Gerald N. Bart, Allergy Care Center, 100004 Kennerly Road, Suite 255, St. Louis, MO 63128; (314) 842-5082.

Lawrence E. Dorman, D.O., 9120 East Thirty-fifth Street, Independence, MO 64052; (816) 358-2712.

William R. Lamb, M.D., Lamb Medical-Psychiatric Associates, Route 2, Box 61-23, Nixa, MO 65714; (417) 869-4833.

Edward W. McDonagh, D.O., 2800-A Kendallwood Parkway, Gladstone, MO 64119; (816) 453-5940.

Kenneth Rall, M.D., 1121 Danforth, Columbia, MO 65201; (314) 443-3577.

James L. Rowland, M.S., D.O., Ph.D., F.A.C.G.P., 8133 Wornall Road, Kansas City, MO 64114; (816) 361-4077.

Charles J. Rudolph, D.O., Ph.D., 2800-A Kendallwood Parkway, Gladstone, MO 64119; (816) 453-5940.

Tipu Sulton, M.D., St. Louis Center for Preventive Medicine, 4585 Washington Street, Florissant, MO 63033; (314) 921-5600.

Harvey Walker, Jr., M.D., Ph.D., 138 North Meramec Avenue, St. Louis, MO 63105; (314) 721-7227.

NEVADA

The Nevada Clinic, 6105 West Tropicana Avenue, Las Vegas, NV 89103; (702) 871-2700.

Robert Bliss Vance, D.O., H.M.D., Vance Medical Center, 801 South Rancho Drive, Suite F2, Las Vegas, NV 89106-3814; (702) 385-7771.

NEW JERSEY

Allan Magaziner, D.O., 8002-A Greentree Commons, Marlton, NJ 08053; (201) 596-3030.

Fiana Munits, M.D., 51 Pleasant Valley Way, West Orange, NJ 07052; (201) 736-3743.

Milan J. Packovich, M.D., 585 Winters Avenue, Paramus, NJ 07652; (201) 967-5081.

Dr. Stanley Skollar, 545 Island Road, Ramsey, NJ 07446; (201) 934-7299.

NEW MEXICO

Annette Stoesser, M.D., 112 South Kentucky, Rosell, NM 88201; (504) 623-2444.

NEW YORK

Migdalia Arnan, M.D., 28 Garfield Place, Poughkeepsie, NY 12601; (914) 473-0048.

Patricia J. Ausman, D.O., 160 Atlantic Avenue, Hempstead, NY 11550; (516) 565-9250.

Ken Bock, M.D., Rhinebeck Health Center, 108 Montgomery Street, Rhinebeck, NY 12572; (914) 876-7082.

Steven Bock, M.D., Rhinebeck Health Center, 108 Montgomery Street, Rhinebeck, NY 12572; (914) 876-7082.

M. L. Boczico, M.D., 12 Greenridge Avenue, White Plains, NY 10583; (914) 949-8817.

Serafina Corsello, M.D., The Stress Center, 152 East Main Street, Huntington, NY 11743; (516) 271-0222.

Allan Cott, M.D., 160 East Thirty-eighth Street, One Murray Hill, New York, NY 10016; (212) 679-5593.

Martin Feldman, M.D., 132 East Seventy-sixth Street, New York, NY 10021; (212) 744-4413.

Leo Galland, M.D., F.A.C.P., F.A.C.N., 41 East Sixtieth Street, New York, NY 10022; (212) 308-6622.

Karl E. Humiston, M.D., 104 East Fortieth Street, Suite 906, New York, NY 10016; (212) 986-9385.

E. M. Levin, M.D., 205 East Seventy-eighth Street, New York, NY 10021; (212) 288-7263.

Warren M. Levin, M.D., World Health Medical Group, 444 Park Avenue South, New York, NY 10016; (212) 696-1900.

H. L. Newbold, M.D., 115 East Thirty-fourth Street, New York, NY 10016; (212) 679-8207.

Frank M. Nochimson, M.D., 157 Eighty-sixth Street, Brooklyn, NY 11209; (718) 630-7195.

Doris J. Rapp, M.D., 1421 Colvin Boulevard, Buffalo, NY 14223; (716) 875-5578.

Stephan Rechtschaffen, M.D., Rhinebeck Health Center, 108 Montgomery Street, Rhinebeck, NY 12572; (914) 876-7082.

Sherry A. Rogers, M.D., 2800 West Genesee Street, Syracuse, NY 13219; (315) 488-2856.

Michael B. Schacter, M.D., Mountain View Medical Bldg., Mountain View Avenue, Nyack, NY 10960; (914) 358-6800.

Morton M. Teich, M.D., 930 Park Avenue, New York, NY 10028; (212) 988-1821.

W. S. Tichenor, M.D., 30 Central Park South, New York, NY 10019; (212) 371-8510.

Juan Wilson, M.D., 1900 Hempstead Turnpike, East Meadow, NY 11554; (516) 794-0404.

Alfred V. Zamm, M.D., 111 Maiden Lane, Kingston, NY 12401-4597; (914) 338-7766.

NORTH CAROLINA

Steve Barrie, M.D., Great Smokies Medical Center, Route 1, Box 7, Leicester, NC 28748; (704) 683-3101.

T. M. Bullock, M.D., 104 Seventh Avenue, Chadbourn, NC 28413; (919) 654-4614.

F. M. Carroll, M.D., 104 Seventh Avenue, Chadbourn, NC 28413; (919) 654-4614.

F. Keels Dickson, M.D., 485 North Wendover Road, Charlotte, NC 28211; (704) 366-7921.

John L. Laird, M.D., Great Smokies Medical Center, Route 1, Box 7, Leicester, NC 28748; (704) 683-3101.

Logan T. Robertson, M.D., Route 2, Canton, NC 28716; (704) 235-8312.

OHIO

L. Terry Chappell, M.D., 122 Thurman Street, Bluffton, OH 45817; (419) 358-4627.

Stuart B. Datt, M.D., 26300 Euclid Avenue, Euclid, OH 44132; (216) 261-3040.

Derrick Lonsdale, M.D., 24700 Center Ridge Road, Westlake, OH 44145; (216) 835-0104.

John W. Rechsteiner, M.D., 1116 South Limestone Street, Springfield, OH 45505; (513) 325-0223.

Charles S. Resseger, D.O., Inc., 853 South Norwalk Road West, Norwalk, OH 44857.

William C. Schmelzer, M.D., 3520 Snouffer Road, Worthington, OH 43235; (614) 761-0555.

Jack E. Slingluff, D.O., 5850 Fulton Road N.W., Canton, OH 44718; (216) 494-8641.

Francis J. Waickman, M.D., M. Ped., F.A.C.A., 1625 West Portage Trail, Cuyahoga Falls, OH 44223; (216) 923-4879.

OKLAHOMA

Leon Anderson, D.O., 121 South Second Street, Jenks, OK 74037; (918) 744-5956.

Howard Hagglund, M.D., 2227 West Lindsey, Suite 1401, Norman, OK 73069; (405) 329-4457.

James W. Hogin, D.O., Brookwood Medical Clinic, 937 Southwest 89, Suite C, Oklahoma City, OK 73139; (405) 631-0524.

Harold G. Sleeper, M.D., 2801 Parklawn Drive, Suite 505, Midwest City, OK 73110; (405) 733-8244.

OREGON

J. W. Fitzsimmons, M.D., P.O. Box 130, Murphy, OR 97533; (503) 474-2166.

John Gambee, M.D., 66 Club Road, Suite 140, Eugene, OR 97401; (503) 686-2536.

John A. Green III, M.D., North Marion Medical Centre, 3674 Pacific Highway, #99-E, Hubbard, OR 97032.

PENNSYLVANIA

Harold R. Buttram, M.D., Route 3, Clymer Road, Quakertown, PA 18951; (215) 536-1890.

Chin Y. Chung, M.D., 210 East Second Street, Erie, PA 16507; (814) 455-4429.

ENT and Allergy Association, 17 Sixth Avenue, Greenville, PA 16125; (412) 588-2600.

Leland J. Green, M.D., P.O. Box 508, Lansdale, PA 19446; (215) 855-9501.

P. Jayalakshmi, M.D., and K. R. Sampathachar, M.D., 6366 Sherwood Road, Philadelphia, PA 19151; (215) 473-4226 and 473-7453.

P. Jayalakshmi, M.D., and K. R. Sampathachar, M.D., Rd. #1, Box 148, Lehighton, PA 18235; (717) 386-3713.

Roy E. Kerry, M.D., 17 Sixth Avenue, Greenville, PA 17022; (412) 588-2600.

Arthur L. Koch, D.O., 57 West Juniper Street, Hazelton, PA 18201; (717) 455-4747.

Donald Mantell, M.D., Mantell Medical Center, 6505 Mars Road, Evans City, PA 16033; (412) 776-5610.

Conrad G. Maulfair, Jr., D.O., Box 71 Main Street, Mertztown, PA 19539; (215) 682-2104.

Ralph A. Miranda, M.D., Holistic Health Center, Route 7, Box 105-B, Greensburg, PA 15601; (412) 838-7632.

M. J. Packovich, M.D., Millcraft Center, 90 West Chestnut Street, Washington, PA 15301; (304) 723-0011 or 723-0013.

Kakkadasam R. Sampathachar, M.D., New Life Center, 6366 Sherwood Road, Philadelphia, PA 19151; (215) 473-4226.

Christiane M. F. Siewers, M.D., Matrix Center for Mental Health and Wellbeing, 135 Freeport Road, Pittsburgh, PA 15215; (412) 782-4700.

Harold C. Walmer, D.O., 50 North Market Street, Elizabethtown, PA 17022; (717) 367-1345.

RHODE ISLAND

Dr. Michael Rosenberg, D.O., 207 Waterman St., Providence, RI 02906; (401) 272-1832.

SOUTH CAROLINA

Mark A. Knipfer, M.D., 1250 Reidville Road, Spartanburg, SC 29301; (803) 576-9201.

Allan Lieberman, M.D., 7510 North Forest Drive, North Charleston, SC 29418; (803) 572-1600.

Robert G. Mahon, M.D., 701 Arlington Avenue, Greenville, SC 29601; (803) 233-6881.

Theodore C. Rozema, M.D., 1000 Rutherford Road, Landrum, SC 29356; (803) 457-4141.

Martin H. Zwerling, M.D., P.O. Box 2456, Aiken, SC 29801; (803) 648-9555.

TENNESSEE

Peter Ballenger, M.D., 1325 Eastmoreland Avenue, Memphis, TN 38104; (901) 725-6853.

James A. Carlson, D.O., 1104 Merchants Road, Knoxville, TN 37912; (615) 688-1141.

William G. Crook, M.D., 657 Skyline Drive, Jackson, TN 38301; (901) 423-1500.

John Curlin, 616 West Forest Avenue, Jackson, TN 38301; (901) 422-0330.

Fred M. Furr, M.D., 9217 Park West Boulevard, Bldg. E, Suite 1, Knoxville, TN 37923; (615) 693-1502.

Cecil E. Pitard, M.D., Newland Professional Building, 2001 Laurel Avenue, Suite 403, Knoxville, TN 37916; (615) 522-7714.

E. William Rosenberg, M.D., Department of Dermatology, 956 Court Avenue, Room 3C-13, University of Tennessee, Memphis, TN 38163; (901) 528-5733.

Robert Skinner, M.D., Department of Dermatology, 956 Court Avenue, Room 3C-13, University of Tennessee, Memphis, TN 38163; (901) 528-5733.

Donald C. Thompson, M.D., P.O. Box 2088, Morristown, TN 37816-2088; (615) 581-6867.

Richard Wanderman, 6584 Poplar, Suite 420, Memphis, TN 38119; (901) 683-2777.

TEXAS

J. W. Bucke, Jr., D.O., Doctors Clinic, 813 Brown Trail, Bedford, TX 76022; (817) 268-4848.

Gary H. Campbell, D.O., Texas College of Osteopathic Medicine, Camp Bowie at Montgomery, Fort Worth, TX 76107; (817) 870-5230.

Steven Cordas, D.O., 1100 West Airport Freeway, Bedford, TX 76022; (817) 267-8181.

William W. Halcomb, D.O., 8311 Shoal Creek Boulevard, Austin, TX 78758; (512) 451-8149.

Charles R. Hamel, M.D., 3801 Hulen, Fort Worth, TX 76107; (817) 731-9531.

George J. Juetersonke, D.O., Camp Bowie at Montgomery, Fort Worth, TX 76107; (817) 735-2252.

A. M. Kincheloe, D.O., Women's Diagnostic Clinic, 620 Matlock Center Circle, Arlington, TX 76015; (817) 265-9928 or 792-3767.

Howard J. Lang, D.O., 1404 Brown Trail, Bedford, TX 76022; (817) 268-1171.

T. M. Lunceford, M.D., 3411 Twentieth Street, Lubbock, TX 79410; (806) 797-3226.

Charles R. Mabray, M.D., 4204 North Laurent, Victoria, TX 77901; (214) 578-5233.

M. C. Maley, M.D., Maley Allergy Clinic, 808 Olive, Suite C, Texarkana, TX 75501; (214) 793-1153.

Don Mannerberg, M.D., 375 Municipal Drive, Richardson, TX 75080; (214) 669-8707.

Linda Martin-Ernst, D.O., Ernst Center of Nutrition and Preventive Medicine 1301 Custer, Suite 828, Plano, TX 75078; (214) 578-1724.

R. W. Noble, M.D., 6757 Arapaho Road, Suite 757, Dallas, TX 75248; (214) 458-9944.

Reginald Platt III, D.O., Platt Osteopathic Clinic, 6804 Bintliff, Houston, TX 77074; (713) 778-1584.

Vladimir Rizov, M.D., Medical Director, 6550 Tarneff, Suite 4, Houston, TX 77036; (713) 771-5506.

Ralph E. Smiley, M.D., 8345 Walnut Hill Lane, Dallas, TX 75231; (214) 368-4132.

Donald Sprague, M.D., 8345 Walnut Hill Lane, Dallas, TX 75231; (214) 368-4132.

John Parks Trowbridge, M.D., Humble Medical Arts Building, 9816 Memorial Boulevard, Suite 205, Humble, TX 77338; (713) 540-2329.

Michael E. Truman, D.O., 1709 Precinct Line Road, Hurst, TX 76054; (817) 281-0402.

Donald R. Whitaker, D.O., P.O. Box 5729, Longview, TX 75608; (214) 759-8333.

UTAH

David J. Harbrecht, M.D., F.A.C.S., 425 Medical Drive, Suite 107, Bountiful, UT 84010; (801) 292-8303.

Robert M. Payne, M.D., 1955 East 5600 South, Salt Lake City, UT 84111; (801) 278-4677.

VIRGINIA

Elmer M. Cranton, M.D., Mt. Rogers Clinic, Box 44, Ripshin Road, Trout Dale, VA 24378; (703) 677-3631.

Lawrence Auburn Plumlee, M.D., 1111 Raymond Avenue, McLean, VA 22101; (703) 821-2144.

WASHINGTON

Murray L. Black, D.O., 609 South Forty-eighth Avenue, Yakima, WA 98908; (509) 966-1780.

Leo J. Bolles, M.D., 15611 Bellevue Redmond Rd., Bellevue, WA 98008; (206) 881-2224.

Jonathan Collin, M.D., 911 Tyler Street, Port Townsend, WA 98368; (206) 385-4555.

Will Corell, M.D., West 508 Sixth Avenue, Spokane, WA 99204; (509) 838-3935.

Jeffrey H. Gelgisser, M.D., The Northwest Center for Holistic Medicine, 4072 Ninth Avenue, N. E., Seattle, WA 98105.

Ralph T. Golan, M.D., 928 Broadway East, Seattle, WA 98102; (206) 324-0593.

T. Daniel Pletsch, M.D., 11012 N.E. Fourth Plain Rd., Vancouver, WA 98662; (206) 256-4118.

Paul Thompson, M.D., 933 North Fifth Avenue, Sequim, WA 98382; (206) 683-1101.

Richard S. Wilkinson, M.D., Yakima Allergy Clinic, 302 South Twelfth Ave., Yakima, WA 98902; (509) 453-5506.

Randall E. Wilkinson, M.D., Yakima Allergy Clinic, 302 South Twelfth Ave., Yakima, WA 98902; (509) 453-5506.

Norman Zucker, M.D., 700 S. 320th Street, Federal Way, WA 98003; (206) 946-0140.

WEST VIRGINIA

Albert V. Jellen, M.D., 2097 National Road, Wheeling, WV 26003; (304) 242-5151.

Anton Ros, D.O., P.C., 135 Palm Drive, Weirton, WV 26062; (304) 723-2929.

WISCONSIN

William J. Faber, D.O., Milwaukee Pain Clinic, 6529 West Fond du Lac, Milwaukee, WI 53228; (414) 464-7246.

George F. Kroker, M.D., 615 South Tenth Street, LaCrosse, WI 54601; (608) 782-2027.

Robert S. Waters, M.D., 320 Race, Wisconsindells, WI 53965; (608) 254-7178.

AUSTRALIA

E. Revai, M.B., B.S., D.P.M., FRANZCP, 253 Oxford Street, Bondi Junction, Sydney 2022; (02) 389-1472.

BRAZIL

Efrain Olszewer, M.D., Clinica Dr. Tuffik Mattar, Rua 7 de Abril 282, Cj 123, 01044 Sao Paulo; (55) 11-255-5855.

CANADA

Ron Greenberg, M.D., 212-2678 West Broadway, Vancouver, BC V6K 2G3; (604) 733-1055.

Abram Hoffer, M.D., Ph.D., 2727 Quadra Street, Suite 3, Victoria, BC V8T 4E5; (604) 386-8756.

ENGLAND

Dr. Hugh J. E. Cox, 46 St. Mary Street, High Wycombe, Buckinghamshire, HP11 2HE; (0494) 31814.

Wayne Perry, M.B., B.S., M.R.C.P., The Chelation Centre, 3 The Glade, Pagham, West Sussex P021 4SD.

PHILIPPINES

P. L. Verzosa, M.D., 26 Ilang-Ilang Street, Cubao, O.C., Philippines; (011) 721-7558.

PUERTO RICO

Ramon Casanova-Roig, M.D., 513 Hostos Avenue, Hato Rey, PR 00918; (809) 764-5715.

INDEX

ABOUT THE AUTHORS

John Parks Trowbridge, M.D., has a simple motto for his Houston, Texas, office practice: "Finally Feeling Better!" Much of his work is pioneering new approaches for troubling problems in patients of all ages.

An Eagle Scout and National Merit Scholar, Dr. Trowbridge trained in biological sciences at Stanford University. He received his medical degree from Case Western Reserve University and did advance studies in general surgery at Mt. Zion Hospital (University of California/San Francisco) and urological surgery at the University of Texas/Houston. He later earned a Diploma in Preventive Medicine Florida State University/Melbourne for graduate studies in nutrition.

An international leader on the frontiers of medicine, he is president-elect of the American College of Advancement in Medicine and is listed in three different editions of *Who's Who*. He is board certified as a specialist by the American Board of Chelation Therapy, for treatment of heart and blood vessel diseases and environmental poisoning. He is a Fellow of the American Society for Laser Medicine and Surgery, performing in-office hemorrhoid surgery with rapid recovery. An attending staff physician at Northeast Medical Center Hospital in Humble (northeast Houston), Dr. Trowbridge also founded and serves as primary lecturer for the Resource Center for Nutrition & Health. He is a private pilot and was appointed by the Federal Air Surgeon in 1983 to serve as a Senior Aviation Medical Examiner.

A sought-after speaker for medical and public meetings and radio/television interviews, he has written dozens of articles on health for national and foreign magazines and, with Dr. Morton Walker, has coauthored three books on topics in complementary (holistic-preventive) medicine.

Morton Walker, D.P.M., works full time as a freelance professional medical journalist and author. Having previously left more than sixteen years of practice as a doctor of podiatric medicine, Dr. Walker has for twenty-one years pursued a second career writing magazine articles and books from his home in Stamford, Connecticut. His byline is on forty-nine published books and over 1,400 consumer magazine articles. Almost all of his research and writing is in the area of holistic health, orthomolecular nutrition, environmental medicine, complementary medicine, and alternative methods of healing.

Dr. Morton Walker has won twenty-two medical research and journalism awards from the health professions, the American medical press, and the American Business Press, Inc. These prizes and citations include two Jesse H. Neal Editorial Achievement Awards for the best series of articles published in all American magazines in 1975, and for creating all the editorial content of the best single issue of any American magazine published in 1976. Of ten recognition medals presented to him by the American Podiatry Association, eight were awarded for his research and writing on *Candida albicans* and allied fungal organisms. He also was bestowed the 1979 Humanitarian Award by the American Academy of Medical Preventics "for informing the public on alternative methods of healing" and the 1981 Orthomolecular Award by the Institute of Preventive Medicine for "outstanding achievement in orthomolecular education."

Bantam's Best in Health and Nutrition

Ask for these books at your local bookstore or use this page to order.

Please send me the books I have checked above. I am enclosing $____ (add $2.50 to cover postage and handling). Send check or money order, no cash or C.O.D.'s, please.

Name _____

Address _____

City/State/Zip _____

Send order to: Bantam Books, Dept. HN 21, 2451 S. Wolf Rd., Des Plaines, IL 60018
Allow four to six weeks for delivery.

Prices and availability subject to change without notice.   HN 21 4/95